豐富多彩的台灣
——林媽利醫師談台灣特有血型及血緣研究

Abundant and Colorful Taiwan
Blood Groups, Heritage and Ups and Downs of Life

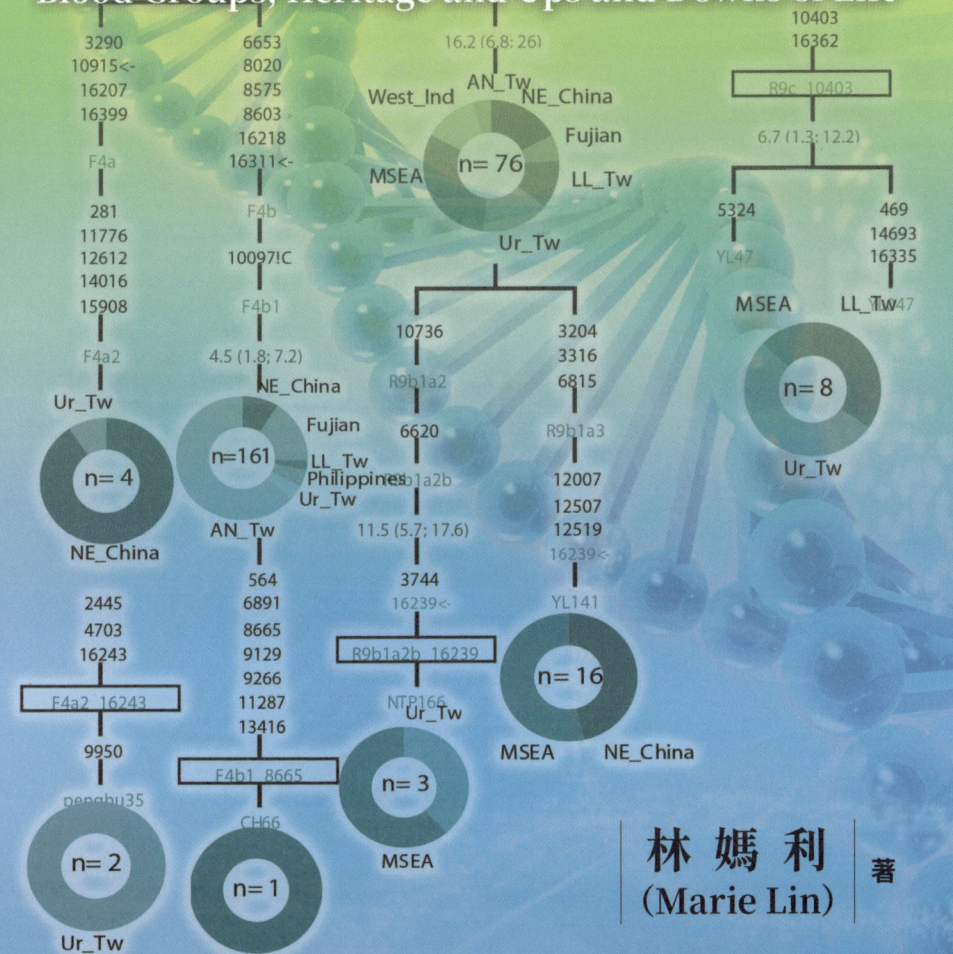

林 媽 利
(Marie Lin) 著

一、內文彩圖

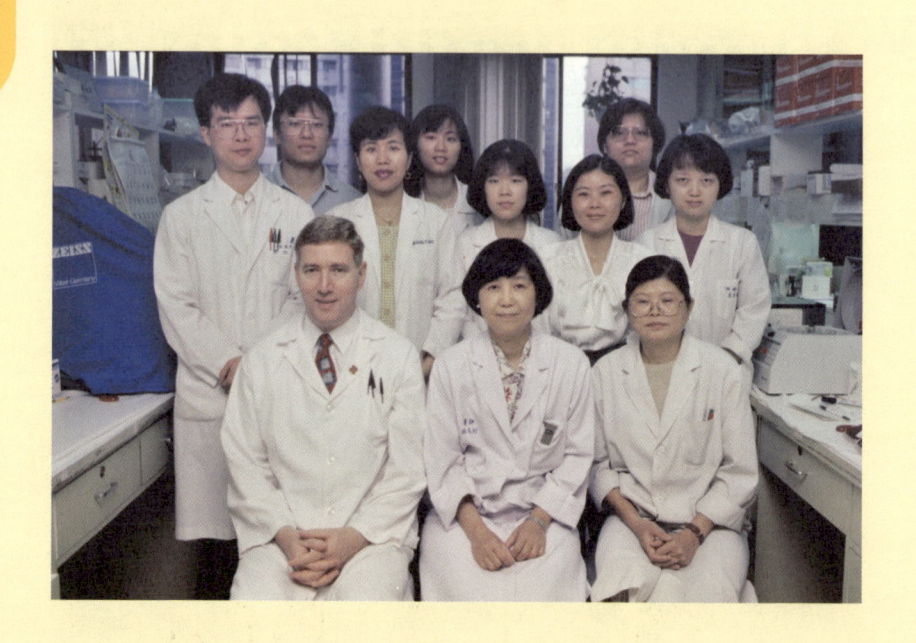

1990年代台北馬偕醫院血庫群英像（馬偕血庫的全盛時代）
後排左起：余榮熾、詹詠絮、鄒佳君，中排左起：陳啓清、王昌玲、李慧玲、陳秀霞、朱志芬，前排左起：Richard Broadberry（鮑博瑞）、林媽利、謝秀花。

1-1

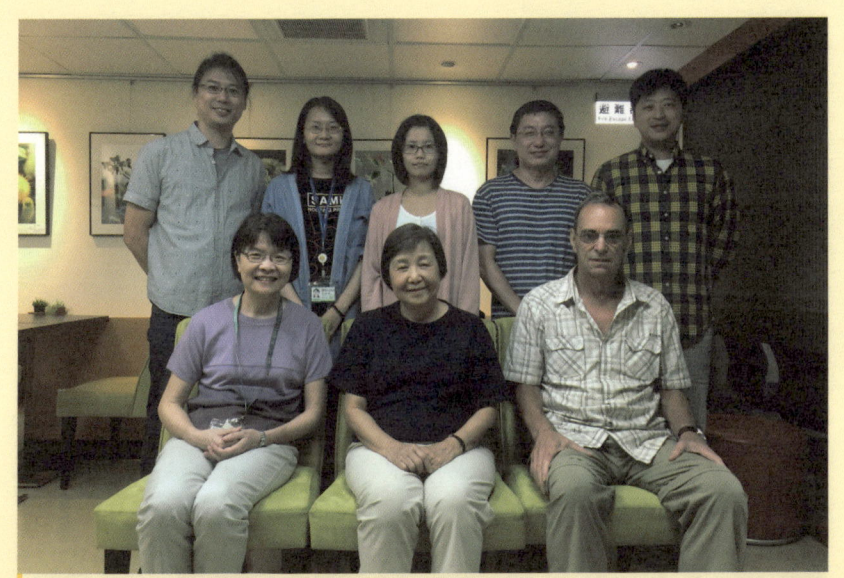

2018 年淡水馬偕醫院分子人類學研究室同工照：
王澤毅、賴穎慧、陳蘭蓉、陳宗賢、黃錦源
陸中衡、林媽利、Jean A. Trejaut (尚特鳩)

1-2

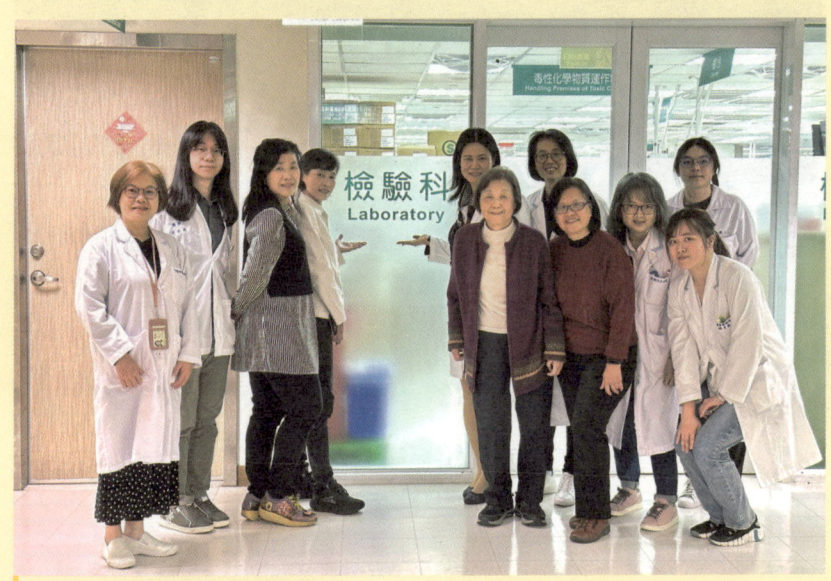

2025 年馬偕醫院血庫群英像
左起：吳乙瀠、姜宸語、王昌玲、張小琳、林媽利、張鳳娟、朱志芬、鍾旻叡，
後排：蔡欣怡、詹詠絮、許嬡真。

1-3

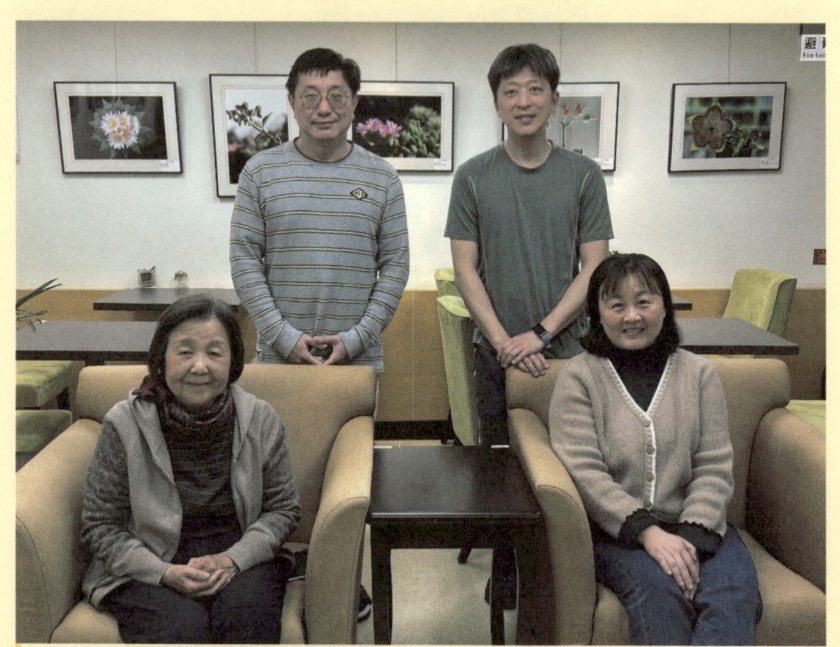

2025 年馬偕醫院分子人類學研究室成員
左下：林媽利醫師，右下：羅韻華助研究員，左上：陳宗賢研究助理，右上：黃錦源研究助理。

1-4

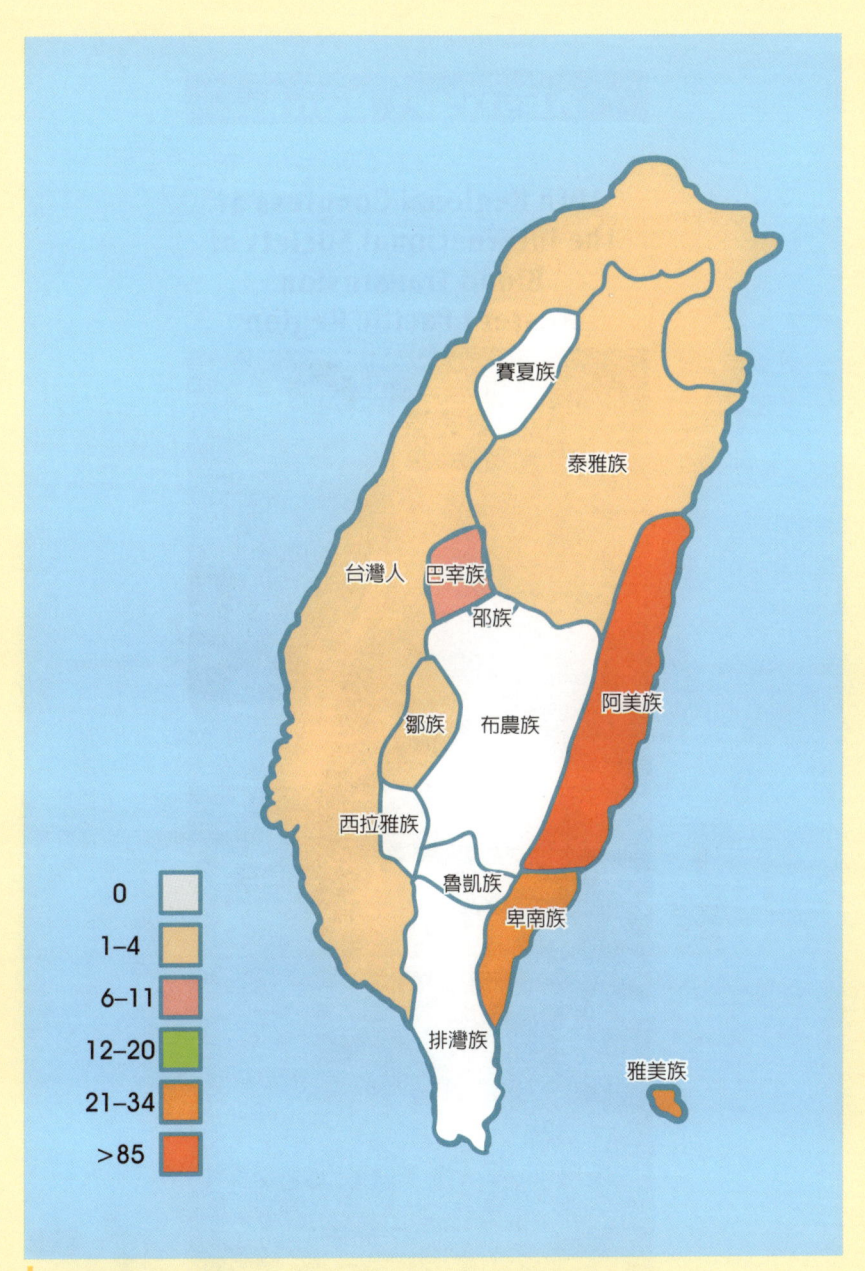

米田堡血型分布圖
阿美族有 95% 的族人帶米田堡血型，雅美族有 34%，卑南族有 21% 屬這血型，但隔壁的布農族、魯凱族及排灣族都沒發現這個血型。

02

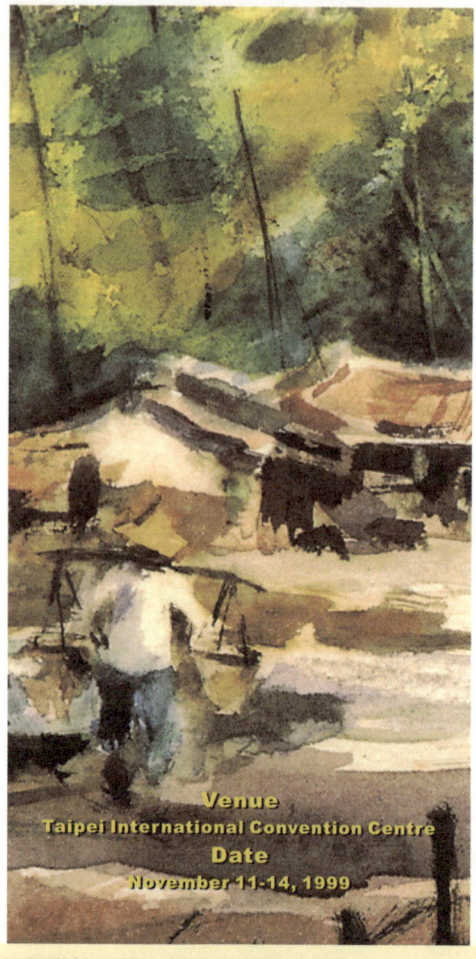

第 10 屆亞太地區國際輸血學會議程摘要集的封面
（中間是名畫家藍蔭鼎先生農家的畫作）

04

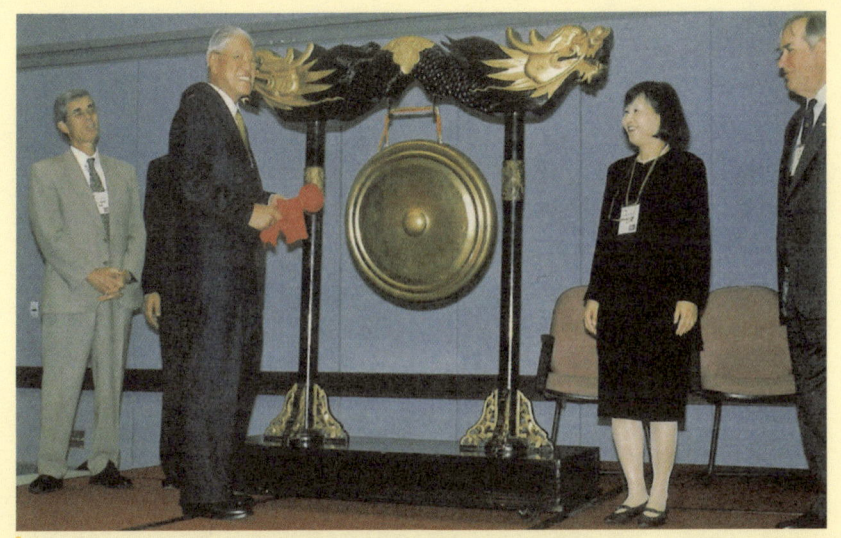

1999年國際輸血學會亞太地區大會首次在台灣舉辦,我擔任大會主席,當時李登輝總統參加開幕典禮,總統擊鑼開啟盛會。兩側分別為前後任國際輸血學會會長。

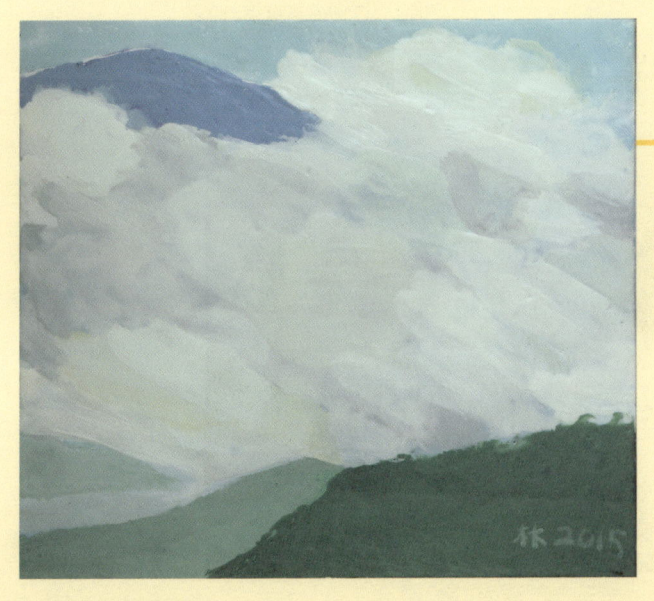

05

1999年台灣輸血學會舉辦國際會議,在籌備的三年間,因缺少資源,讓我失眠三年,事後我常常想起當時的焦慮,所以我在2021年1月舉辦了為台灣輸血學會義賣的畫展,畫展是在台中市凡亞藝術空間舉辦,感謝蔡正一先生慷慨提供場地,這幅〈雲海〉是當時參展的作品之一。

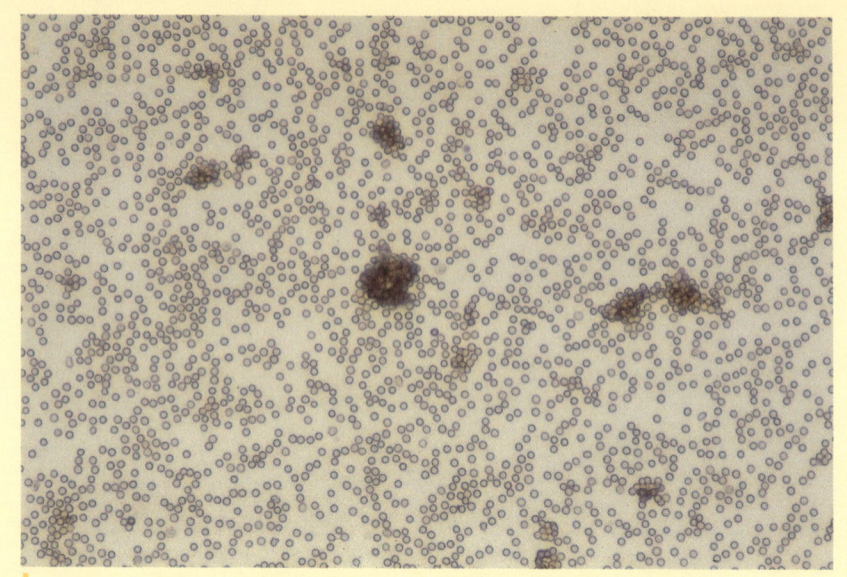

B₃ 血型：血球與 anti-B 反應，有些血球有反應呈小凝塊，有些沒反應，稱紅血球的混合反應。

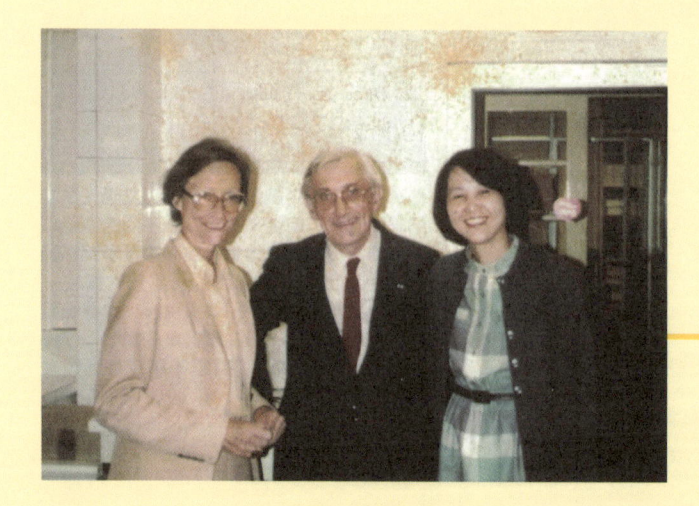

06

1984 年我（右）與法國巴黎血液中心的 Salmon 教授（中）合影

07

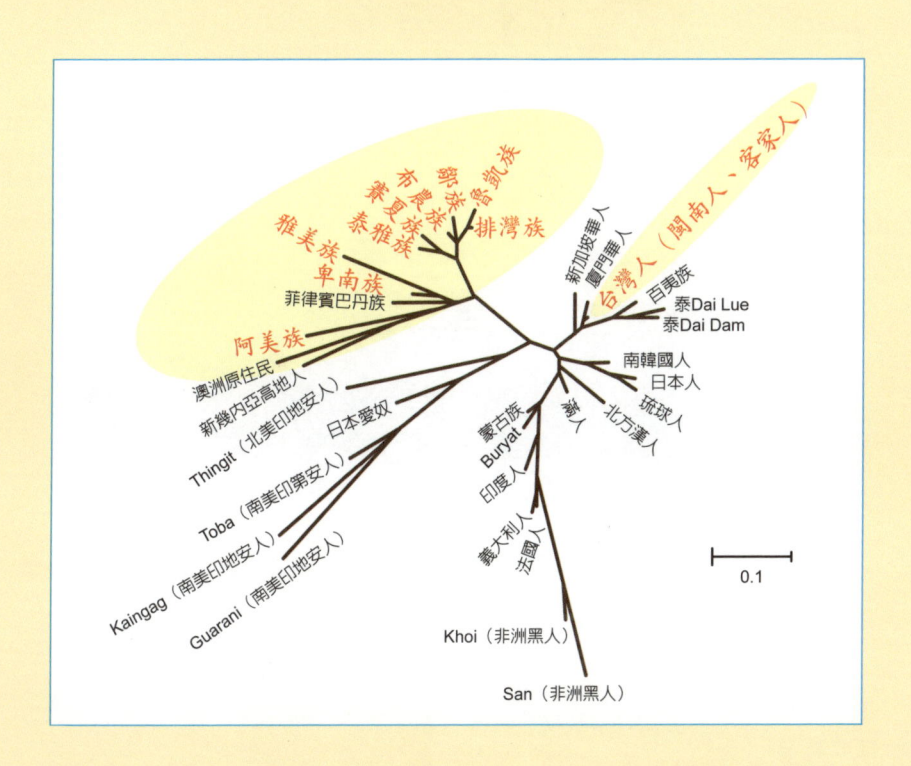

台灣族群的血緣關係樹

透過組織抗原（HLA-A, B, DRB1 基因頻率）的研究，可以知道台灣族群（紅字所示）間及與台灣以外族群的關係及基因距離，台灣高山原住民與其他亞洲族群包括閩南人、客家人分開並有顯著的基因距離。黑線表示基因距離，黑線的長短，表示基因距離的長短。

08

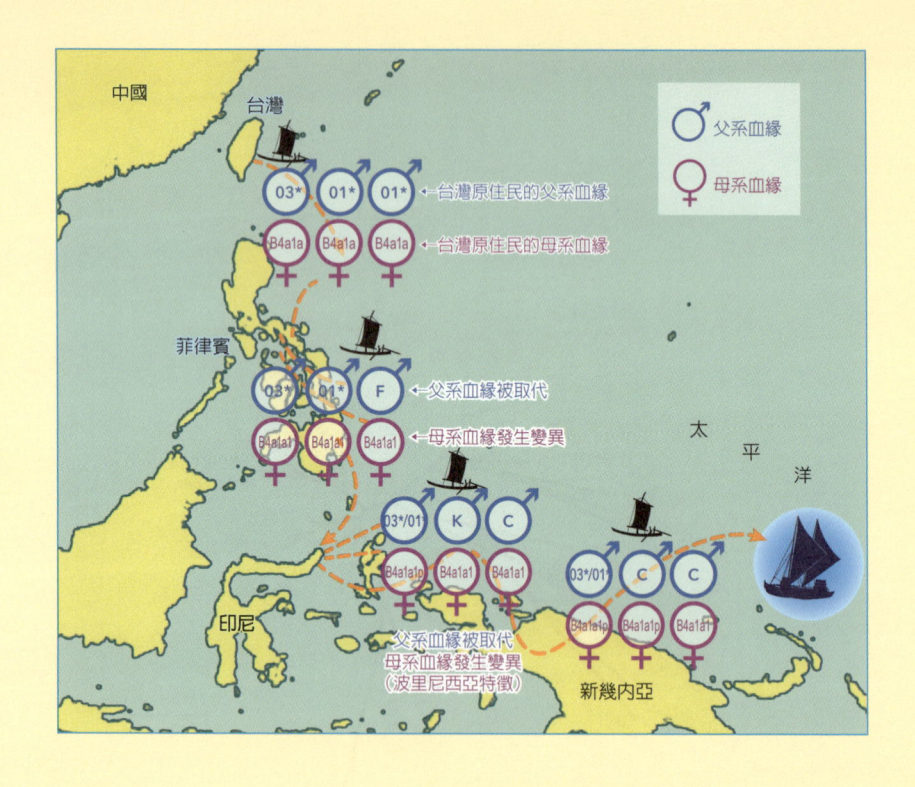

B4a1a 血緣的遷移

B4a1a 血緣的遷移起始於台灣，沿著圖中的橘色虛線遷移。帶 B4a1a 台灣原住民的祖先從台灣出發，先後經過菲律賓、東邊的印尼群島，再到達新幾內亞，途中發生基因的突變，到達新幾內亞形成波里尼西亞人的特徵血緣 B4a1a1a，再擴散到太平洋的島嶼。台灣原住民的父系血緣，在遷移過程中，大部分被美拉尼西亞的血緣所取代。所以波里尼西亞人是台灣原住民的母系血緣與美拉尼西亞人的父系血緣混合的人種。

09

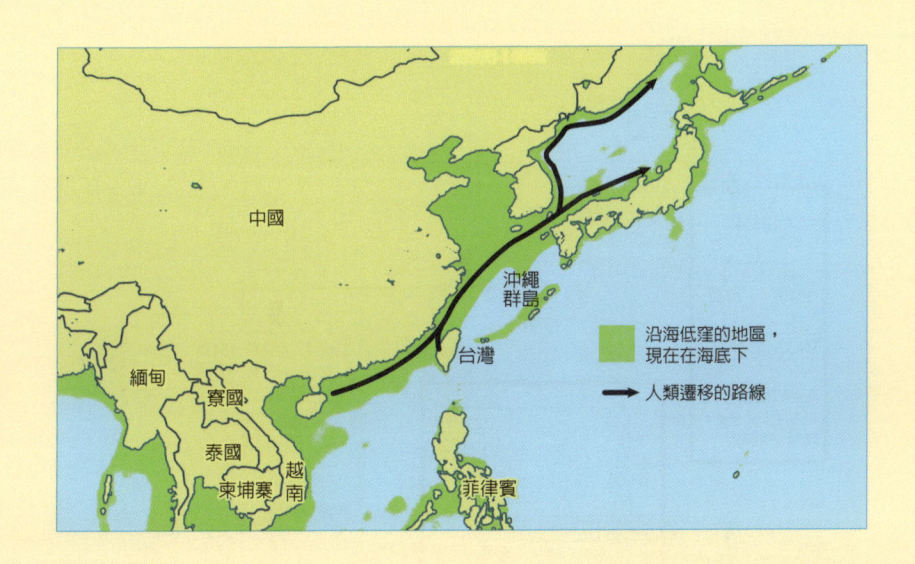

A24-B48 血緣的可能遷移路線
台灣高山原住民帶高頻率東北亞特徵的 A24-B48 血緣，紐西蘭的毛利人也同樣帶 A24-B48 血緣，從組織抗原單倍型（HLA haplotype）A24-B48 的分布，可推測在 50,000-10,000 年前，東亞人類的祖先，沿著海岸遷移的可能路線。

10

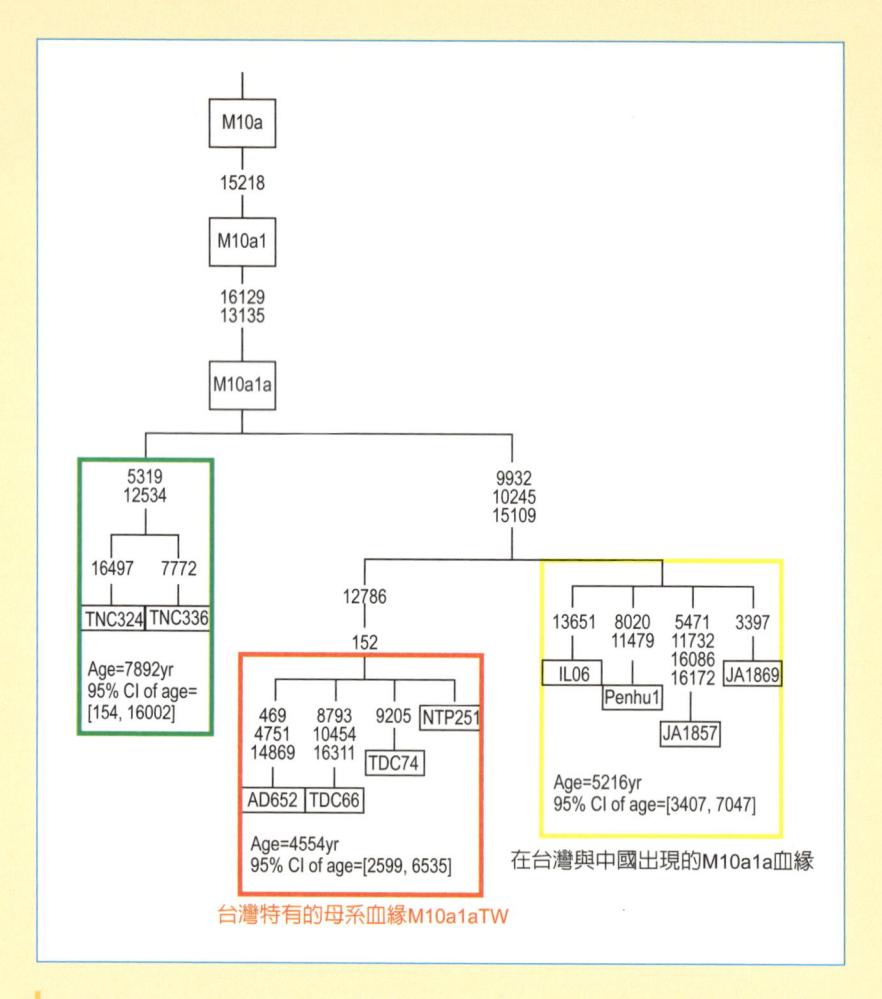

```
                    ┌─────┐
                    │ M10a│
                    └──┬──┘
                     15218
                    ┌──┴──┐
                    │M10a1│
                    └──┬──┘
                     16129
                     13135
                   ┌───┴───┐
                   │ M10a1a│
                   └───┬───┘
            ┌──────────┴──────────┐
          5319                   9932
         12534                  10245
                                15109
```

綠色框:
5319 12534
16497   7772
TNC324 TNC336
Age=7892yr
95% CI of age=
[154, 16002]

紅色框 (12786 152):
469   8793   9205   NTP251
4751 10454 16311
14869   TDC74
AD652 TDC66
Age=4554yr
95% CI of age=[2599, 6535]
台灣特有的母系血緣 M10a1aTW

黃色框:
13651 8020   5471   3397
       11479 11732
IL06   16086 JA1869
       Penhu1 16172
              JA1857
Age=5216yr
95% CI of age=[3407, 7047]
在台灣與中國出現的 M10a1a 血緣

M10a1a 血緣的演化

在人類的遷移過程中，M 血緣在 44,000 年前在阿拉伯半島形成，在 22,000 年前演化成 M10 血緣，15,000 年前演化成 M10a 血緣，14,000 多年前演化成 M10a1，11,000 多年前演化成 M10a1a 血緣，經過三個鹼基位置 9932、10245、15109 的突變，演化成 M10a1a-9932 血緣（黃色框），發生的年代是 5216 年前，這時 M10a1a 血緣從亞洲大陸開始遷移到台灣，所以這個血緣有兩個是中國人、兩個是台灣人。M10a1a-9932 血緣發生 12786、152 突變而形成在中央的紅色框 M10a1a-12786 血緣，發生的年代是 4554 年前，因為四個帶這血緣的人都是台灣人，所以是台灣特有的血緣，我們稱之為 TW 血緣。M10a1a 血緣分布情形是：韓國最多，佔人口的 2%，其次是中國 1%，其他日本、俄國、越南都是少於 1%。（M10a1a-9932、M10a1a-12786 血緣均為暫用的名字）

11

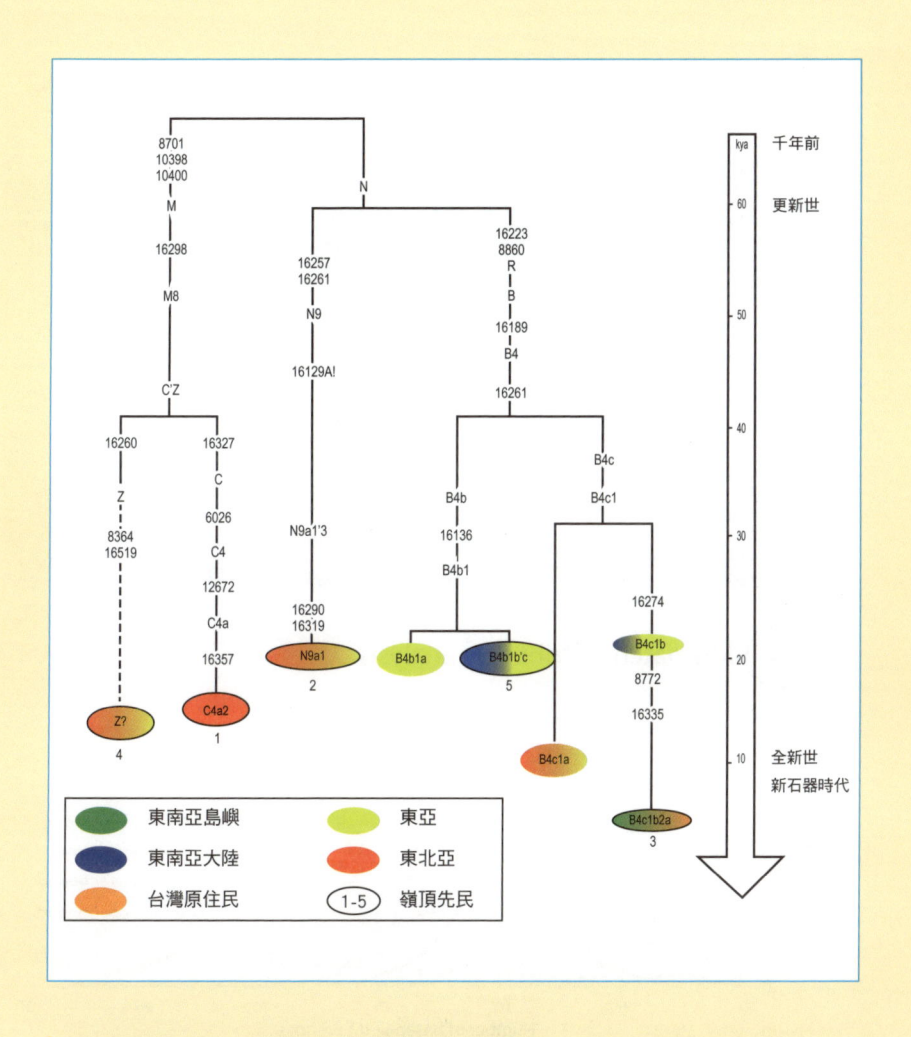

嶺頂遺址先民粒線體 DNA 單倍群的親緣關係樹

我們成功的定出 5 個先民（編號 1-5）母系血緣的型別（單倍群 Haplogroup），分別是 C4a2、N9a1、B4c1b2a、Z 和 B4b1 血緣。這 5 個血緣皆常見於現今台灣人，除了 B4c1b2a 血緣常見於台灣中部高山原住民（編號 3），其他 C4a2（編號 1）、N9a1（編號 2）、Z（編號 4）和 B4b1（編號 5）血緣屬於東亞大陸血緣。其中代表台灣原住民的 B4c1b2a （編號 3）血緣在台灣的分布狀況，很有趣的是，北部與中部原住民的頻率是高於南部原住民與非原住民，也見於少數的非原住民的台灣人。C4a2 和 Z 血緣常見於現代東北亞人群，表示新石器時代晚期在台灣東海岸有東北亞的血緣。相反的，B4b1 血緣屬於東南亞大陸血緣，N9a1 血緣屬於東北亞及東亞的血緣。

12

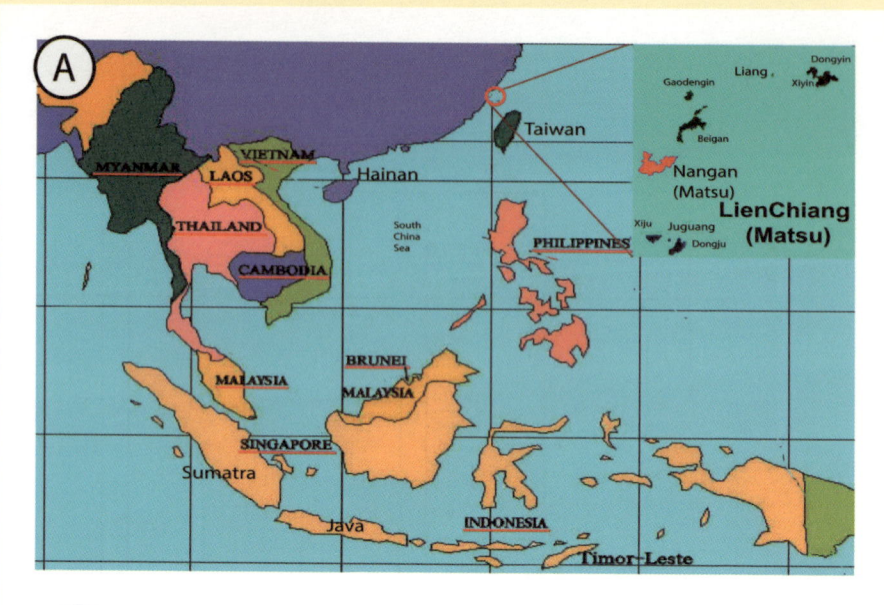

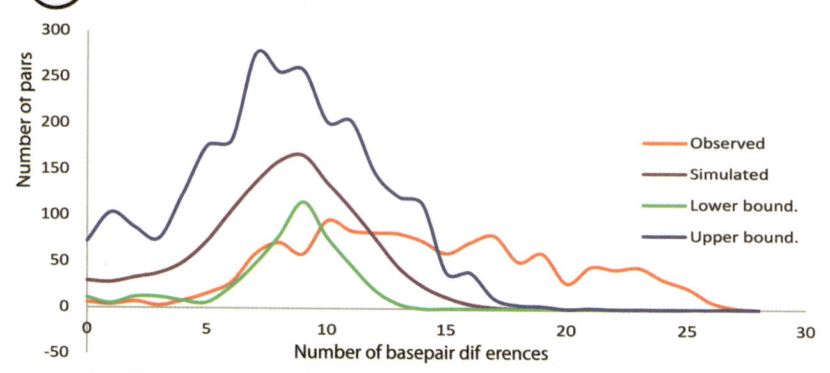

A) 馬祖人群與周邊東亞人群的關係研究中之檢體含括位置。
B) 錯配分布分析顯示，在 5 至 25 個鹼基對差異間呈現平坦且寬的單峰曲線，其平均差異為 14.5 鹼基對。這些結果顯示馬祖人群血緣的歧異，來自多個亞洲起源群體的基因混合，而非由單一人口擴張引起的。

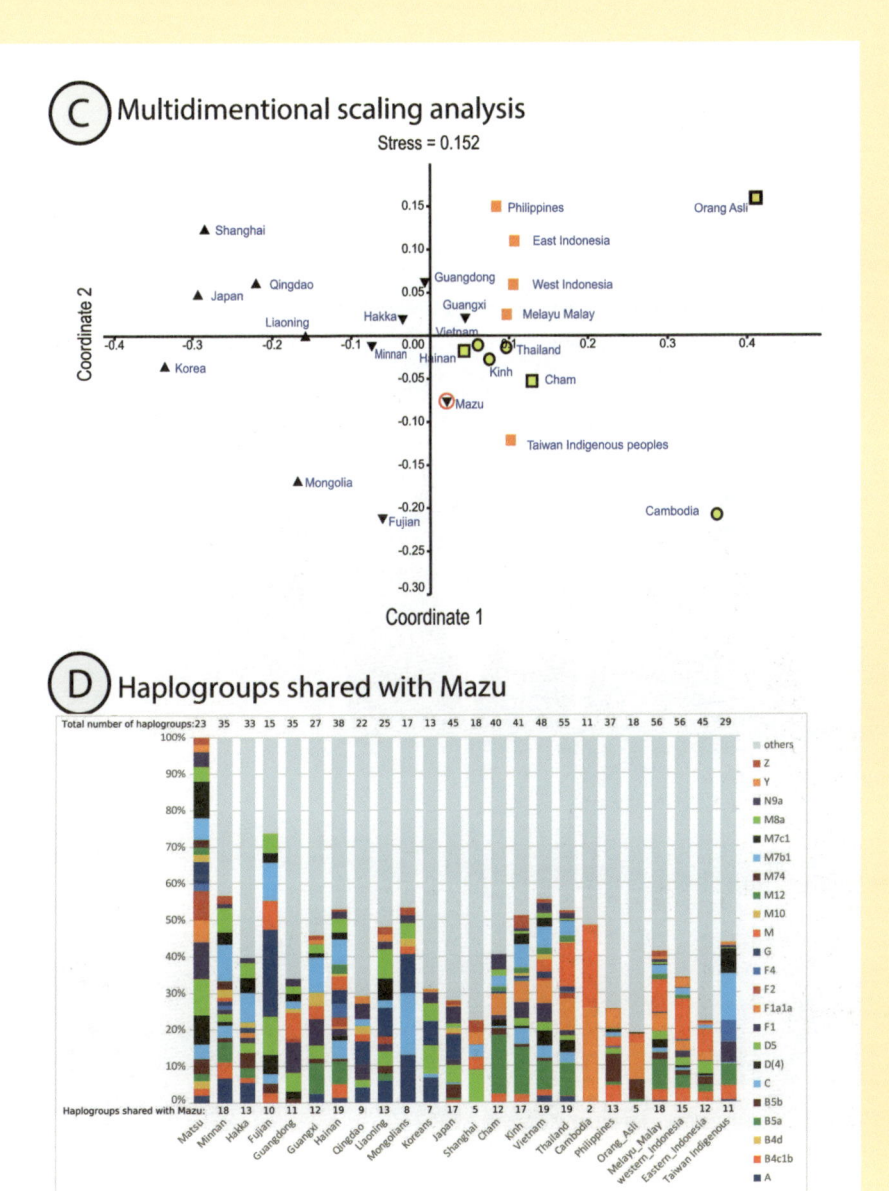

# C) Multidimentional scaling analysis
Stress = 0.152

D) Haplogroups shared with Mazu

C) 通過多維尺度分析（PCA 分析）檢測馬祖與其他亞洲人群之間的母系遺傳分布。馬祖人群高單倍群多樣性及大量獨特單倍型表明，其基因結構中存在相對高比例的核苷酸差異，顯示這是一個自新石器時代以來，經歷多次基因流動的不同種族人群。

D) 8 個單倍群（D4、D5、F1、F2、G 和 M7）出現的頻率超過 5%。其中，D4、D5、F2 和 G 的亞型在現代東北亞人群中較為常見，而 F1 和 M7 的亞型則多見於東南亞地區。馬祖人與台灣原住民的母系血緣並沒有特別的關係。

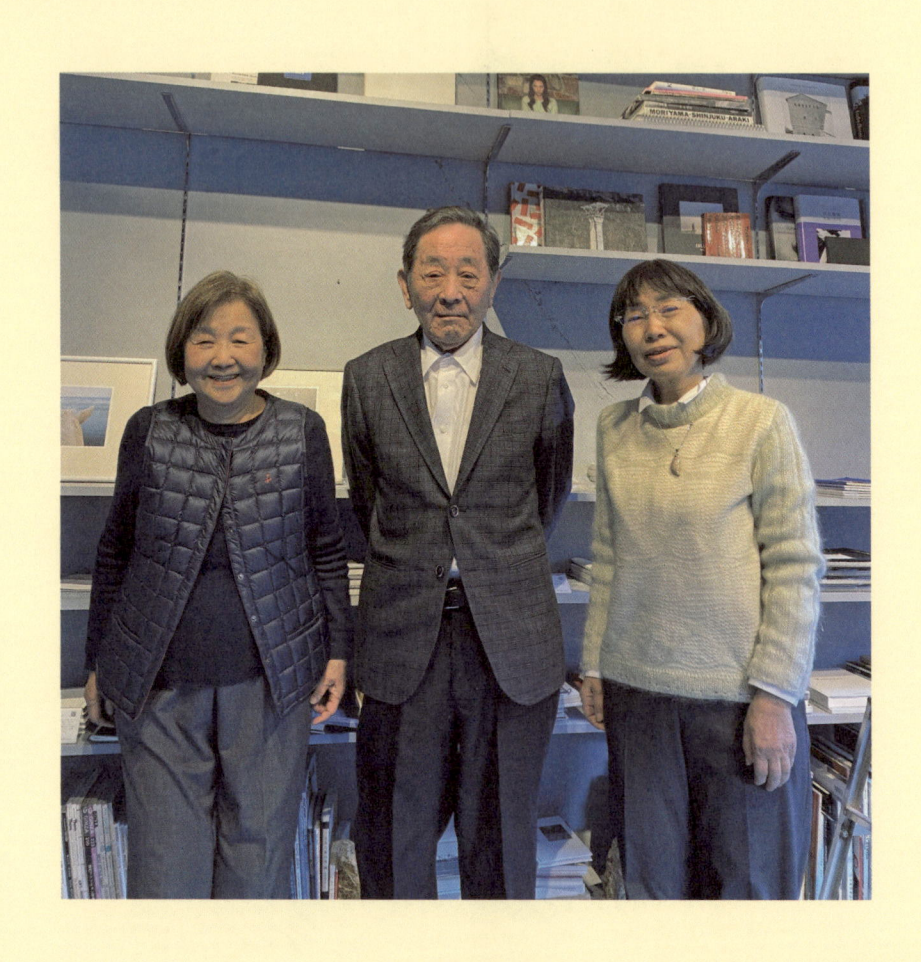

2024年3月5日,我重返東京去探望十字猛夫教授,向他30年前義無反顧的幫助我們成立組織抗原實驗室道謝,左起:我、十字教授、十字教授前秘書。

二、高雄醫學院年代

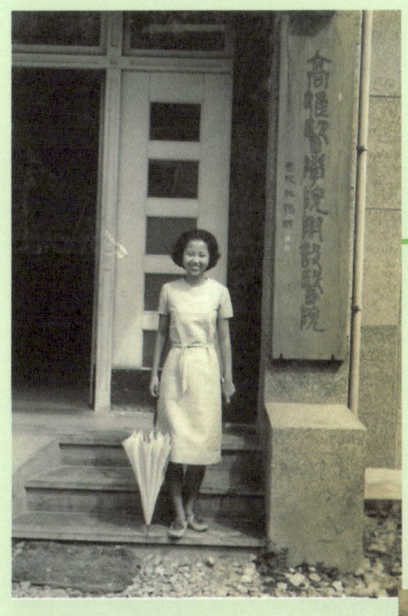

1959年攝於當時的高醫教室門口,高雄天氣炎熱。在我右後方,有杜聰明老師寫的字「高雄醫學院附設醫院」牌子。

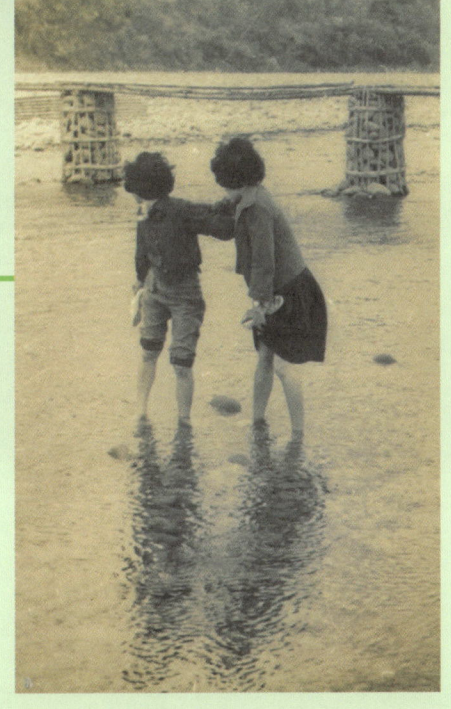

高醫時代,在週末常去附近的大小山爬山,1959年我與李憓理爬完大岡山後,涉溪去找公車回學校。

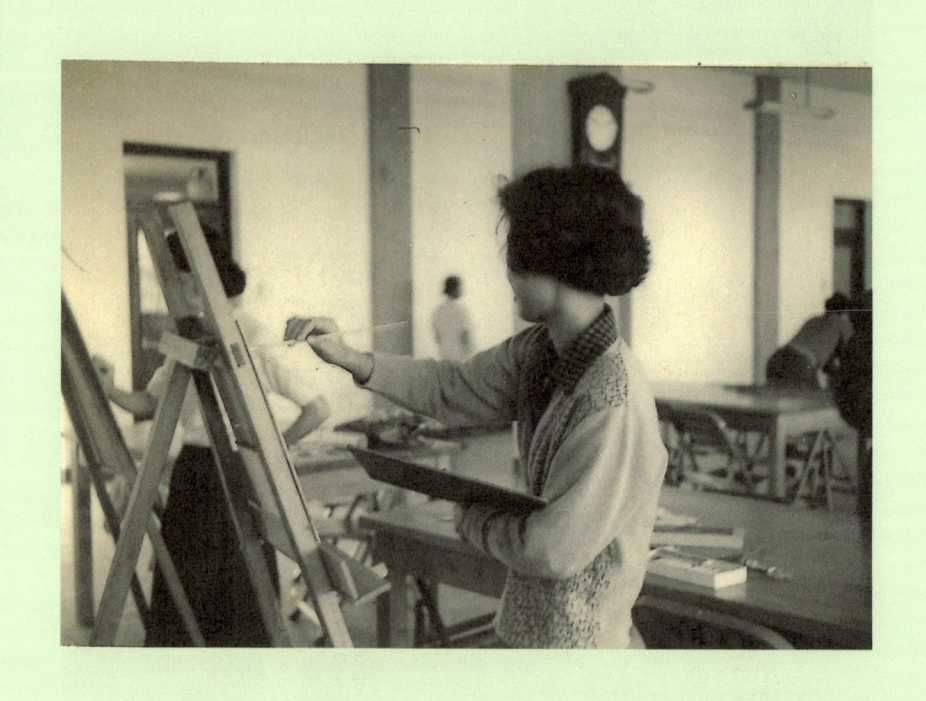

我們的杜聰明院長主張,醫師要懂藝術、文學,所以我和幾個朋友參加高雄醫學院「星期六畫會」學習繪畫,師劉啓祥老師。

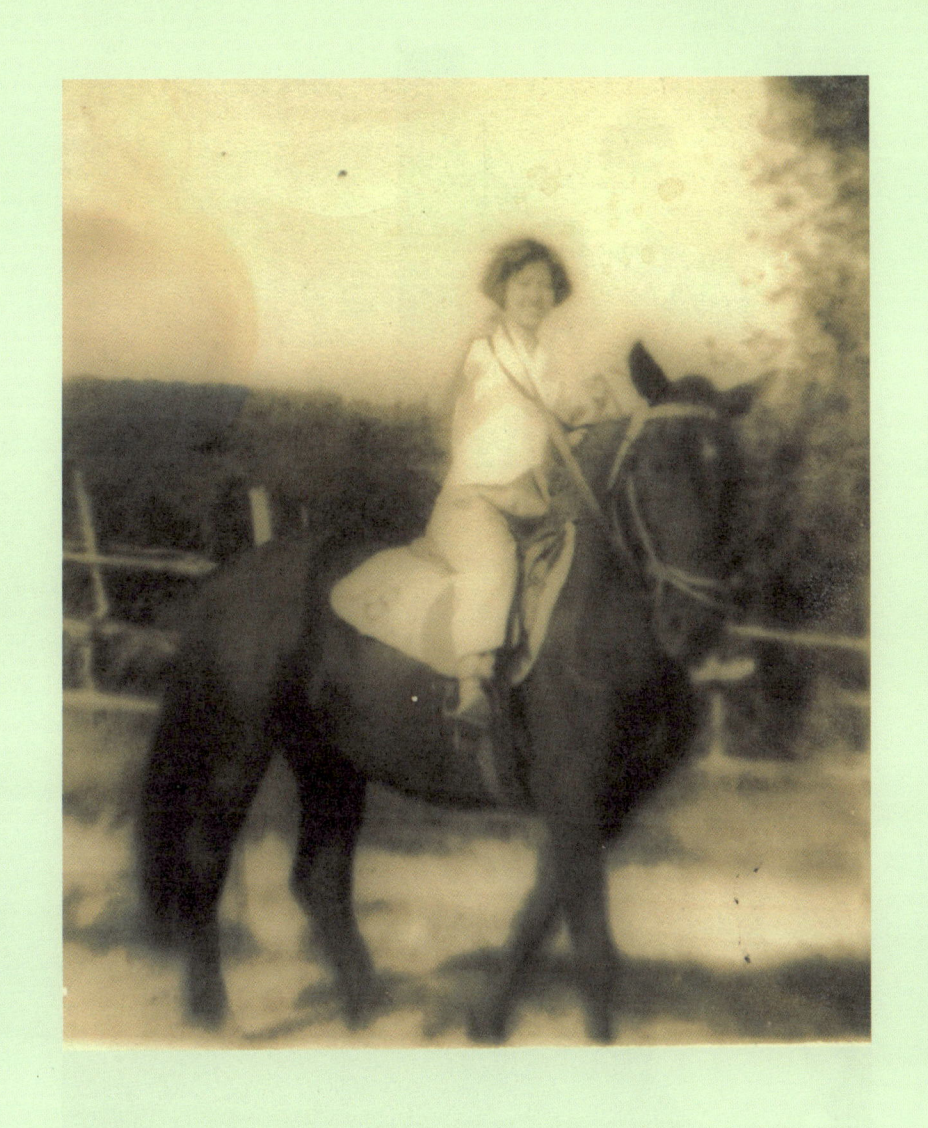

年輕時異想天開，1959 年我與同學林竹信、林安石、林梅圃、吳幸雄，到台中后里的騎馬場騎馬。

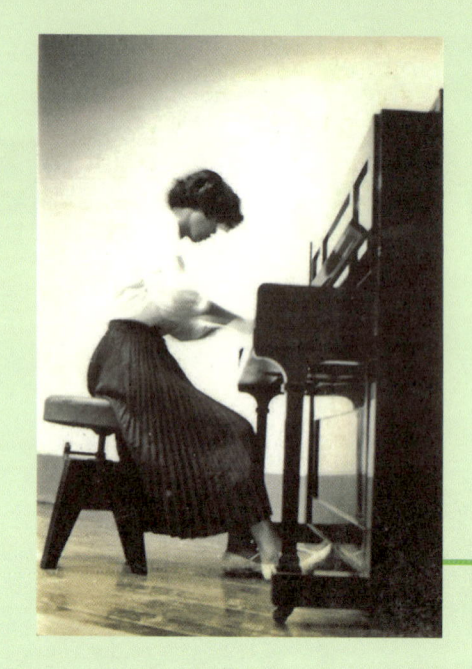

1962 年，我在高醫校慶晚會演奏蕭邦的曲子（幻想即興曲）。

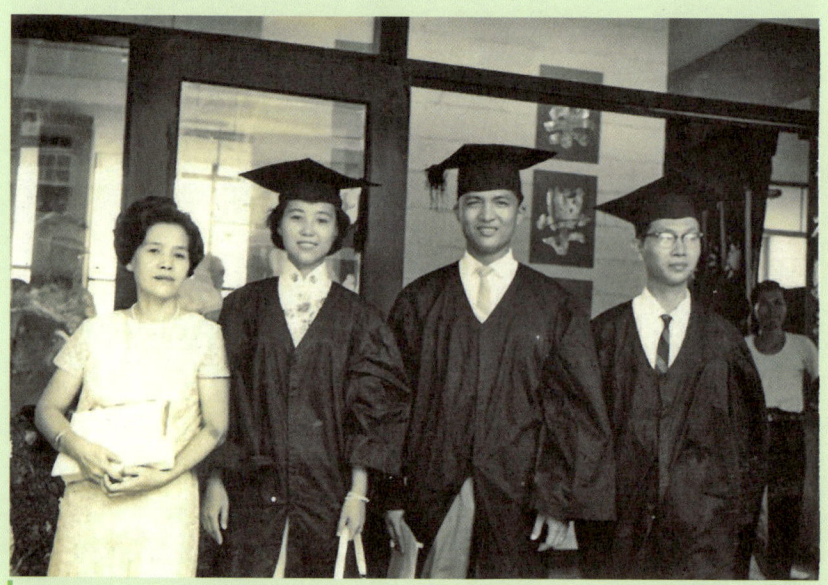

1964 年從高雄醫學院畢業，畢業典禮後，我與同學合照，自右：王啓釧同學、張簡俊一同學、我、我的母親。

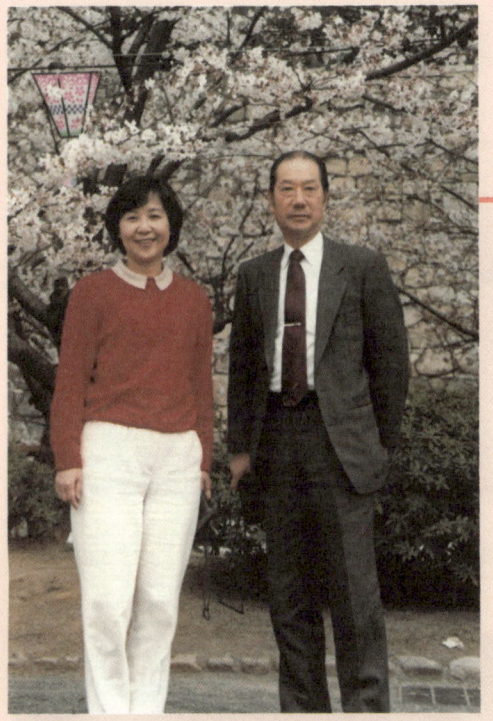

三、馬偕醫院輸血醫學暨分子人類學組時期

日本春天全地盛開著櫻花，在1990年代台灣還是沒有多少櫻花可欣賞，為了重溫日本童年在櫻花樹下漫遊的喜悅，1991年我在櫻花季節，專程去拜訪日本大阪府紅十字會副會長大久保康人教授，他是國際著名的血型專家，感謝他長期提供台灣研究所需要的稀有血型的血球和血清（攝於日本古蹟大阪城）。

1991年我與恩師西岡久壽彌教授（川村明義教授未能參與）（中）參觀高雄醫學院與謝獻臣老師（右）合影。

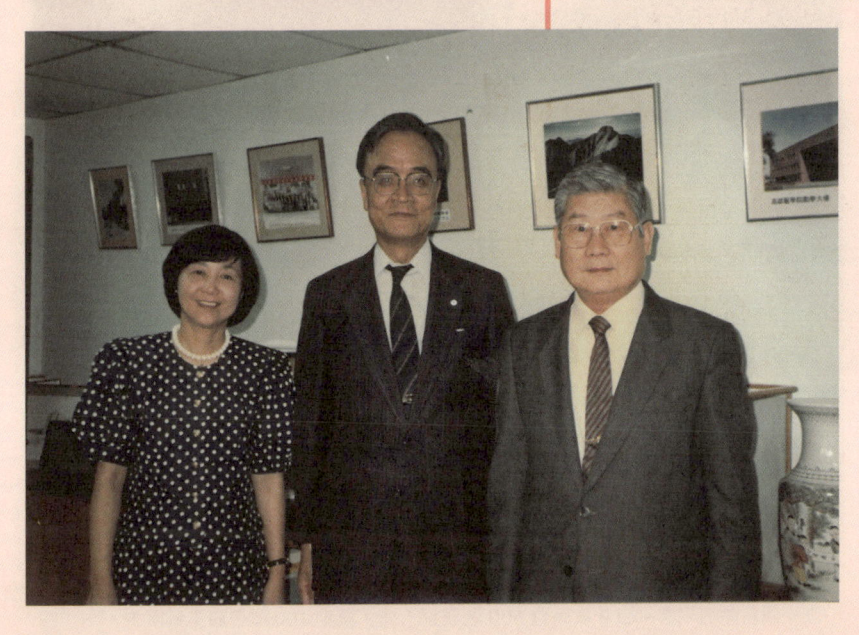

21

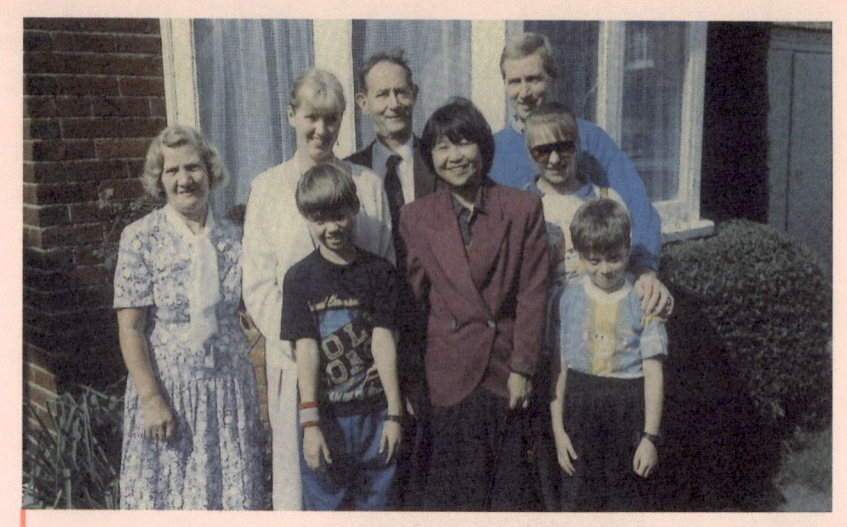

1992 年藉著參加倫敦 1992 年國際輸血學會之便去拜訪鮑伯瑞先生的家人，後排自左：鮑先生父親、鮑先生，中排：鮑先生母親、妹妹、鮑先生太太，前排：鮑先生甥兒、我、鮑先生甥兒。

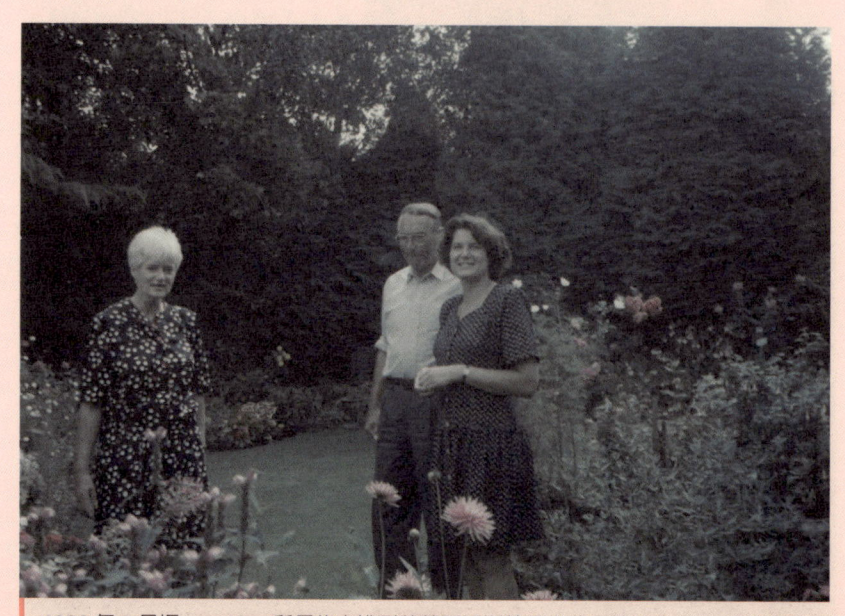

1992 年 7 月經 van Alen 所長的安排到荷蘭阿姆斯特丹血液實驗中心（CLB）為期一個月，與研究白血球的 Judith Heermans（右一）研究用放射性同位素法測量顆粒性白血球的抗體，以解決當時偶爾在台灣出現的輸血引起的呼吸窘困症（TRALI）的問題，週末被邀到前所長家，前所長是著名的學者 Paul Engelfriet（中間），左邊是秘書，他家有一個美麗的花園。CLB 當時有 500 個研究人員，其中 100 個是醫生或博士。

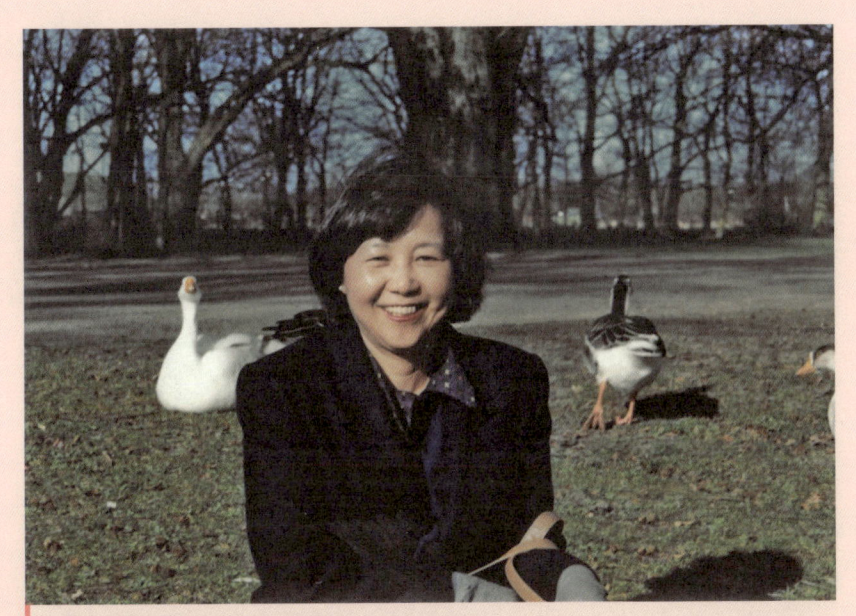

1990 年攝於阿姆斯特丹一處鄰近 CLB 的公園。

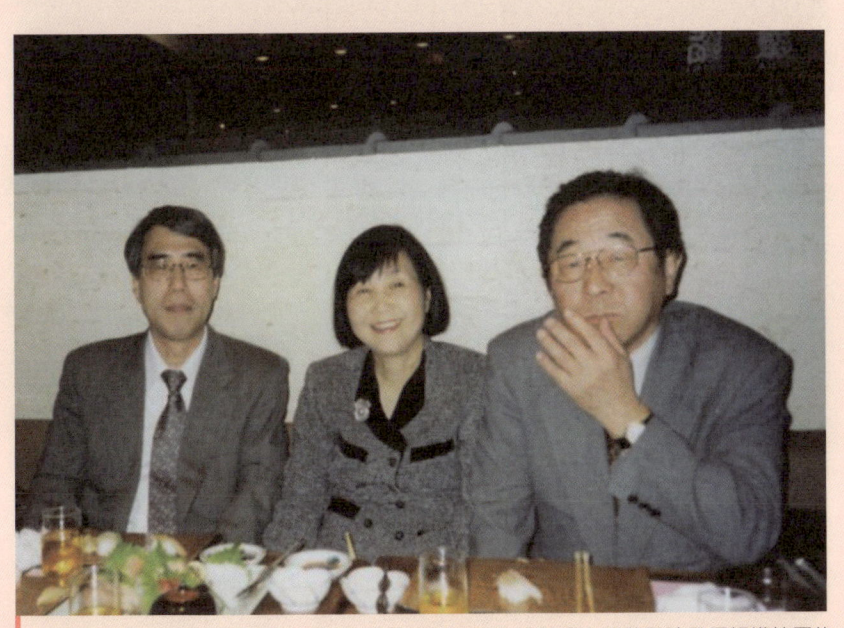

1994 年與日本紅十字會血液中心的友人聚餐，右為協助我在馬偕醫院發展組織抗原的十字猛夫教授，左為松田教授（Mazda Toshio）。

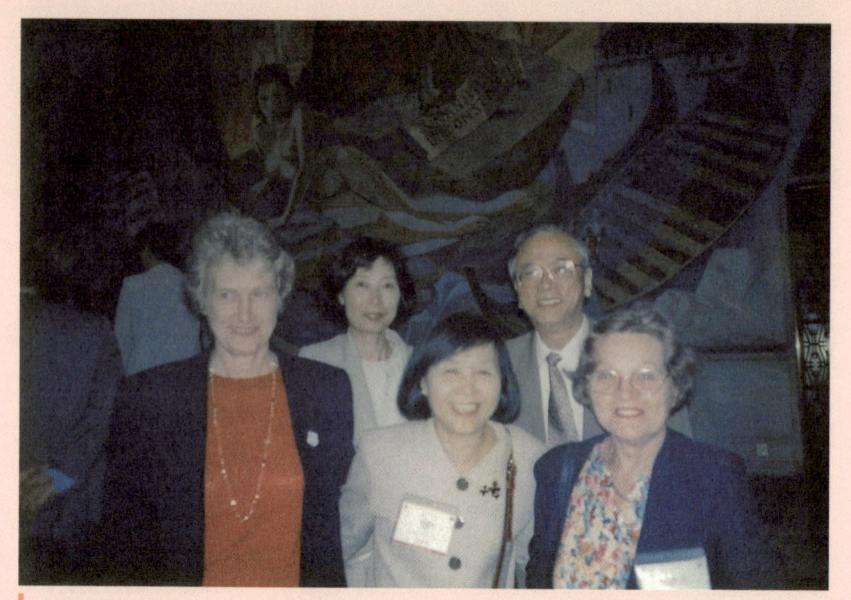

在國際會議中，我與許多別國的朋友相見歡，台灣的血液醫學能有先進國家的水準，是許多人的功勞，右一為 Patricia Tippett，右二是我，左一為 Marion Reid，後排為清水教授夫婦。

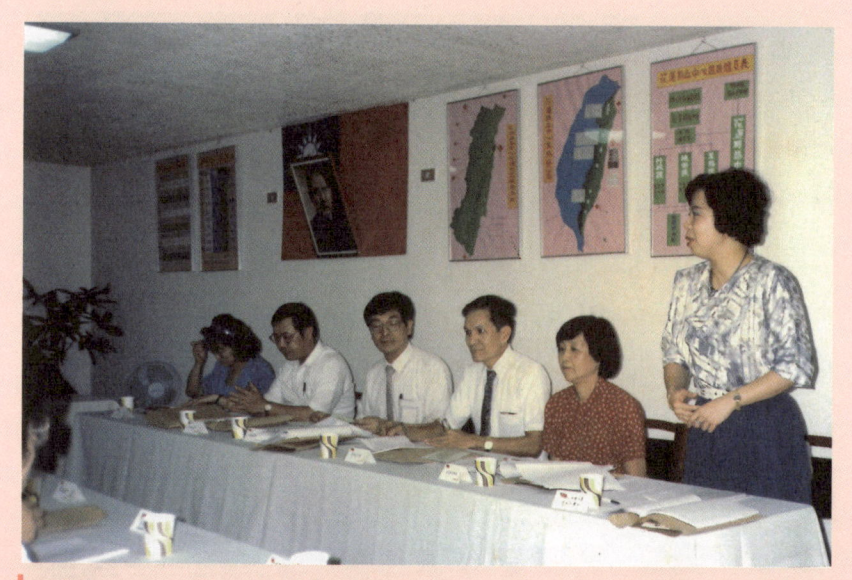

台灣在 1985 年開始了全台醫院血庫及捐血機構的評鑑。這是 1991 年捐血中心的評鑑，評鑑委員共有四人：左二為李正華，左三為孫建峰，左四為高原祥，左五是我等四人，右一為衛生署蔡素玲。

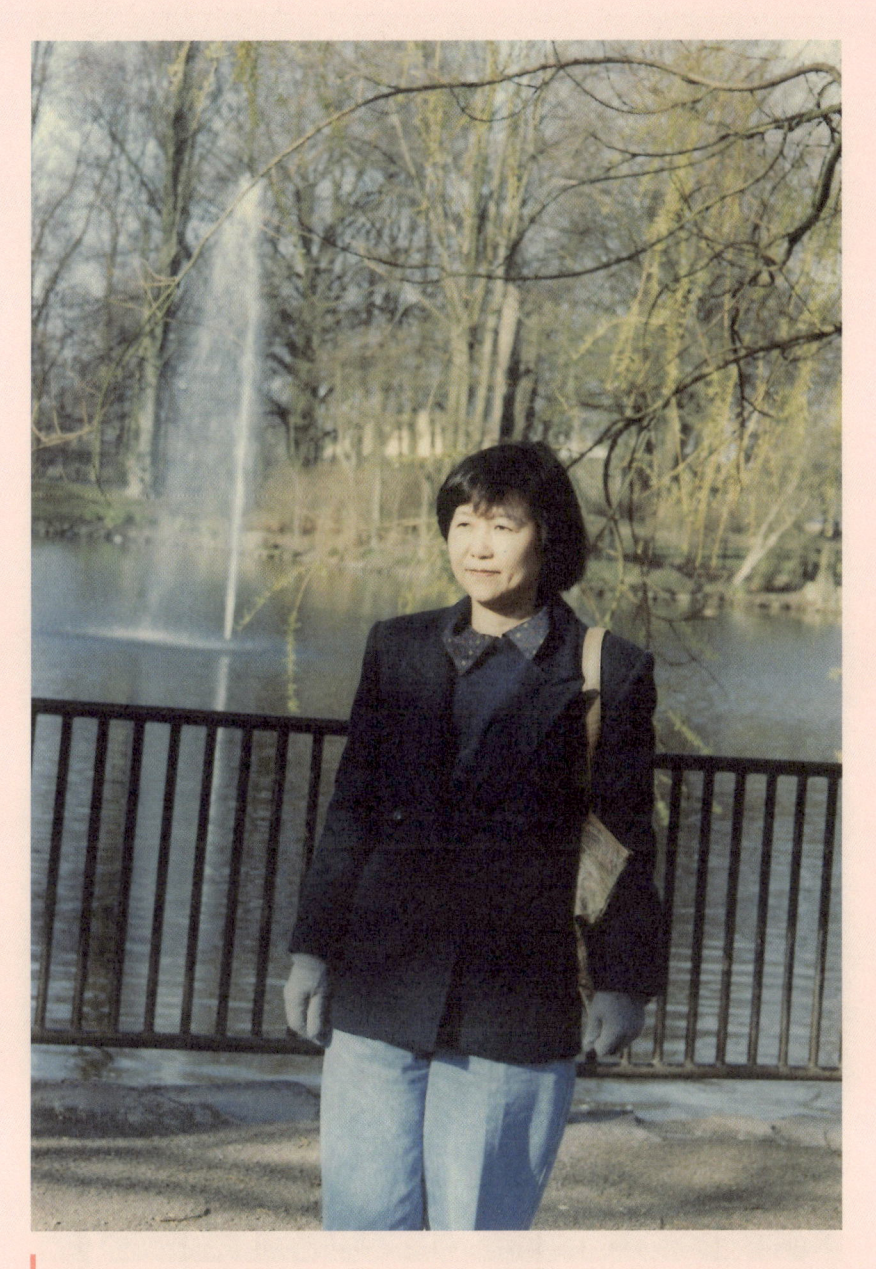

1986 年,我與鮑博瑞赴瑞典 Lund 參加第一屆國際血型單株抗體的會議,我們發現只見於亞洲的 Le(a+b+) 血型而震驚國際。照片攝於會場外。

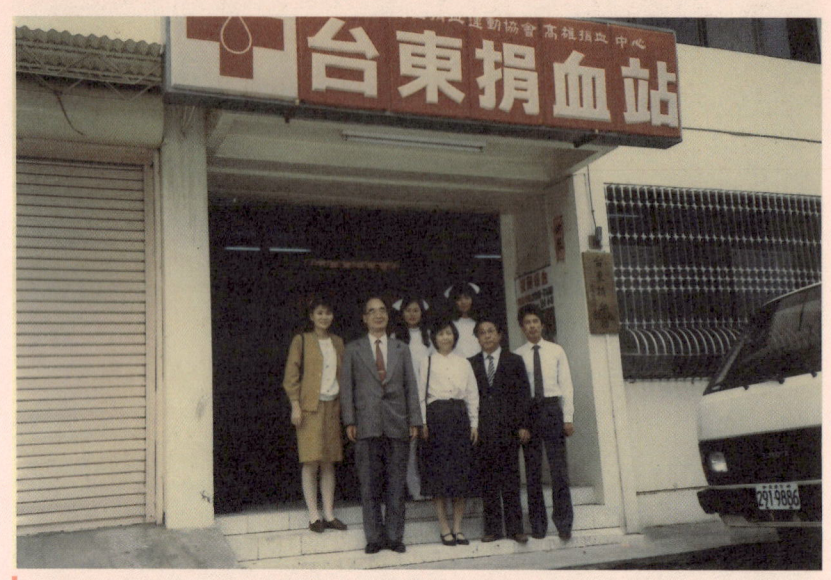

1991 年，到台東捐血站評鑑，左一為衛生署石美春，左二為榮總雍建輝，左三是我，右二為高雄捐血中心主任王鏡山。

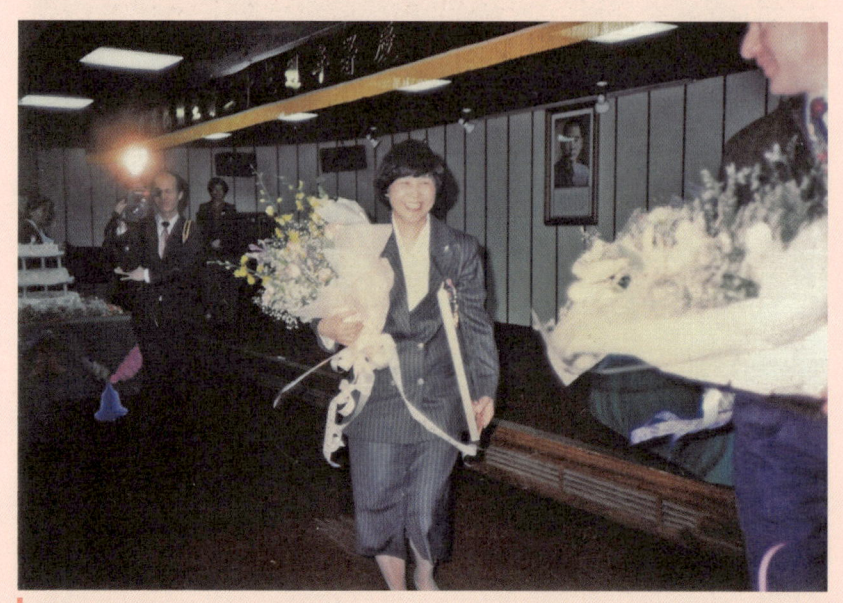

1994 年衛生署頒發衛生獎章給我，獎勵我「制定血液政策，改進血庫作業方法，貢獻至鉅」。

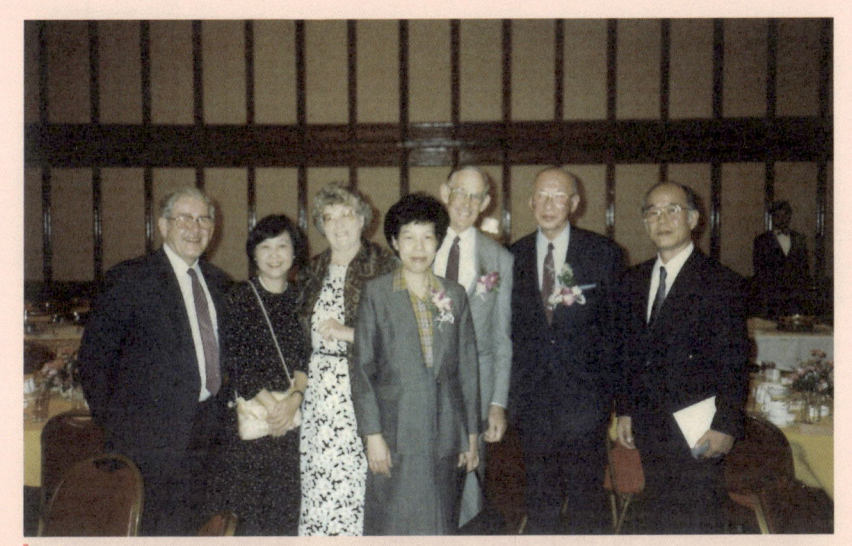

1991 年,輸血學會年會邀請國際輸血學會會長 H. Gunson（左一）及其夫人（左三）、左二是我,當時衛生署署長張博雅（右四）,前會長 Archer（右三）及日本輸血學會前會長遠山博（右二）與日本輸血學會會長湯淺晉（右一）來台演講。

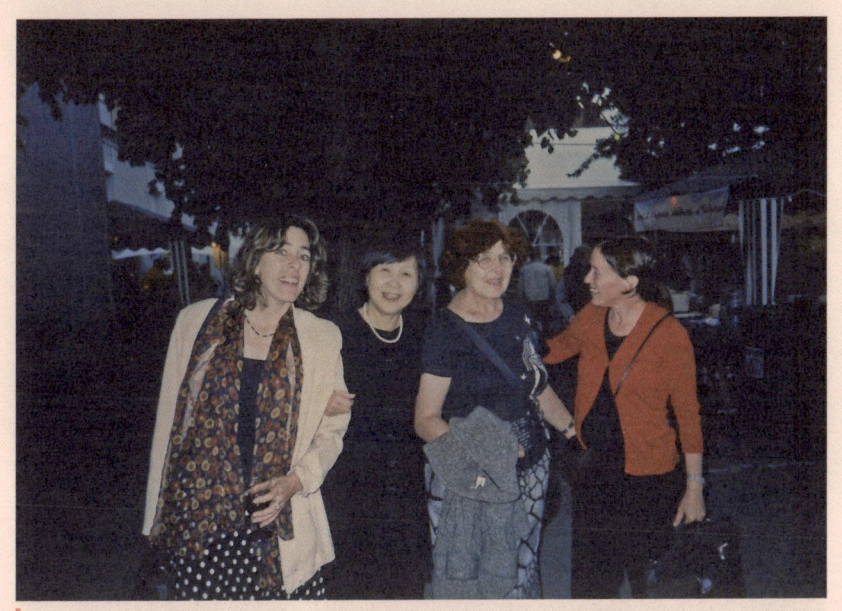

2004 年,在瑞士日內瓦大學我（左二）與日內瓦大學人類學教授 Alicia Sanchez-Mazas（左一）及 Roger Blench 等合辦「從基因、語言及考古看東亞大陸及台灣島上人類的遷移」研討會,與參加研討會的俄國學者 Ludmilla Osipova（右二）及挪威的 Erica Hagelberg（右一）合照。

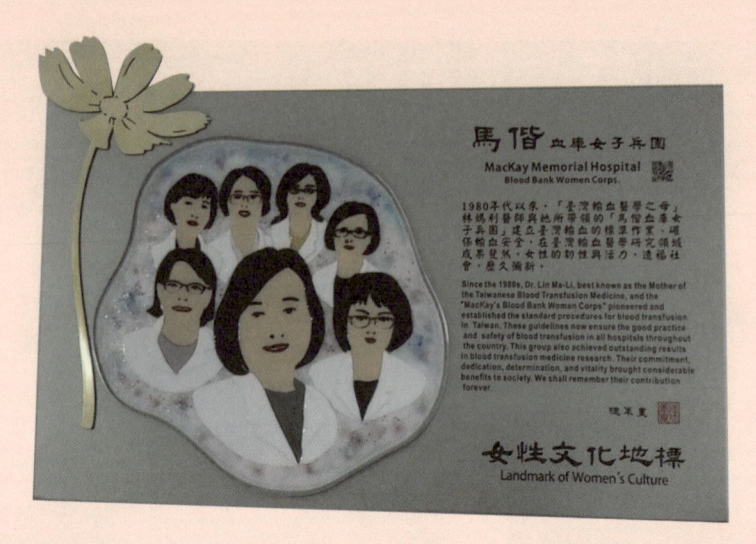

「馬偕血庫女子兵團」女性文化地標：自 1980 年代，「台灣輸血醫學之母」林媽利醫師與所帶領的「馬偕血庫女子兵團」，建立台灣輸血的標準作業，確保輸血安全，在台灣醫學研究領域成果斐然，女性文化地標總策劃陳秀惠女士為感謝林媽利醫師貢獻，特贈由藝術家陳彥君創作的「馬偕血庫女子兵團」女性文化地標。

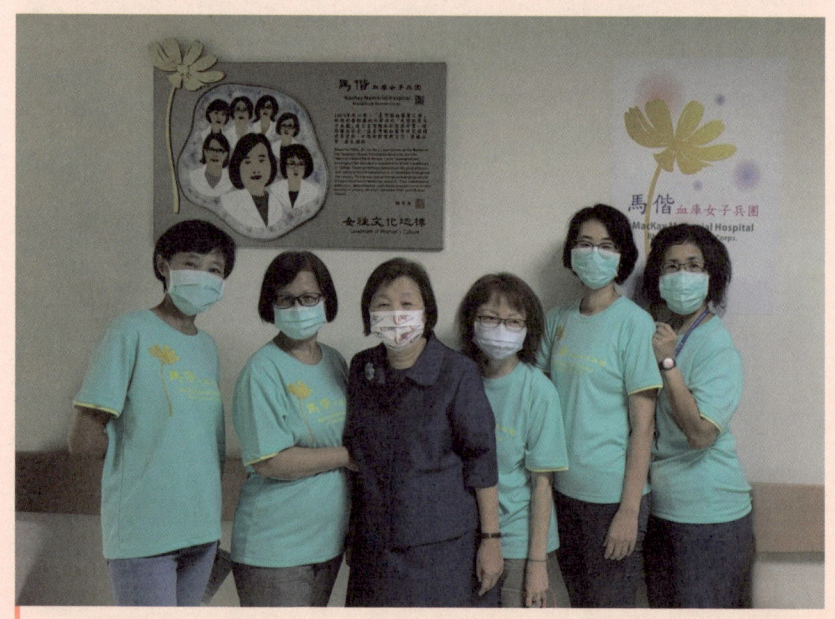

我與馬偕血庫女子兵團於女性文化地標前合影，由左至右：張小琳、張鳳娟、林媽利、朱志芬、詹詠絮、王昌玲。

28

四、家人

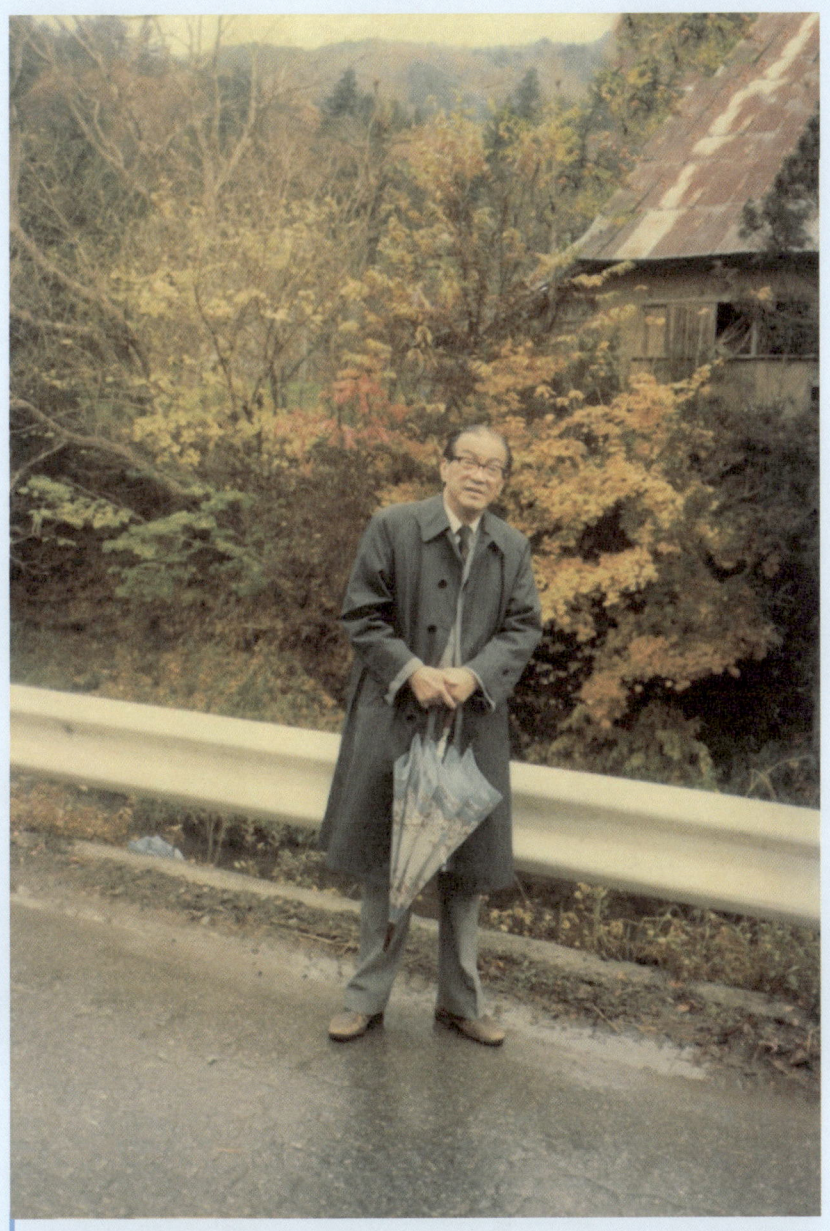

1983年秋天，我到日本東北的陸前高田，探望在日本無醫村執業行醫的年邁父親林新振醫師。1987年黑名單解禁，他才又回到故鄉台灣。

1954 年攝於台南家中
前排左起：
母親吉武牧野、弟弟林秀人、父親林新振
後排左起：
姊姊林聆利、林媽利

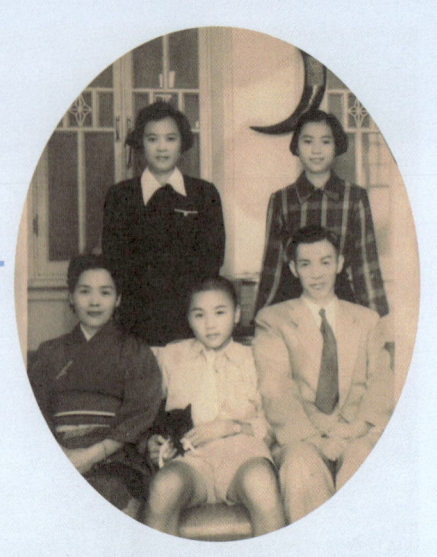

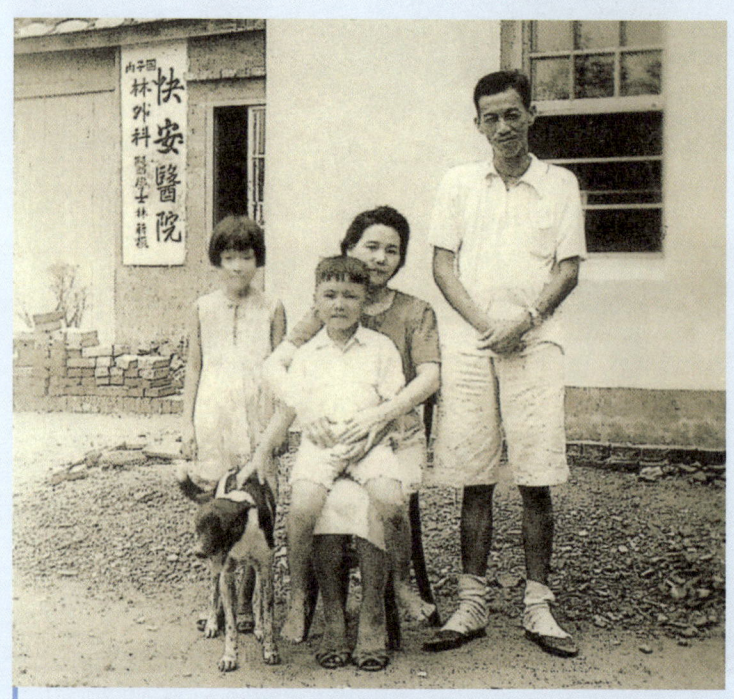

1947 年隨著父母從中國東北（滿洲）回到台灣。1948 年，我在父親的故鄉高雄縣湖內鄉圍仔內的診所快安醫院外，與父母親及弟弟和愛犬合照。

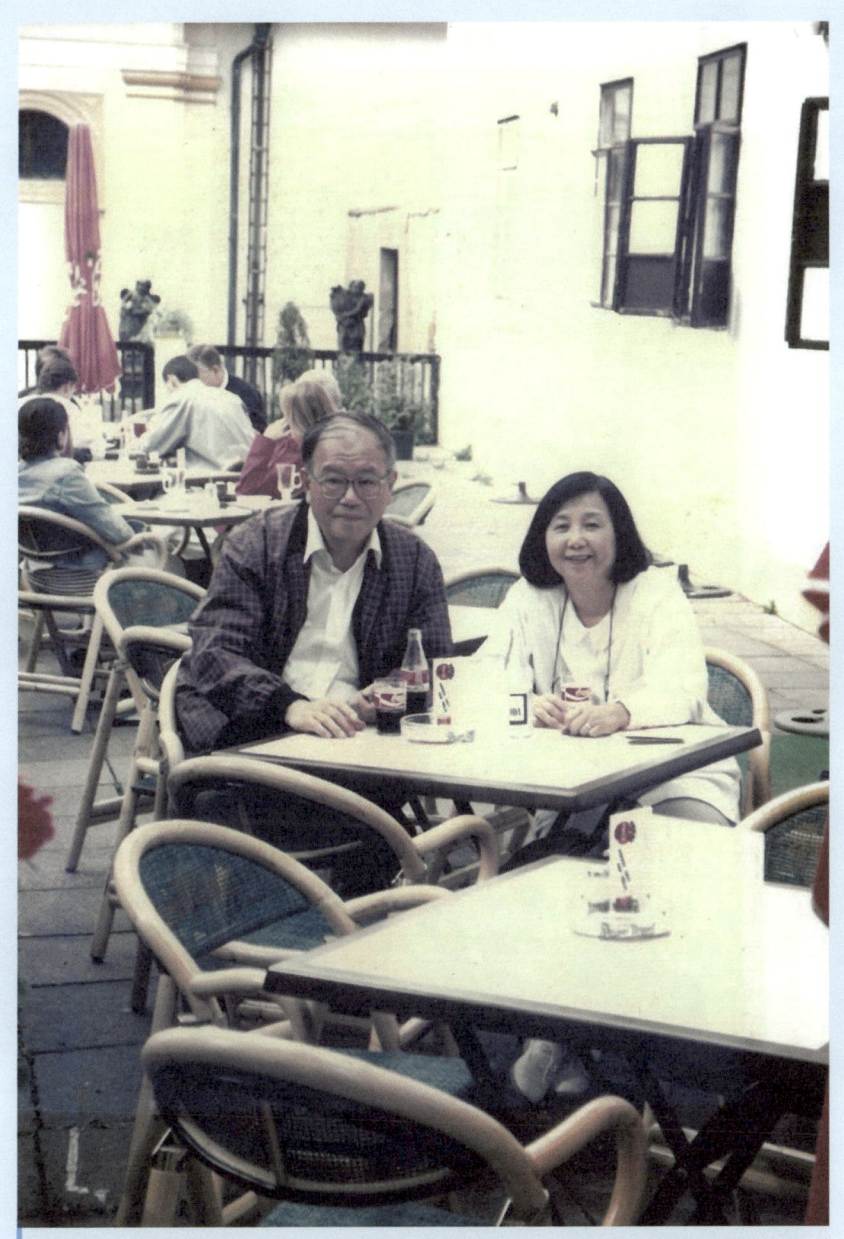

1995 年，參加國際輸血學會後，我與先夫郭惠二攝於羅浮宮屋頂的陽台休息處。

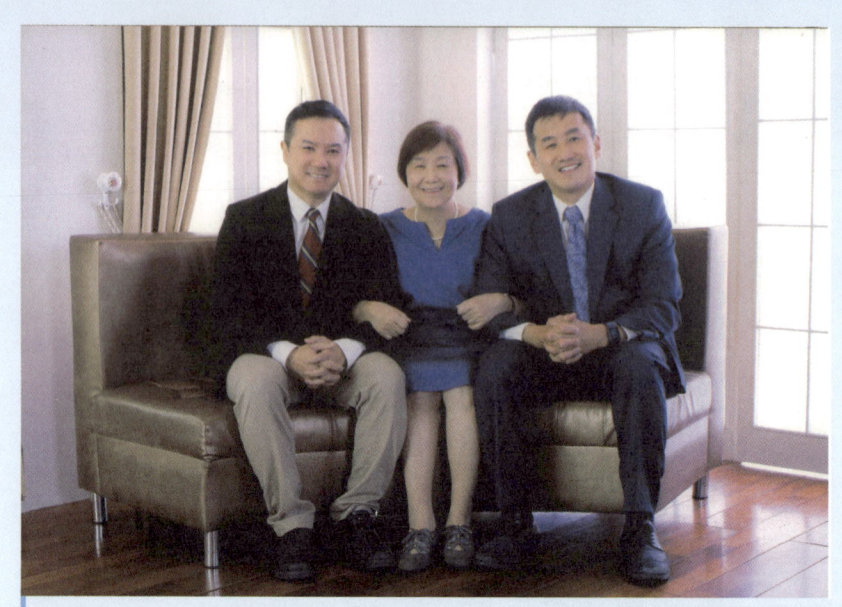

2018 年，我八十歲生日，與兩個孩子合影，左為大兒子暐濤，右為小兒子暐崧。

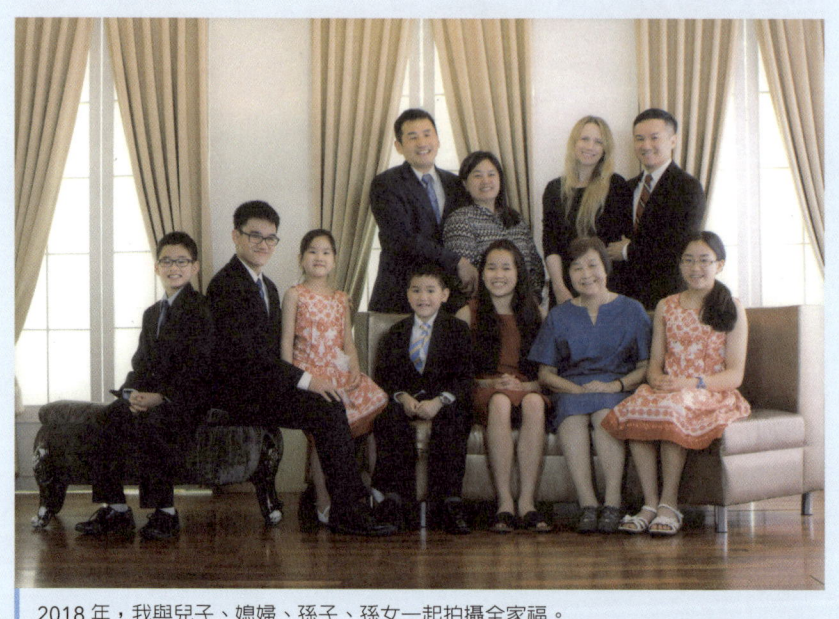

2018 年，我與兒子、媳婦、孫子、孫女一起拍攝全家福。

| 目 次 |

寫在前面 — 38

一、談台灣的輸血與血型

1. 革新發展台灣的輸血醫學；協助建立台灣的國家血液政策；健全捐血系統 — 54

    A. 建立全台的血庫標準作業 — 54

    B. 米田堡血型的發現 — 56

    C. 建議刪除輸血前 RhD 的篩檢 — 58

    D. 健全捐血系統 — 60

    E. 舉辦 1999 年第 10 屆亞太地區國際輸血學會 — 62

2. 台灣血型的研究 — 65

    A. 台灣的分泌型亞孟買血型 — 65

    B. 有關亞孟買血型的輸血 — 68

    C. B_3 血型 — 69

    D. 台灣的成人 i 血型 — 72

    E. 台灣的路易士血型 — 75

    F. K_{null} 稀有血型 — 78

    G. Jk(a-b-) 血型 — 80

H. Diego 血型系統 — 81

　　I. 努力七年證明「只和新鮮血小板」反應的抗體 — 83

　　J. HLA-class I 與 2003 年 SARS 冠狀病毒感染的關係 — 85

二、談台灣的血緣

1. 台灣南島語族（高山原住民）的研究 — 90

　　A. 南島語族母系血緣（mtDNA）B4a1a 遷移的研究 — 90

　　B. 台灣南島語族群和南北亞洲的族群共有相同的 HLA haplotypes — 92

2. 台灣非南島語族（台灣人）的研究 — 94

　　A. 2001 年 HLA 基因的研究 — 94

　　B. 2010 年代台灣母系血緣的研究 — 98

　　C. 2023 年台灣母系血緣的研究 — 98

　　D. 談台灣的父系血緣 — 102

3. 古代 DNA（Ancient DNA, aDNA）的研究 — 108

Review of Professor Dr. Marie Lin Research Career（英文版）

Foreword — *116*

I. About Blood Transfusion and Blood Groups

1. Assistance in Formulating Taiwan's National Blood Program — *127*

　　A. Development and Evolution of Taiwan Transfusion Medicine — *127*

　　B. Enhancing the Blood Donation System — *129*

2. Extensive Taiwanese Blood Groups Studies — *130*

II. Research on the Molecular Anthropology of Taiwan Ethnic Groups

1. Studies of the Austronesian Speakers in Taiwan (1994-2014) — *134*

　　A. Research on the Migration of Maternal Lineage (mtDNA) B4a1a among the Austronesian Speakers — *134*

　　B. Shared HLA Haplotypes between Austronesian Language Family Groups in Taiwan and South/North Asian Populations — *135*

2. **Studies of Non-Austronesian Speakers in Taiwan (2000-2023)** — *136*

    A. HLA Research in 2001 — *136*

    B. Research on Maternal Lineages in the 2010s — *137*

    C. Research in 2023 and Ancient DNA Study — *137*

    D. The Paternal Lineage in Taiwan — *139*

【附件】

附件 1. ｜ Dr. A. Kellner 的信（台灣的國家血液政策，1983）— *150*

附件 2. ｜ 前國際輸血學會會長 Contreras 的信，鼓勵別的國家效法台灣血庫的作業 — *162*

附件 3. ｜ 台灣從事常規 Rh 血型篩檢的爭議，及馬偕醫院血庫的堅持 — *163*

附件 4. ｜ 捐血運動 50 週年貢獻獎及得獎感言 — *165*

附件 5. ｜ 2003 年 SARS 期間，我們發現台灣人帶有使 SARS 病人容易轉重症基因的論文，引起國際的重視及評論 — *167*

附件 6. ｜《經濟學人》2005 年評論我們「台灣南島語族（高山原住民）母系血緣粒線體（mtDNA）B4a1a 與波里尼西亞人有直接血緣關係」的發現 — *175*

【附錄】談悲歡人生

附錄 1. | 馬偕醫院的親子鑑定
　　　　──台灣親子鑑定檢驗工作的發展史 — *178*

附錄 2. | 「讓二二八受難者遺骸找到回家的路」
　　　　工作始末（2011-2019）— *182*

附錄 3. | 從事族群研究的無奈：噶瑪蘭口水事件
　　　　──還原歷史真相 — *192*

附錄 4. | 台灣人可能沒有古老的 M174 父系血緣 — *221*

附錄 5. | 馬祖居民的粒線體 DNA 遺傳多樣性及其歷史淵源 — *223*

附錄 6. | 1990 年代與國際輸血專家學者的討論往返書信，可以看到台灣在 10 年當中，輸血醫學趕上歐美國家的軌跡 — *226*

附錄 7. | 演講記錄（2006-2016）— *247*

林媽利教授簡介 — *250*
About Professor Dr. Marie Lin — *252*
林媽利教授（Marie Lin, Lin M）學術著作 — *254*

一、專書 — *254*

二、期刊論文集（* 責任作者）— *254*

三、學術研討會摘要集（1983-2009）— *271*

寫在前面

　　1981年，我在美國德州大學做完四年美國病理專科醫師訓練，並考取美國病理專科醫師執照，同年10月1日，帶著台大醫學院病理研究所副教授及美國病理專科醫師的光環，到馬偕醫院的檢驗科（臨床病理）報到，我很快發現並不能在馬偕醫院同時也做熟悉的（之前在台大病理研究所做了16年）的組織病理（解剖病理），而在檢驗科只能做血庫。因為當時血庫（immunohematology, 免疫血液學）是一個新的學門，許多人並不是很了解，而我在美國四年的訓練主要在血庫，於是我勉強接受這個工作。和大部分的醫院一樣，當時血庫只有兩三坪大，有一台冰箱、一個離心機、一張桌子和一位醫檢師，害得我台大的同事看到這個情形就說：「妳在這裡做什麼血庫？」

投身血液政策與血型研究

　　我每天上班，只是看到醫檢師忙著抽血牛（有價供血者）的血，當時捐血量非常少，所以只能提供給醫院一小部分的病人使用。我試著教醫檢師最基本的交叉實驗，從教她如何搖試管，如何看結果開始。我同時也發現，台灣有關血型的資料，除了ABO、Rh以外，好像只有一點點MN血型的資料而已，一切需要從頭開始！

當時全台為盛行的高 B 型肝炎帶原率所不安，我一有空就往衛生署跑，因為我受到高醫時代的老師許子秋衛生署長邀請，參與制定國家的血液政策 [國家的血液政策，見附件1]。台灣的捐血輸血在 1980 年代初期都很混亂，於是我偕同台灣輸血學會會員孫建峰、李正華和美國的高源祥等醫師，衛生署的長官葉金川、蔡素玲及助理石美春等，做了全台捐血機構及醫院輸血單位（血庫）的評鑑及督導，再根據評鑑的結果，擬定制度及規範。所以從 1984 到 1992 年，在八年之中，把台灣的捐輸血制度建立起來。在 1992 年，台灣的捐血量足夠提供全台醫院所需要的用血，有價供血（血牛）從此消失。1992 年台灣變成一個沒有血液買賣的國家，在短短八年，把買賣血液的國家變成捐血的國家，應該是世界上前所未有的。

　　另一方面，在 1983 年，英國血庫專家、宣教師鮑博瑞先生（Richard E. Broadberry, FIMLS）應上帝的呼召，來到台北的馬偕醫院血庫工作，他變成我最好的工作夥伴，從此展開了 1-20 年燦爛非凡的台灣血型的拓荒研究工作。後來加入年輕的生力軍余榮熾博士，繼續做後續的血型基因的研究，使得許多亞洲，尤其是東南亞特有的血型及新的血型，不斷地被發現。同時大家驚訝的發現，不只是白種人和黃種人的血型分布不同，連東北亞的日本（中國很晚才做血型的研究，所以 1980 年代沒有資料可以做比較）和屬於東南亞的台灣，兩者的血型也有所不同。

　　台灣血型的發現，使歐美輸血醫學先進國家的專家、科學家，張大眼睛觀看台灣，特別是我們團隊一連串的發現，於是台灣的血型在 1980、1990 年代，在國際上喧騰一時。我們跟國際專家的討論信件，也就好幾年每年約有 100 封，包括和國際專家討

論的往返信件,和國際友人做稀有血型血液的交換,常常使我們的信件滿天飛 [見附錄 6]。同時我們的年輕人也在國際輸血學界佔有一席之地。

我們著名的發現之一,是分泌型亞孟買血型,這血型讓親子間 ABO 血型不配合。如 1985 年馬偕醫院的嬰兒室,發生一對 O 型的父母親生出一個 B 型的男嬰而引起家庭糾紛,我們很快地證明,嬰兒的父親是帶 B 基因的亞孟買血型者,而他給男嬰的 B 基因,經過嬰兒母親所帶正常的 H 基因傳給嬰兒而表現出來,而生出 B 型的小孩。原來 ABO 血型的表現,必須有兩個基因(見頁 66 的圖 1),一個是 ABO 血型的基因,另外一個是為要表現 ABO 基因,須要有的另一個 H 基因。亞孟買血型的人並沒有正常的 H 基因,所以沒有辦法表現他的 A 或者是 B 的基因,因此表現成 O 血型。在台灣,每 8,000 個人有一個是屬於亞孟買血型,所以全台應該至少有 3,000 個亞孟買血型的人。

另外,台灣的亞孟買血型和白種人的亞孟買血型不同,可輸一般 ABO 血型的血,可能因亞洲的亞孟買血型全部是分泌型,所以血漿中出現 ABO 血型物質,而阻止了 ABO 血型抗體的產生,因此可輸一般 ABO 血型的血,我們也經人體試驗證實了這個結果。白種人的亞孟買血型或孟買血型,是一定要輸相同的孟買血型的血,我還記得小時候讀了一本小說,說一個孟買血型的車手要出去賽車,就必須帶同一血型的妹妹一起去,以防失事受傷沒血輸,現在想來,這個故事應該是白種人的故事。

此外,我們也發現台灣的路易士血型中,出現只在亞洲出現的血型 Le(a+b+) 血型。因為歐美血型專家沒看過這血型,所以開始時以為我們做錯,經過不斷的交換測試血液檢體以及試藥,最

後說服國際學者接受亞洲有這個 Le(a+b+) 血型。而且我們比著名的瑞典頒發諾貝爾獎的 Karolinska Institute，早一年找到 Le(a+b+) 血型的相對基因 Se^w 基因，震撼國際。

我們也發現稀有血型 i 血型與先天性白內障的關連，進而發現 I 血型的基因，而促成 I 血型變成國際上第 27 個血型系統（這是台灣的努力促成的），*Blood* 期刊將這報告當成當期的傑出論文，說：「i to I and the eye」[109]，翻成中文是「從小我到大我，再到靈魂之窗眼睛」。這血型的發現，最大的協助，來自日本大阪府紅十字會血液中心的大久保康人教授的幫助及提供稀有的抗體及細胞。

我們在 2003 年 SARS 流行期間發現，組織抗原 HLA-B*4601（越族的主要血緣）使帶這血緣的病人容易轉成重症。我們從 SARS 在台灣流行時，開始研究收集血液檢體，因為我的工作人員的家人，也怕他們把病毒從醫院帶回家，許多人變成有家歸不得，所以不少人就因此辭職。我希望可以找出一個和 SARS 相關的檢查方法，來篩檢工作人員，讓工作人員較安全的照顧 SARS 的病人。所以我把收集到的血液做組織抗原的研究，因為抗原系統是和人體的感染和免疫反應有關的。我一共收集到 166 位和 SARS 感染相關的血液檢體（有些是曾暴露在 SARS 病毒），因為 SARS 的感染力很強，所以我全副武裝在負壓的工作台上，完成血液檢體前半部白血球分離的危險工作。從 5 月中開始收集血液檢體，在短短的一個半月，完成 SARS 相關人員 HLA 的檢測，分析結果，寫成報告，馬上投稿，很快的在三個月後（9 月中），出現在國際期刊上，結果各大媒體爭相報導，變成國際上重要的醫藥新聞 [見附件 5]。最讓人不解的是，我們的發現在《華爾街

日報》（*The Wall Street Journal*）有半版的介紹，路透社、日本的《朝日新聞》也有報導，我的朋友從馬來西亞剪了一塊有關我們發現的報紙寄來給我，甚至我和先夫在加德滿都的候機室，還遇到一個德國的復健師對我們說：「你們台灣發現了 SARS 相關的病毒。」但是我們國內的新聞只有半天講一講，就全部消音，我不太知道背後是什麼因素，只是我知道，當時的衛生署長到立法院報告的時候，說我的 SARS 研究的個案數不夠，但是《華爾街日報》上說，他們的記者去訪問歐洲的一位教授，該名教授說有 37 個病人已經足夠來分析了。2003 年的 SARS 流行，顯然和 2019 年爆發的全球 COVID-19 的流行有很大的差異，因為後者看不到前者的族群傾向。

另外讓國際友人絕倒的是，1983 年（不是 1986 年）在馬偕醫院病人身上找到米田堡血型（Miltenberger blood group）的抗體，這個重要血型的發現，是 1983-1986 年的三年間，經馬偕醫院血庫、北倫敦血液中心、英國醫學研究委員會（MRC）、日本紅十字會東京血液中心及大阪府紅十字會血液中心、泰國 Siriraj 醫院的 Chandanayingyong 的共同努力定出的血型。這種血型，在歐美白種人的國家是沒有看過的稀有血型，在台灣人有 4.5% 是這個血型，更令人驚訝的是，台灣原住民的頻率是從零到 95%。後來證明，這個血型在台灣是繼 ABO 血型之後，最重要的血型，因為米田堡血型抗體危險，可引起溶血性輸血反應及新生兒溶血症，而我們的病人有 2% 帶這個抗體，所幸全台血庫在 1990 年就開始做輸血前米田堡血型抗體的篩檢。很快的，東南亞國家也發現這是最重要的抗體，所以紛紛學習台灣的作業。

我也發現了在華人的第一個 ABO 亞血型的 B_3 血型，這血型

在白種人是稀有血型，各國專家紛紛向我要 B_3 的血球。至於其他重要的發現，詳見內文（〈一、談台灣的輸血與血型〉）。

最讓我覺得遺憾的是，我畢生主張「廢除常規的 Rh 血型的篩檢，來解決在台灣屬於稀有血型 Rh 陰性（RhD–）者輸血的問題」，並沒得到適當的結果。我看到過去 RhD– 的人死亡的主要原因，是緊急需要輸血的時候沒有血輸，因為許多醫護人員並不太懂血型，不知道台灣絕大部分 RhD– 的病人因沒帶抗體，可以安全的輸入陽性的血，詳見內文（〈一、談台灣的輸血與血型〉）。

許多人一定會覺得奇怪，為什麼在亞洲，會是台灣獨領風騷？因為在亞洲，除了北亞洲的日本有好的血型研究及健全的捐血輸血系統外，東南亞的國家，當時大部分處於開發中國家，輸血醫學須在更開發的社會才可能發生，輸血醫學也叫做免疫血液學，所以須要加上有免疫血液學的專家才能做成，因為血型必須先從血清學的發現做起，再做基因的研究，剛好馬偕有血清學及基因研究最強的陣容。我們血型基因的研究，開始於 1993 年，台大生化研究所博士班剛畢業的余榮熾博士參加我們的團隊，當時我們剛好用免疫血清學的方法發現了許多新的血型，在接下來的近九年中，余榮熾努力做新血型基因的研究，因此重要的論文紛紛刊登在國際刊物上面。他在 2001 年被台大生化研究所以副教授聘回，讓我們很高興，記得我在推薦函中寫說「我們為這件事覺得很光榮」。之後的近 20 年，余榮熾繼續和我們合作研究，後來才會有重要的 Se^w 及 I 基因的相繼發現。

至於中國，因為之前經過紅衛兵之亂，所以 1990 年代當我被中國輸血協會邀請去中國講學（在國際輸血學會安排下），發現

中國情況和1983年之前的台灣差不多。東南亞除了泰國,當時其他的國家都還沒發展輸血醫學,所以東南亞的血型大部分沒有被研究過,因此給馬偕的團隊一大片未開發的大地,以致著名的紐約血液中心從事輸血醫學研究的學者 Dr. Laurence Marsh,看到我就羨慕的說:「林醫師是坐在金礦上的人,有挖不完的寶!」

在大家的努力下,台灣在短短的十年當中,趕上歐美的輸血醫學。除了天時、地利、人和,還加上馬偕團隊的努力,這可以從每一年馬偕醫院血庫約有100封的往返國際信件看到。我們的發現及研究的結果,很快的也變成東南亞國家輸血醫學重要的參考資料。

研發本土的組織抗原測定盤

1993年在台北的組織抗原研討會,邀請了日本東京紅十字會血液中心主任十字猛夫教授(Dr. Takeo Juji)來演講。因為我們都是國際輸血學會的會員,在研討會常常見面,所以很熟悉。他在會後表示,實在是不了解為什麼台灣政府花了很多經費,請台灣幾個研究單位從事組織抗原測定盤的研發,已經有幾年了,卻都做不出來。於是他鼓勵我來做,他說他願意用日本紅十字會的全國組織抗原團隊做我的後盾,協助我在馬偕醫院成立組織抗原的實驗室,同時研發台灣的測定盤。雖然沒有計劃的支援,我馬上請馬偕醫院婦產科留下原本要銷毀的胎盤,讓我可以收取胎盤裡面的血清來研發測定盤。

正確的組織抗原測定結果,對疾病的診斷、治療(包括骨髓移植)非常重要,在1980及90年代,全球都用血清學的方法來做組織抗原的測定,但是如要得到正確的測定結果,必須靠當地

血清中的抗體來完成測定,所以當時先進國家都努力的用當地的血清中的抗體來做測定盤。十字教授在1994年8月派遣日本東京紅十字會血液中心的赤座達也醫師(Dr. Akaza)帶助理、試藥、日本測定盤等來台一個月,幫我們設立了一個全台最好的組織抗原研究室。

隨後我們寫了好幾篇相當令人注目的論文,包括2000年的[89]「Heterogeneity of Taiwan's indigenous population: possible relation to prehistoric Mongoloid dispersals」,及2001年的[92]「Diversity of HLA among Taiwan's indigenous tribes and the Ivatans in the Philippines」,文中有關台灣原住民血緣的圖9(見彩圖8),讓我驚訝的發現,台灣人與原住民之間有很明顯且大的基因距離,在百思不解後,從台灣古代的地理及氣候變遷的記錄,了解到舊石器時代的晚期,約一萬多年前冰河時期,台灣還是陸連到歐亞大陸時,人類可能沿著近海的低地遷徙,後來地球暖化,融解的冰河流到海裡,海水上升,低地變成海底,也使台灣變成一個島嶼,有些古代的先民被隔離孤立在台灣,長期的隔離,造成與歐亞大陸間的基因距離,這些也促成我漸漸的轉向人類學。後來有關台灣人的2001年的[94]「The origin of Minnan and Hakka, the so-called "Taiwanese", inferred by HLA study」,這篇論文的內容是:「從組織抗原來看,台灣人是屬於南方的亞洲人,而不是北方漢人。」這篇除了引起台灣島內許多人欣喜外,也引發一陣騷動,及一些批判,更招來中國國務院正式的譴責,說是「可恥、有政治目的」。可能因為期刊的編輯委員當中有中國的代表,所以延遲一年以後,文章才勉強經由別的編輯委員們強行通過而刊登。

因為做測定盤必須要先知道台灣所有族群組織抗原分布的情形，因此讓我們慢慢地轉進族群組織抗原的研究，進而從事台灣族群 DNA 的研究。2024 年 3 月 5 日，我重返東京去探望十字教授，向他 30 年前義無反顧的幫助我們成立組織抗原實驗室道謝（見彩圖 14）。這個實驗室的成立，使我有機會做台灣人的 DNA（台灣人血緣研究），而我們團隊的研究結果對台灣產生了深遠的影響。1990 年代初期，台灣人的台灣認同（認為自己是台灣人）不到 20%。我從 1994 年開始做組織抗原的研究，在 2001 年發表台灣人不是北方漢人，導致許多人罵我，然而台灣的認同慢慢爬升來到 40% 左右。

2003 年到 2005 年我重新編輯修改我的第二版教科書成第三版的《輸血醫學》，把台灣發現的新血型全部寫進去。我看到當時台灣的輸血醫學蓬勃發展，許多醫院血庫的作業及研究能力，因著輸血學會持續的舉辦血庫工作人員在職訓練，加上馬偕血庫團隊 20 年來，熱心、免費的提供許多醫療院所輸血遇到困難的個案時，即時給予的諮詢及協助，大大的提升全台血庫的工作能力及士氣。我也看到許多年輕的研究者，如余榮熾、陳定平等，活躍在國際上，而且台灣血型的研究，從血清學的研究，更上層樓，繼續做到血型基因的研究，全台的血庫差不多上了軌道，這時我知道上帝給我的階段性使命已經完成，我可以放心的去做台灣血緣的研究了。我把原本十四章的第三版《輸血醫學》，分送給十四位當時活躍在台灣輸血醫學的工作者，預先請他們準備寫新版中的一章，因為我知道做台灣血緣的研究有時空的急迫性，我無法再分心去寫第四版了。

揭開台灣各族群血緣之謎

　　台灣血緣的研究，最熱門的是台灣原住民的研究，因為國際上有關南島語族的遷移，被認為是人類史上重要的議題，受到重視，加上在國內原住民的研究不太會受到政治的干擾，研究計劃也比較容易通過，所以許多學者紛紛去做台灣原住民的研究，我們也不例外，最開始也是做台灣原住民的血緣研究。我們在2005年參加中央研究院有關台灣原住民的大型研究計劃，因為申請到計劃的時候，重要的DNA定序價錢在市面上已減半，結果讓我們多出不少的經費，讓我們決定用這筆經費來做佔有台灣人口98%的台灣人（非高山原住民，非南島語族）血緣的研究。

　　我們在2010年代從事台灣人父母系血緣的研究，也做了台灣周邊地區族群的血緣研究，分析資料，陸中衡發現非原住民台灣人的母系血緣中，不少血緣是屬於台灣特有的血緣，這是個重要的發現，也就是這些血緣是鄰近地區（包括中國）看不到，推測是台灣人的祖先（台灣先民）到達台灣以後發展出來的血緣，稱為「台灣特有的血緣」（TW血緣）。

　　我們在2023年已經收集到，且分析了7,000多人的父母系血緣，希望幫助追溯台灣人的來源。同時，我們另外收集及分析三代以上父母親的祖先都是原居住在台灣的767名沒有親緣關係的居民，我們分析這767人的母系血緣，發現台灣人的祖先有部分是來自東北亞，大部分是來自東亞及東南亞，包括東南亞島嶼。且今日台灣人大部分的人口，是近一千年內移民到台灣的後代，部分是古代的移民（台灣先民）的後代，來到台灣的時間可能遠到距今五千年之前的久遠。這個時間，在考古學上屬於新石器時

代晚期，我們的發現，呼應了考古學家劉益昌教授發表的「在相近時間，台灣在不同的地方有不同成熟的文化突然出現」。我們的文章發表的期刊（Nature 旗下的新期刊 Human Genome Variation）編輯的評論：「研究分析台灣人的母系血緣，發現台灣人已於新石器時代晚期從東南亞大陸定居台灣，隨後歷經隔離和遺傳擴張，林媽利等確定了台灣人許多不同的遺傳譜系，包括許多屬於台灣的血緣，可以追溯『可能發生的年代』到幾千年前，這結果表明台灣人史前定居於台灣和擴張的時間，遠在近代唐山公抵達台灣之前。」

我們的團隊在 2000 年代有法裔尚特鳩博士（Jean A. Trejaut, PhD）的參與，使我們更順利的轉移到分子人類學的領域，而且在台灣原住民（台灣南島語族）的研究也有亮麗的成績，Jean 做了貢獻。我們經台灣原住民特有的母系血緣 B4a1a 與東南亞、大洋洲、太平洋上波里尼西亞人的血緣相比較，發現台灣原住民的祖先約 4,000-5,000 年前從台灣出發（Out of Taiwan），經過東南亞、大洋洲，到達新幾內亞，然後再擴散到太平洋上的島嶼，變成波里尼西亞人的祖先。長久以來，台灣是不是南島語族的故鄉的問題，經過我們追蹤高山原住民母系血緣 B4a1a 基因的流向，得到肯定，所以從分子人類學的研究，我們肯定了台灣還是南島語族的故鄉。我們這一篇 2005 年的論文，引起國際很大的迴響，在當時 Yahoo 的網路上出現 605 篇的評論（英文），到 2023 年有 305 篇論文討論到我們這篇文章，甚至《經濟學人》（The Economist）在 2005 年 7 月 9 日的文章說「台灣人與夏威夷人是雙胞胎」[見附件6]。

「平埔公」並沒有消失，而是意氣風發的生活著，台灣男性

人口不一定全是「唐山公」的後代。「平埔公」的後代，從古至今繼續存活著。「平埔公」的父系血緣，最多源自可能原發自台灣的 O1-M119 的 O1a1* 及古代 O3-M122 的移民，這兩個血緣也是構成近代移民「唐山公」的血緣 [188]。關於台灣的父系血緣，詳見內文（〈D. 談台灣的父系血緣〉）。

我們當前面臨的困境

台灣是多族群的島嶼，有南島語族（高山原住民）與非南島語族（所謂的台灣人）。馬偕醫院分子人類學研究室自 1990 年代就開始從事「台灣人」族群的分子人類學（基因）的研究，希望解決台灣人來源的問題，特別是台灣男性是不是全是唐山公的後代？所以近年來全力做台灣人 DNA 的研究。但是馬偕醫院原本就是一個教會醫院，服務一般的民眾，對於尖端高科技 DNA 的研究，尤其是對於我們另外還做的古代 DNA（即古代遺骸 DNA）的研究，並沒有辦法做多餘的支持，現在研究人員越來越少（見彩圖 1-4），我們雖然尚無實驗室關門的危機，但是我認為，我們這個實驗室為台灣長期負擔的責任，實在是很難再繼續下去。

反觀中國，近 20 年來用龐大的國家力量，積極的邀請許多在國際上從事分子人類學的專家（主要是華裔），回到中國成立許多分子人類學研究所（包括古代 DNA 的研究），現在這些研究所在國際上已成為有名的研究所。這些研究所也積極的派人到歐美分子人類學的研究所訓練（如到 2022 年諾貝爾醫學獎得主 Svante Paabo 在德國萊比錫 Max Planck Institute 的古代 DNA 實驗室），現在中國做古代 DNA 的實驗室很多，除了在中科院有古脊椎動物與古人類研究所外，尚有北京大學等約十所大學。

至於台灣，我在 1993 年在日本紅十字會全力的支持下（經費及實驗室的資源），在馬偕醫院成立了 HLA 的實驗室，後來這個實驗室轉換為現在的分子人類學的實驗室。2005 年因為參與中央研究院史語所李壬癸教授所主持的南島語族的研究，申請到一筆經費和一個古代 DNA 實驗室，但這個研究計劃只有三年，接下來我們就沒有經費了。因為在台灣，一般的情形是，除了原住民（南島語族）的研究外，很難從國科會申請到研究的經費。有關非南島語族（也就是台灣人）的研究，本來就很難，如同 2001 年本人寫的上述報告 [94]「The origin of Minnan and Hakka, the so-called "Taiwanese", inferred by HLA study」，招來許多的指責。因為意識形態的問題，所以從事台灣人的研究是非常困難的。至於全台原住民的研究，後來全面停止，所以經費的來源變得更加困難。

　　從前因為戒嚴，沒有人敢做台灣人的研究，所以所有的資料和研究都必須從零開始，加上當時也找不到台灣近代史，所以我們對台灣的認識實在是非常有限，我們像瞎子摸象，拼湊我們做出的結果和資料，希望從各項研究的結果找到一些線索，在模糊的祖先的面貌之下，希望看出台灣人是誰？我們研究分析台灣人的母系血緣，發現台灣人已於新石器時代晚期，自東南亞大陸定居台灣，隨後歷經隔離和遺傳擴張血緣，可以追溯可能發生的年代到幾千年前（最多在 1,000-2,600 年），甚至可能到 5,000 年前。這結果表明，台灣人史前定居於台灣和擴張的時間，遠在近代唐山公抵達台灣之前。

　　我希望這本書能幫助大家更認識台灣，同時我也希望在我們繼續從事血緣及古代 DNA 的研究時，不用再去面對資源及人員

的匱乏。希望我的呼籲能夠引起大家的注意，積極改善現在台灣研究單位對分子人類學及古代 DNA 研究的忽視。現生的分子人類學及古代 DNA 研究，關係到台灣的主權及歷史的話語權，甚至可影響到國安。

我希望政府能協助加強馬偕醫院分子人類學暨古代 DNA 實驗室（後者是台灣唯一的實驗室）。現在台灣分子人類學的研究團隊，只有兩個單位在做，一爲馬偕醫院（共有四人），另一則在陽明交通大學（三人）。希望別的研究單位能分別設立分子人類學及古代 DNA 實驗室。

最後我要感謝台灣的社會和天上的父神，讓我參與了漫長的探索台灣之旅，讓我的生命充滿了意義，願榮耀歸與上帝，天祐台灣。

一、
談台灣的輸血與血型

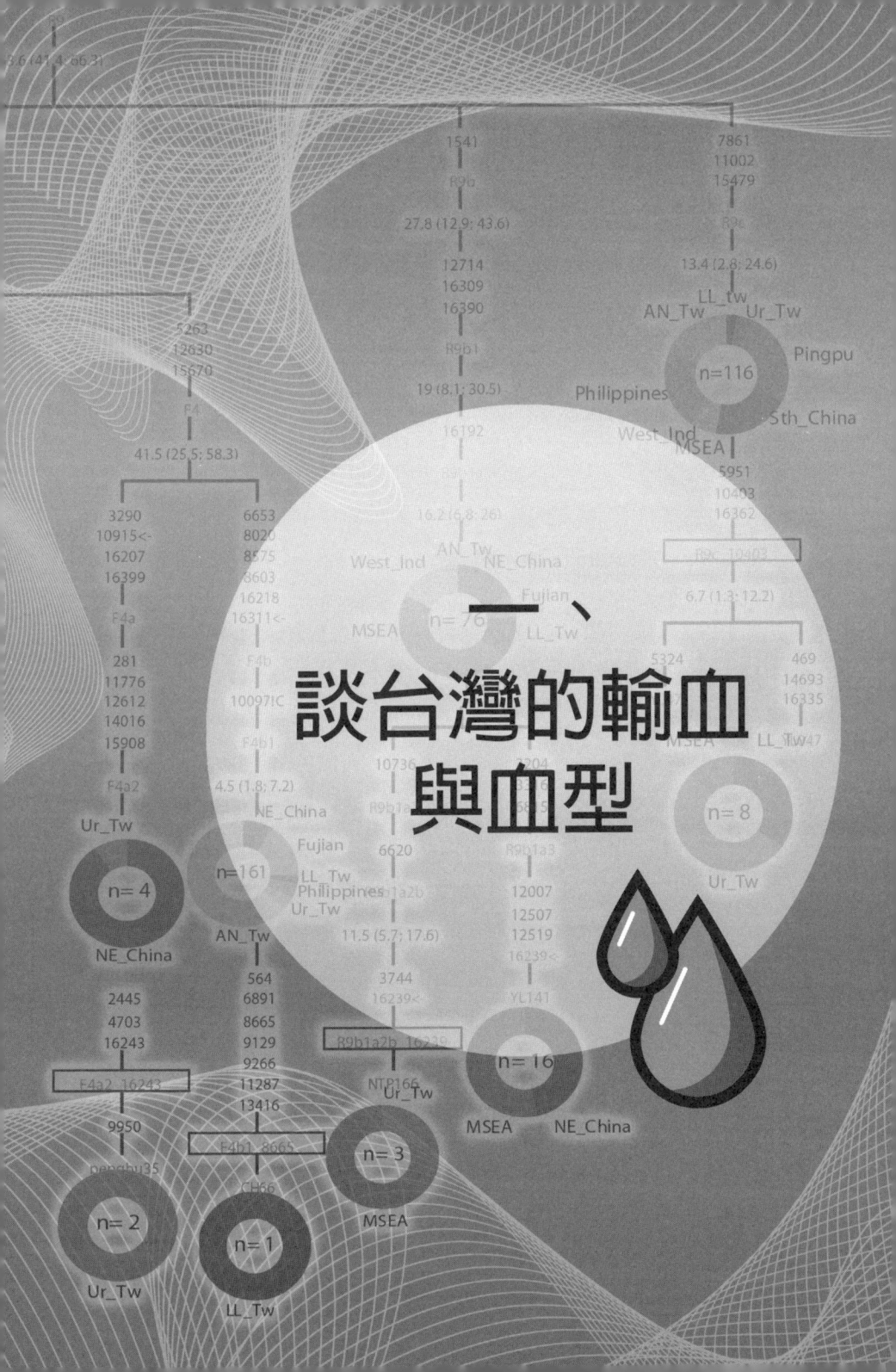

1. 革新發展台灣的輸血醫學;協助建立台灣的國家血液政策 [見附件1];健全捐血系統 [見期刊論文集 54]

A. 建立全台的血庫標準作業

　　1980 年代台灣國內醫院血庫輸血前的檢驗（也叫交叉、配合試驗），大概全部都使用不安全的鹽水玻片法，全台血庫作業混亂，需要做大修正，也需要建立全台標準的作業。1984 年我及團隊（見彩圖 1），發現 manual Polybrene (MP) 不加做抗球蛋白試驗的方法，是最適合國人的作業，MP 法敏感，增加了輸血的安全，快速可節省人力，作業所需的時間，是白種人傳統方法的十分之一，尤其是在 1980 年代輸血醫學不受重視，以致工作人員人力缺乏，MP 法有很大的幫助 [17]。MP 法不必使用昂貴進口的試藥（抗球蛋白試劑），MP 法試藥可以自行泡製，試藥的品質可以自己管控，而且所需費用約白種人傳統方法的 1%，這大大的幫助了 1980 年代開發中國家的台灣的輸血安全。

　　經過我帶領的台灣輸血學會持續的在職訓練 [33]，很快的 MP 法在 1980-1990 年代，變成全台血庫輸血前檢查的標準作業，台灣血庫首次有了標準作業。原來全球的輸血作業，都是根據歐美

的標準作業，所以歐美的作業成爲全球標準的作業，這主要因爲輸血醫學最開始是從歐美發展出來的，所以歐美的輸血標準變成全球的標準，亞洲包括台灣也不例外。但是在 1980 年代的台灣，因爲資源及專業人材的缺乏，所以我們做最簡單的玻片法，談不上標準作業。

我開始做血型的研究，就發現亞洲人和白種人在血型上有很大的不同，比如 K 血型抗原，在白種人有 9%，這個 K 抗原的抗體可以引起危險的輸血反應，這抗體不容易用 MP 法找到，但是台灣沒有人有 K 抗原，所以也不會有人帶 K 的抗體，因 MP 法較不容易找到 K 抗體，所以雖然在歐美發展出 MP 法，但歐美不太能使用 MP 法，在台灣，剛好我們沒有 K 抗體的問題，所以我們把這個最輕易、最好的方法，好好的應用在台灣，把 MP 法發揚光大。MP 不只適用在台灣，也可以在別的國家應用，如東南亞的國家及中國。

1994 年，我將 MP 法及 Rh 的問題，發表在 [55]「The modification of standard Western pretransfusion testing procedures for Taiwan（修改西方的輸血作業來配合台灣的需要）」，刊登在國際輸血學會的會刊 *Vox Sanguinis*。*Vox Sang* 的總編輯 M. Contreras「讚許林醫師爲台灣整體的輸血作業所做的傑出決策及實踐」，台灣經驗可供別的國家參考，建議不同的族群應該像台灣那樣，發展適合自己國家的輸血作業 [附件2]。

除了輸血作業的革新外，我於 1988 年在馬偕醫院成立「台灣血庫諮詢中心」，約二十年期間，義務性免費協助全台醫療院所的血庫從事即時的協助（電話或檢體），解決困難的輸血個案，因此在短短十年之內，大大提升了全台灣輸血工作人員的能力及

素質,提高了全台血庫的水準,確保了輸血的安全。

B. 米田堡血型(Miltenberger, MiIII, GP.Mur)的發現

　　1983年華人的米田堡血型,首次在馬偕醫院的病人身上發現,當時我發現病人的血清和不少台灣捐血人的血球反應,但是和馬偕醫院血庫儲存的近100人白種人的血球完全沒有反應,於是我把這帶有一團迷霧的血液,先和有Vw抗原經驗的鮑博瑞先生,先在馬偕醫院內的血庫做了一番的測試及分析,懷疑是米田堡血型。然後寄到英國北倫敦血液中心的Contreras處(當時檢體有細菌汙染),也懷疑是米田堡血型,1986年再寄到英國的醫學研究委員會(MRC)的血型研究單位Patricia Tippett處,得到肯定。

　　能夠有這個結果,不只是我們的努力,還有泰國Dasnayanee Chandanayingyong、日本大阪府紅十字會血液中心的大久保康人(Yasuto Okubo)及日本東京血液中心內川誠的協助,不只幫我們確認為米田堡血型,甚至於幫助我們把台灣的這一型米田堡血型,在複雜的米田堡血型分類中,找到所屬的米田堡第三型。

　　米田堡血型名字由來,是在1966年Cleghorn收集了一群相關的抗原而成。屬於MN血型系統變異型的米田堡血型的抗體(首先在米田堡太太身上找到,因此得名),只和幾個白種人的血球反應,因此經過許多的研究才定義的這個血型系統,後來在英國測試了兩三萬人,只找到一個人和我們一樣的反應(米田堡血型者),後來等到我在台灣找到不少這種血型的人,就跌破許多歐美科學家的眼鏡,發現台灣豐富的族群有很多不同的分布,如非

原住民台灣人的頻率大概是在 4.5% 左右（我最先測試 1,000 多個捐血人，得到的頻率是 7.3%）。讓人驚訝的是，米田堡血型在原住民有很不同的分布（見彩圖 2），有低頻率 0% 的布農族等，到世界上最高的頻率的阿美族 88-95%。

　　台灣人是屬於米田堡第三血型，大部分東南亞的人也都是屬於第三型的米田堡血型。台灣人口的頻率，由我們原先測出的 7.3%，修改到最近的 4.5%，香港是 6.3%，泰國 9.6%，日本人 0.006%，在台灣的中國人（北方人）0%（0/78）。所以台灣在族群上是屬於東南亞的族群。米田堡血型的英文是 Miltenberger blood group，Milten 在西班牙是小米的意思，因為 Hamburger 在中文是寫成漢堡，所以我把這個在台灣除了 ABO 血型以外最重要的血型 Miltenberger 血型，在台灣取名為「米田堡血型」，希望這樣子會讓大家比較容易記得。

　　米田堡血型是繼 ABO 血型之後，在台灣（後來證明也在東南亞）是最重要的血型，因為相對抗體 anti-'Mi^a' 是台灣最常見的異體抗體（2% 病人陽性），不只可引起血管內溶血的輸血反應，也可以引起新生兒溶血症，所幸台灣的血庫從 1990 年就做 anti-'Mi^a' 篩檢。後來證明，這問題也是整個東南亞的問題，米田堡血型變成西太平洋區最熱門的血型，東南亞紛紛學習台灣的血庫作業 [53,57,73]。anti-'Mi^a' 自 1990 年成為全台（現在也是大部分東亞國家）輸血前常規篩檢的項目。

　　anti-'Mi^a' 自 1990 年成為全台輸血前常規篩檢的項目後，輸血前是否須要增加這一項篩檢，曾在國際論壇（*Transfusion*）上討論一時，1994 年我和香港衛生部 C. Feng 有一番論戰 [57]，現在大部分東亞國家紛紛學習台灣的血庫作業，將 anti-'Mi^a' 的篩檢當

一、談台灣的輸血與血型

作輸血前常規篩檢的項目。

馬偕醫院許淳欣發現，米田堡血型使 CO_2 較易跑出血球，使帶這血型的人較能容忍較耗氣的工作，阿美族米田堡陽性率高達 88% 到 95% 等，所以許多著名的運動選手是阿美族人，如楊傳廣、古金水及陽岱鋼等。

C. 建議刪除輸血前 RhD 的篩檢（解決台灣 RhD 陰性輸血的問題）

Rh 血型的被重視，是因為 1950、1960 年代歐美盛行 RhD 陰性（RhD–）的媽媽生出 RhD 陽性新生兒時，引起新生兒溶血症，不少新生兒因此死亡，而引起注意。因 RhD– 佔白種人口的 15%，為了避免經輸 RhD+ 的血的婦女產生 RhD 的抗體，P. L. Mollison 教授等主張做輸血前 RhD 的篩檢，歐美的情況因而改善。但輸血前 RhD 的篩檢，從此變成全球的作業，台灣也不例外，不管在台灣 RhD– 是屬於稀有血型，頻率只有 0.3%，意味著輸血前常規的檢驗在尋找稀有血型。雖然屬於稀有血型，輸血前 RhD 的篩檢還是照做，因此 RhD– 病人在台灣緊急需要輸血時，常找不到 RhD– 血，結果 RhD– 在台灣死亡主要的原因是缺血。即使白種人的國家（頻率有 15%）也曾發生同樣的找不到血，因此國際上的共識「不管膚色，RhD– 者，如果不帶 RhD 的抗體 anti-D，可安全的輸 RhD 陽性的血」，經我詢問國際 Rh 專家英國 P. L. Mollison，他也贊同台灣不需要做輸血前 Rh 的篩檢。

北倫敦血液中心主任 M. Contreras 和 P. L. Mollison 教授討論後，在 1985 年寫來：「... that it is not logical in your population to type for D when E-typing and c-typing are not done. The same applies to anti-Rh(D) immunoglobulin (Rhogam) administration as there is no anti-E or anti-c immunoglobulin available. Your problem (or "nonproblem") with D is less than our problem with K and c and yet we do not type antenatal patients for K and c. <u>My conscience is quite clear when I give you this advice that it is ethical to discontinue routine Rh(D) typing of recipient and antenatal patients.</u> I agree with you that you should selectively test "a proportion" of your donors for Rh(D), E, c, Fya, Jka, Jkb in order to have "antigen negative" blood available for patients with atypical red cell antibodies in need of transfusion ... 」〔信件詳見附件 3，RhD– 的爭議〕M. Contreras 也贊同台灣不需要做輸血前 Rh 的篩檢。

　　因為種族不同，在台灣，RhD 的表現型和白種人不同，孫建峰的研究也發現，台灣 RhD 基因結構和白種人不同，可能因此在台灣罕見 RhD 的抗體 anti-D，也罕見 anti-D 引起的新生兒溶血症。相反的，在 1983 年連續看到兩個病人因找不到 RhD– 的血而死亡。我曾處理過帶高力價 anti-D 的 RhD– 病人輸 RhD+ 的血的輸血反應，病人輸入 500、500、750ml RhD+ 的血，病人發生發冷、發熱、嘔吐的輸血反應，經輸入 RhD– 血，病人復原出院。RhD– 帶 anti-D 病人的輸血反應，在文獻上很可能找不到死亡的案例，2023 年馬偕醫院的 RhD– 病人，帶 anti-D 的頻率是 0.03%，相較米田堡血型危險的抗體的 2% 低很多，但是很少聽到米田堡血型抗體的討論。

　　為了減少社會越來越重視 Rh 血型及對 RhD– 的恐慌，讓 RhD– 不帶 anti-D 者可以安心（醫護人員及病人）的輸到血，自 1988 年起，經馬偕醫院及在國際輸血學會同意及認可下，我在

馬偕醫院刪除輸血前 RhD 的篩檢 [22,58]。30 年後，2017 年回顧及統計 30 年中沒做 RhD 篩檢病人發生 anti-D 的頻率，發現並沒有改變，就是說沒有做 RhD 篩檢，病人發生 anti-D 的頻率和有做篩檢時的頻率相同，也和捐血人的統計頻率一樣（就是和一般台灣人的統計頻率一樣，並沒有增加），肯定了馬偕醫院的作業 [142,200]。這前瞻性的做法，解決了台灣 RhD– 輸血的問題，也拯救了無數 RhD– 的病人，更為台灣的血型檢驗節省人力和資源。比較遺憾的是，全台只有馬偕醫院系統刪除病人輸血前 RhD 的篩檢，其他醫院照樣做，這可能和 RhD 篩檢有不錯的健保給付有關。雖然這樣，但是較欣慰的是，捐血機構的進步，建立起 RhD 陰性捐血人的檔案，同時 RhD 陰性的病人如果突然需要大量的輸血，會安心的輸到 RhD+ 的血，而不引起無謂的擔心及煩惱 [見附件 3，RhD– 的爭議，參考資料 22,58,142,200]。

D. 健全捐血系統 [54]

　　1974 年 4 月，紅十字會台灣省分會會長蔡培火先生與熱心公益的機關、社團、人士，共同發起愛心無償捐血運動，成立中華民國捐血運動協會，為有效執行捐供血作業，相繼成立台北、台中、台南、高雄四個捐血中心。1978 年捐血中心開始提供血液的成分，但很少醫院使用。到 1984 年，經過積極的醫師在職訓練，血液成分的使用明顯的增加，紅血球及全血的使用比例變成 1:1。另一方面，醫院血庫也在 1980 年代初，從簡陋的設備和簡單的作業慢慢改革，1984 年因著衛生署的要求，我和馬偕醫院的英國血庫專家鮑博瑞先生，聯合從美國受訓回來的孫建峰醫師和

李正華醫師，開始舉辦為期一個禮拜的血庫工作人員在職訓練，這個在職訓練後來縮短為兩天，接下來的 2-30 年，甚至到現在，全台血庫工作人員在職訓練還繼續在舉辦，全台血庫工作人員差不多全接受過在職訓練。

1985 年，衛生署隨即開始全台醫學中心、區域醫院（1986 年加入國立醫院）的評鑑，也是由我、孫建峰醫師和李正華醫師等三人，以及後來加入的美國路易斯安那州立醫院的高源祥醫師，完成衛生署的第一次全台血庫的評鑑，這個評鑑也成了幾年後衛生署做醫院全部作業評鑑的開端。1985 年血庫及捐血機構評鑑後，根據評鑑的結果，設立了血庫的設置標準，隨即設立捐血機構設置標準和捐血人的健康標準。捐血機構也在衛生署的要求下，免費提供台灣所有醫院「血型的判定標準細胞和抗體篩檢細胞」。1987 年成立台灣輸血學會，1988 年由學會開始做全台醫療院所血庫的精確度（能力）調查。

另一方面，當時的捐血系統屬於內政部，不在衛生署的監督之下，所以缺少監督捐血機構從事正確作業的機制，加上沒有開拓血源的規劃和計劃，捐血量非常不足，再加上早期台灣 B 型肝炎的帶原比例非常高（約 15%），所以發展健全的捐血系統，提供安全的血液（來自捐血）來取代當時盛行的有價供血（沒有監控、不安全的血牛供血），變成是國家醫療政策重要的方向。從許子秋署長任內的 1984 年開始，我與輸血學會孫建峰、李正華等會員，及衛生署長官葉金川等，經過長時間全台捐血機構及醫療院所血庫的評鑑監督，擬定捐血機構設置標準及作業標準 [33]，1990 年促成台灣血液基金會的成立，使得捐血系統歸在衛生署的管轄之下，捐血的品質受到衛生署的監督及管制，醫院輸血也在

評鑑的要求下,優先使用捐贈的血液。醫院漸漸捨棄使用有價供血,捐血系統在有效的開拓血源及醫院需求的增加之下,在 1992 年捐血量達到 1,180,000 多單位,捐血提供了近 100% 國內醫院用血的需要,有價供血自然消失。1992 年台灣消滅血液的買賣,台灣捐輸血的成就,受到國際的肯定,1996 年被置於「已開發國家的血液政策」,與美、英、日等 15 個已開發的國家並列評比（*Transfusion* 1996; 36: 1019-32）[附件 4]。

E. 舉辦 1999 年第 10 屆亞太地區國際輸血學會

我在 1983 年成為國際輸血學會的會員,1987 年台灣輸血學會（開始是中華民國輸血學會）成立,我在 1992 年到 1996 年,被選為國際輸血學會的理事（當時台灣的國際輸血學會會員,大概不到五個）,我在 1995 年威尼斯舉辦的歐洲地區國際輸血學會理事會上,提出台灣有意申辦 1999 年亞太地區國際輸血學會的提案,隨即通過台灣的申請案。回國後,發現台灣輸血學會會員大概不到 100 人,而且是一個很窮的學會,這讓我接下來的幾年因為擔心資源不夠無法辦好國際會議而長期失眠。沒想到在接下來的四年,我們大家努力工作、研究,積極參與各處舉辦的國際輸血學會下,1999 年 11 月 11-14 日在台北國際會議中心舉辦第 10 屆國際輸血學會亞太地區大會,是一次成功圓滿的國際會議。

國際輸血學會每兩年定期舉辦區域性學術研討會,這個會議由各國輪流召開,已成為國際輸血醫學界的一大盛事,這個會議的召開,不但成功的促成與會國家在輸血醫學相關領域的學術交流,更可以藉由經驗的分享,提供更多國際化、更多元的思考空

間。這次亞太地區的國際輸血學會,由台灣輸血學會主辦,1997年設立會議的籌備委員會,委員會的主席是馬偕紀念醫院林媽利教授,副主席是長庚醫院孫建峰主任,秘書長是三軍總院萬祥麟醫師。

  兩天半的會期中,共有11個專題演講,13項專題討論,口頭與壁報論文發表共120篇。台灣有369個血庫工作人員、研究人員、捐血機構人員參加這場大會。另外從29個國家:日本、比利時、加拿大、印度、西班牙、法國、芬蘭、南斯拉夫、美國、英國、香港、挪威、泰國、紐西蘭、馬來西亞、捷克、荷蘭、菲律賓、越南、奧地利、新加坡、義大利、葡萄牙、德國、澳洲、盧森堡和韓國,共155人來參與,其中日本最踴躍,有49人。受邀的貴賓都是輸血醫學界一時之選,既有國外知名專家學者(多為輸血醫學有關雜誌的編輯及各國紅十字會主管或實驗室負責人),也有41位國內相關領域領導者,其中13位受邀於會中演講。

  這次大會是台灣第一次主辦有關輸血醫學的國際性會議,其中所討論的議題,都是當今輸血醫學重要及熱門的議題,而專題演講的內容,涵蓋台灣的輸血醫學現況,各國的捐血國家計劃,輸血的安全性及如何安全有效使用血漿及血漿的衍生物,輸血醫學在人類學上的應用,以及血液幹細胞的製備跟使用等。

  這次大會,是台灣血液事業25年來一個重要的里程碑,在台灣血液事業的發展的重要過程中,期間歷經的25年間,中華捐血運動協會的成立,衛生主管機關主導介入血液事業之發展及政策,台灣輸血學會的全程熱心參與與推動,民眾的熱心支持跟付出,終至今日的燦爛成就。這次大會能爭取到由台灣主辦,意義不再只是一個國內外學者專家齊聚一堂的學術交流,更是對台灣

血液事業（國家的血液政策）從草創到蓬勃發展，乃至積極參與國際學術交流的一項回應與肯定。（見彩圖3、4、5）

2. 台灣血型的研究 [83]

我們長期研究台灣血型,發現許多台灣(同時也可能是華人)新血型及相關的新基因,我同時也研究相關新的稀有血型輸血的可行方案[83],被國際學者喻為坐在金礦上的人。除了下面5項(亞孟買血型,B_3, i 血型,Le(a+b+),K_{null})外,尚發現 A_2, A_3, A_{el}, A_m, A_x, B_{el}, B_m, B_x, B(A), D_{el}, Jk(a-b-), Lu(a-b-), Di(a+b-), D^{v1}, Dc-, St^a, Tj^a 等 17 項新或稀有血型及相關的新基因的發現,加上 Tn, Cad 多重凝集的發現,使我的台灣資料,變成東南亞國家如越南、緬甸、印度、中國等國家血庫作業的重要參考資料。

A. 台灣的分泌型亞孟買血型(H 抗原缺乏分泌型);O_h-secretor; O_{Hm}

亞孟買血型,也叫「H 缺乏的血型」,台灣(也是華人)的第一例亞孟買血型,是 1985 年在馬偕醫院的開刀病人備血時發現的。這個病人在備血時,ABO 血型測定上,血球與血清的型別互不相配合(即血球像 O 型、血清像 B 型),後來證明這個病

圖1　紅血球上 ABO 血型抗原的遺傳

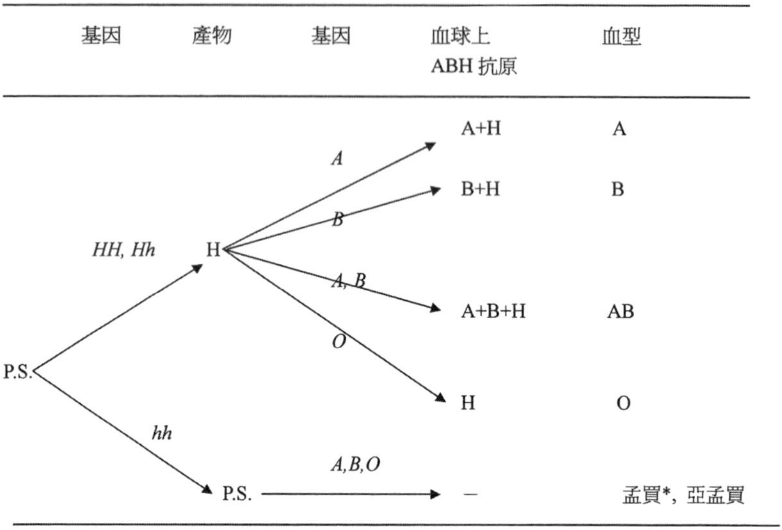

基因	產物	基因	血球上 ABH 抗原	血型

```
                            A
                          ─────→  A+H      A
                            B
                          ─────→  B+H      B
          HH, Hh    H
                           A, B
                          ─────→  A+B+H    AB
                            O
   P.S.                   ─────→  H        O
          hh
                          A, B, O
           →   P.S.      ─────→   —       孟買*, 亞孟買
```

　　人是帶 B 基因的稀有血型亞孟買血型，因他沒有正常的 H 基因，無法表現 B 基因，所以病人本身表現像 O 血型，因此這個帶 B 基因的亞孟買血型的 B 基因，就借太太正常的 H 基因，表現在他兒子身上，成 AB 血型，即太太是 A 型，他們有一個 AB 型的兒子（圖1）。這個亞孟買血型的雙親是正常的血型，顯然亞孟買血型的基因的遺傳，是隱性的遺傳。這第一例是由北倫敦血液中心的 Marcela Contreras 及紐約血液中心 Laurence Marsh 來確定我們的結果。

　　這種亞孟買血型是1965年 Solomon 首先在美國印地安人發現，1990年長庚醫院孫建峰等篩檢約 50,000 個病人，發現六個是亞孟買血型，所以國人較精確的頻率是每 8,000 個人有一個，到

2005年台灣共發現86個亞孟買血型的人,台灣23,000,000的人口,估計總共約有3,000個亞孟買血型。泰國的Chandanayingyong用植物的種子萃取液叫Ulex,篩檢捐血人,發現每5,000個捐血人有一個是屬於這個血型。日本大阪府紅十字會大久保康人到1983年,一共發現日本有82個亞孟買血型,所以日本人的頻率是,每120,000個人中有一個是亞孟買血型。

在〈寫在前面〉講到,亞孟買血型最有趣的是,這個血型的遺傳,會讓父母與小孩的ABO血型不配合,而亞孟買血型本人都以為自己是O型,如果另一方是正常O型,可以生出A或B血型的小孩,常引起家庭糾紛。歐洲的孟買或亞孟買血型,在1975年由英國Race and Sanger分類為三類,認為由一個基因來控制血球及分泌物中ABH抗原的表現,但隨著台灣分泌型亞孟買血型的發現,及隨之進行的台灣基因研究(余榮熾),就推翻了歐洲的理論,而知道是由 *H* 及 *Se* 基因分別來控制血球及分泌物中的ABH抗原的表現。到2005年,國際上一共發現27個相關亞

表1　H缺乏的血型

型	標誌		抗原 血球 A	B	H	分泌液 A	B	H	血清中抗體
H缺乏非分泌型 (孟買血型)	O$_h$	O$_h^O$	−	−	−	−	−	−	Anti-H
		O$_h^A$	−	−	−	−	−	−	Anti-H
		O$_h^B$	−	−	−	−	−	−	Anti-H
H部分缺乏非分泌型 (亞孟買血型)	O$_h$		−	−	−/w	−	−	−	Anti-H
	A$_h$		+/w	−	−/w	−	−	−	Anti-H
	B$_h$		−	+/w	−/w	−	−	−	Anti-H
H部分缺乏分泌型 (亞孟買血型)	O$_h^B$-secretor (O$^B_{Hm}$)		−	−	−/w	−	−	+	Anti-HI
	O$_h^A$-secretor (O$^A_{Hm}$)		+/w	−	−/w	+	−	+	Anti-HI
	O$_h^B$-secretor (O$^B_{Hm}$)		−	+/w	−/w	−	+	+	Anti-HI

圖2　台灣亞孟買血型者的家譜

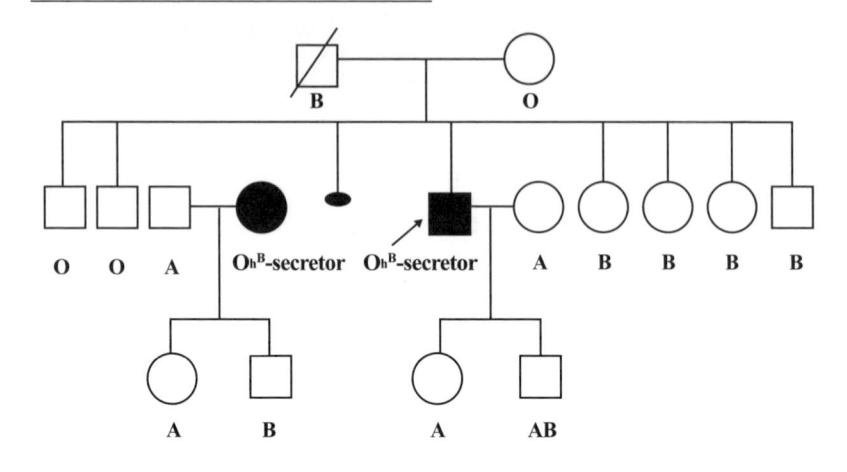

```
             ┌─────────┐     ┌─────────┐
             │    B    │─────│    O    │
             └─────────┘     └─────────┘
    ┌────┬────┬────┬─────┬─────┬─────┬─────┬─────┬─────┐
    □    □    △    ●     ⬬    ■     ○     ○     ○     ○
    O    O    A  Oh^B-   Oh^B- A     B     B     B     B
              secretor secretor
         ┌────┴────┐         ┌────┴────┐
         ○         □         ○         □
         A         B         A         AB
```

孟買血型的基因（h），其中7個是在台灣發現的。

B. 有關亞孟買血型（O_h-secretor）的輸血

　　因傳統的觀念認為，孟買血型者需輸孟買血型的血，因如表1所示，第一型孟買血型（O_h）的血清中出現強力 anti-H，再加上強力 anti-A 及 anti-B，所以孟買血型者須輸同血型的血。一般認為，第二型亞孟買血型也可能要輸孟買或亞孟買血型的血。但我們發現，第三型台灣的分泌型亞孟買血型，可能因為帶 Se 基因，所以血清中的相對抗體弱，如帶 B 基因的分泌型亞孟買血型（O_h^B-secretor），血清中 anti-B 的力價低，同樣的 anti-H/HI 的力價也低，這些抗體在37℃常無反應，所以理應可輸一般 B 及 O 型血。實際的情況是，在臨床上已有四例報告這種血型的病人，在緊急狀況下，成功的輸入一般 ABO 血型的血，一例在法國，一

68　豐富多彩的台灣

例在美國，兩例在台灣（彰化基督教醫院，1,500ml 一般的 B 型的血輸給一個帶 B 基因的亞孟買血型，500ml O 型血給另一個帶 B 基因的分泌型亞孟買血型），這些病人的血紅素有預期的上升，無任何不良反應，haptoglobin（連接血紅素的蛋白）在輸血後保持正常，表示沒溶血。

亞孟買血型者在緊急或需要大量輸血時，很難找到同樣血型的血，在此情形下，應可以用預溫技術法（IAT）找適合的血，如帶 A 基因的亞孟買血型的人，可輸入 A 或 O 型的血。以台灣 2,300 萬的人口，總共約有 3,000 個亞孟買血型，捐血中心平常只備少數亞孟買血型的冷凍紅血球以供開刀的需要（緊急輸血則來不及供應）。我們經人體試驗，證明了分泌型亞孟買血型可輸入一般人的血，讓一般的醫院在緊急情況下，放心的輸一般人的血給分泌型亞孟買血型的病人。我們是先用 ^{51}Cr 去標誌 54ml 一般 B 血型的紅血球濃厚液，再把這標誌好的血液輸給帶 B 基因的分泌型亞孟買血型，輸血過程順利，無輸血反應，輸入的 B 型血，在這個亞孟買血型者的體內存活接近正常，由此可以說在緊急狀況下，亞孟買血型者可以輸交叉試驗適合的血 [詳見參考資料 30,40,81]。顯然早年在台灣流傳的，孟買血型的賽車手每次要出賽，就要帶同是孟買血型的妹妹去的故事，應該是白種人的故事。

C. B_3 血型，在華人發現的第一個 ABO 亞血型 B_3 血型

長久以來，台灣醫學界都知道白種人最常見的 ABO 亞血型是 A_2 血型，大家都不知道台灣人有沒有 A_2 血型？如果沒有的話，

到底有沒有別的亞血型？在 1983 年，我從一個捐血人找到 B 的亞血型，這個 B 亞血型的血球在和抗體 anti-B 反應時，沒有正常強度凝塊的反應，而是在沒凝集散開的紅血球中混雜著紅血球的小凝集塊，稱紅血球的混合反應（見彩圖 6），經過使用當時從我參與的「ABO 血型國際單株抗體工作研討會」得到的單株抗體反應後，才知道是屬於 B 型陽性弱反應的亞血型，如同曾被報告過的 B_3 血型，1984 年經送血液到法國巴黎血液中心的 Salmon 教授處（見彩圖 7），得到肯定。這個血型是台灣最常見的 ABO 亞血型，頻率是每 900 個 B 型人有一個 B_3 血型，每 10,000 個台灣人有三個 B_3 血型，這和北歐每 1,000 個 A 型者有一個 A_3 血型，成對比。在 1983 年我們發表之前，曾經在新加坡發現弱反應的血球，但是沒有訂出一個名字。因為 B_3 血型在白種人罕見，所以國際友人紛紛來要血球。經過余榮熾分子生物學的研究，發現是 B 基因的突變，B 基因的 intron 3 的 +5 鹼基發生 G>A 突變（IVS3+5G>A），exon 3 成 pseudoexon，造成缺少 19 個氨基酸的 B 轉化酶，結果造成 B 轉化酶的功能減弱和改變 [見參考資料 105]。B_3 血型有時候不小心會被誤認為是 O 血型，而輸給 O 型病人，可能引起輸血反應。

除了發現 B_3 血型以外，我也發現了許多別的 ABO 亞血型，有 A_2、A_3、A_{el}、A_m、A_x、B_{el}、B_m、B_x，加上因 A 及 B 單株抗體的應用而發現 B 型血球帶有很弱 A 抗原的 B(A) 血型。尚發現 ABO 血型可發生後天性的改變，即 A 血型者因腸道阻塞及感染，細菌的繁殖，細菌酵素將部分 A 抗原改變成似 B 抗原，而成像 AB 型的「後天 B 抗原」。另有因白血病，使血球的 A 或 B 抗原弱化成亞型或 O 型（見圖 3）。這麼多新血型的發現，就要感謝「國際單株抗

體研討會」發給我們的許多不同國際研究單位製成的單株抗體，讓我們很「奢侈的」從事了許多亞血型及ABO相關血型的研究。

除了多樣的ABO血型外，我們也發現台灣人ABO血型抗原的形成，台灣嬰兒比白種人早，相對抗體的形成也比白種人早，台灣ABO抗體形成的高峰，在小孩的時期就達到了，但是在白種人要等到青春期才會到高峰，是很有趣的事。而且我也發現，抗體的力價，在1980年代台灣人明顯的比白種人高，會不會是因為當時我們居住的環境有更多的細菌抗原的刺激而引起的？[見台灣血型的研究, 83]或是遺傳的因素？台灣的新生兒，因母子ABO血型的不配合（特別是O型媽媽有A或B型的嬰兒），較易見到新生兒溶血症，當時甚至歐美的國家也注意到，黃種人的新生兒黃疸較明顯，這應該與國人當時血型抗體的力價高有關。在1980年代，常見ABO血型母子的不配合而發生新生兒黃疸而須要換血，很奇怪的是，在2000年代已逐漸減少，現在已少見到了。

圖3　A$_1$血型病人的家譜（在第一行病人為急性骨髓性白血病病人，A抗原減弱呈A$_3$血型）

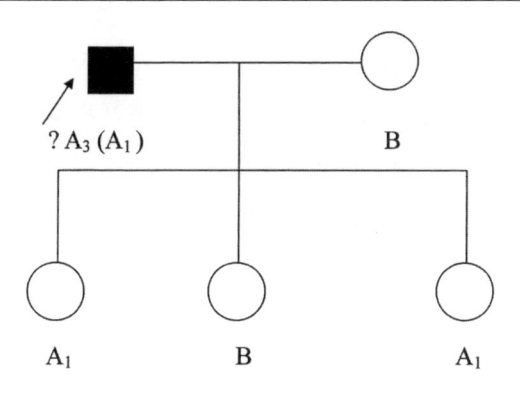

D. 台灣的成人 i 血型，證明 I 血型基因及 i 血型與先天性白內障部分連結的分子遺傳學機制；同時也證明了 I 血型基因，促使國際輸血學會於 2003 年將 I 抗原升格為人類第 27 個血型系統

「台灣的成人 i 血型」者的血球，在成人血球沒有應該有的 I 抗原，而只有血球胎兒期 I 原始抗原的 i 抗原，稱為成人 i 血型，或 i 血型。為稀有血型，基因型為 *ii*。1970 年日本大阪府紅十字會血液中心山口英夫、大久保康人等人發現，i 血型與先天性白內障一起發生，推測 *Ii* 基因及先天性白內障的隱性基因一起遺傳（close linkage）。1990 年台灣第一例 i 血型合併先天性白內障，是發現在台中捐血中心送給我的個案，因血清中出現強力 anti-I（因血球缺少 I 抗原），所以引起捐血中心 ABO 血型鑑定的困難（血球的血型為 B 型，但血清因 anti-I 與所有的血球反應，呈 O 血型反應）。後來我們證明是 i 血型，且查出捐血人有先天型白內障，就讀啟明學校。做家族的篩檢，發現他的姊姊也是 i 血型，且合併先天性白內障，他的雙親和四個兄弟均為一般的 I 血型且有正常的視力（見圖 4 的第 1 家）。隨即做 100 個同校學生 I 血型的測定，發現另一個 i 血型的學生合併先天性白內障，家族的檢查，發現一個妹妹和她的情形一樣，她的父母及另外一個妹妹有正常的視力及屬於一般的 I 血型（見圖 4 的第 2 家）。篩檢北部的啟明學校 32 個患有先天性白內障的學生，發現另一個 i 血型合併先天性白內障，這個案的父母親為近親結婚，家中沒有其他人有相同的情況（見圖 4 第 3 家）。i 血型的鑑定，是用 anti-I（日本大阪府紅十字會血液中心大久保康人博士提供）和血球反應，沒反應者為 i 血型。

圖4　成人i血型合併先天性白內障的三個家譜

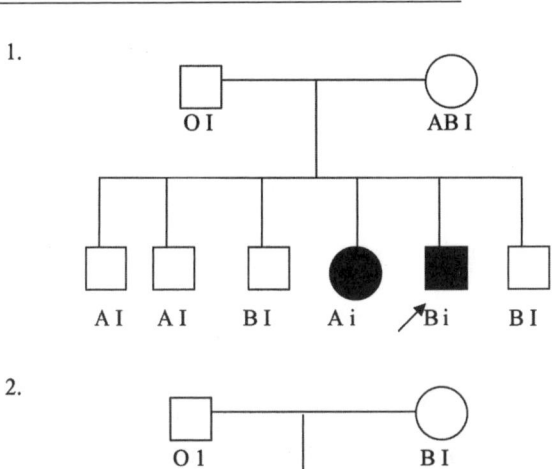

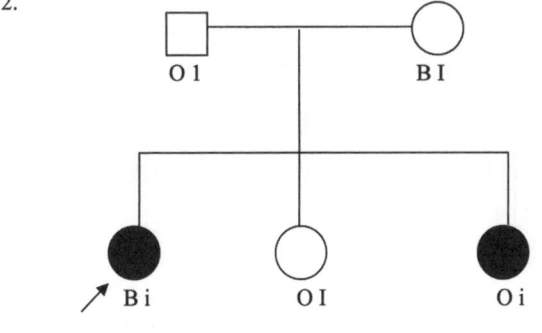

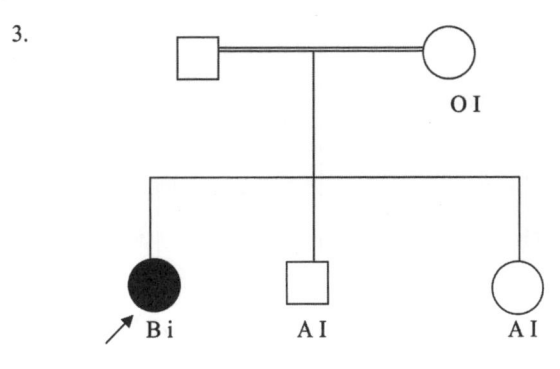

1.
- 父：OI　母：ABI
- 子女：AI、AI、BI、Ai（實心）、Bi（實心，箭頭）、BI

2.
- 父：OI　母：BI
- 子女：Bi（實心，箭頭）、OI、Oi（實心）

3.
- 父母：OI（近親）
- 子女：Bi（實心，箭頭）、AI、AI

■ ●：實心為先天性白內障

一、談台灣的輸血與血型　73

我們發現，台灣先天性白內障的視障者中，出現 i 血型的機會約為 2%，而在白內障者中，同時有 i 血型及先天性白內障的機會為 1%，這頻率遠較日本高，山口英夫篩檢 382 個日本視障者並沒發現 i 血型，國人的頻率可能是現有的最高頻率。白種人 i 血型合併先天性白內障的報告，只在澳洲發現一家族，Marsh 篩檢紐約捐血人，發現 6 個 i 血型，都沒有合併先天性白內障。

　　i 血型血清中均出現 anti-I，可能不具多少臨床意義，所以可以輸一般人的血。因為 i 血型為稀有血型，當 i 血型需要大量輸血，如果因有 anti-I 弱抗體而要輸 i 血型的血，可能無法提供輸血。三軍總院萬祥麟曾為 i 血型的病人輸血，雖然病人的 anti-I 在 37°C 有弱反應，病人輸注 6 單位來自病人兒子（*Ii* 基因型）的血液後，Hb（血紅素）自 4.6gm/dl 上升到 7gm/dl，且無輸血反應。這配合 Mollison 的發現，i 血型帶 anti-I 者，輸入 II 血型血球，血球存活期間不超過 15 分鐘，但輸入 Ii 血型血球則可存活正常。另外一例發生在南部的病人就沒有那麼幸運，在 2005 年有一個 80 歲白血病的病人，發現是 i 血型，他需要長期輸血，但無家屬，他的血液中出現很強的 anti-I，對抗所有的人的血球，所以輸入一般人的血球（II 血型血球）很快地被破壞，他在後來的 376 天，共輸入 153 袋血，平均每 2.5 天需要輸一袋血，最後他的病情惡化而死亡。2005 年血液基金會還沒有稀有血型的捐血人名冊，所以沒有辦法提供稀有血型 i 血型的血袋。病人本身沒有小孩，也沒有兄弟姐妹，所以沒有 Ii 血型的血可輸。2020 年血液基金會發表稀有血型的名冊檔案，其中 i 血型有 19 袋冷凍血，希望這個名單可以繼續擴大下去，去服務需要的病人。

　　台大生化所余榮熾教授團隊，在 2001 年、2003 年分子生物

圖5 *I*血型基因有特殊基因結構，突變位置決定 i 血型是否連結先天性白內障發生

I血型基因有特殊基因結構；突變位置決定小i血型是否連結先天性白內障發生

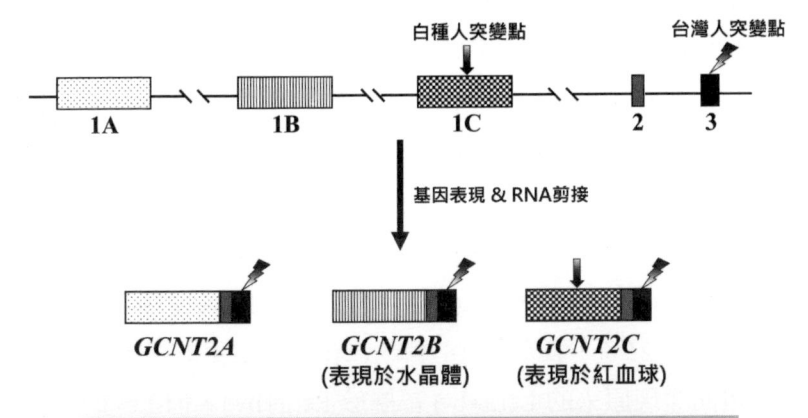

白種人突變點　　　　台灣人突變點

1A　　1B　　1C　　　2　　3

基因表現 & RNA剪接

GCNT2A　　GCNT2B　　GCNT2C
　　　　　(表現於水晶體)　(表現於紅血球)

台灣人的突變，位於三基因共有區，一個突變破壞掉三個基因產物的酵素活性。
白種人的突變，僅破壞了表現於紅血球的一個基因。

學的研究，證明 *I/i* 基因有 3 個不同的 *GCNT2* 基因，因 *GCNT2* 基因結構的突變所致，台灣人的先天性白內障和 i 血型的共同的出現，是因突變發生在三個 *GCNT2* 基因共有區，因此一個突變破壞掉三個基因產物的酵素活性引起的。白種人的 i 血型，是突變僅破壞了表現於紅血球的 *GCNT2C* 基因 [98,109,182]，如圖5。

2003 年的論文 [109]，因此獲選為 *Blood* 當期期刊的 Plenary paper，編輯推薦並撰文：「i to I and the eye」。

E. 台灣的路易士（Lewis）血型

1980 年代，在馬偕醫院、榮民總醫院、長庚醫院及捐血中

心，共做約 4,000 人血球的路易士血型，結果均發現，除了三種國際上認定的表現型 Le(a+b-)、Le(a-b+) 及 Le(a-b-) 血型外，很意外的，台灣人尚出現在歐美沒看過的 Le(a+b+) 血型。1988 年在馬偕醫院，這四種血型的頻率為 Le(a+b-) 10%、Le(a-b+) 67%、Le(a-b-) 10% 及 Le(a+b+) 13%。

我為參加 1990 年第二屆國際紅血球單株抗體研討會，我用研討會提供的 anti-Le^a、anti-Le^b 單株抗體，加上優良的輸血製劑公司 Ortho 的 anti-Le^a、anti-Le^b 多株抗體，在馬偕醫院測 100 個健康國人血球及口水中 ABO 及 Le^a、Le^b 抗原出現的情形，結果很意外的發現，台灣人沒有 Le(a+b-) 血型，但歐美沒有的 Le(a+b+) 血型竟高達 25%，我在 1988 年的 Le(a+b-) 個案的冷凍保存紅血球，重測發現原來的 Le(a+b-) 都屬於 Le(a+b+)，但 Le^b 的抗原為弱反應，所以 1988 年誤辨為 Le(a+b-)，因此台灣人的 Le(a+b-)、Le(a+b+) 血型的血球上 Le^b 的抗原強度，因人不同而不同，反應的強度 ±~4+，Le^b 的抗原強度很弱時呈現為 Le(a+b-)。Le(a+b+) 口水中，Le 抗原有正常的含量的 Le^a 及 Le^b，但 ABH 呈不定量的減少，這種減少的現象，Sturgeon 在 1970 年解釋為由弱分泌基因 Se^w 引起的，所以 Le(a+b+) 血型的出現，一般認為由 Se^w 基因引起的。口水中均出現 ABH 抗原，所以台灣人 100%（或接近 100%）為分泌型。Le(a+b+) 血型也在紐澳原住民發現（Henry 及 Woodfield，1989）。

我們的結果及紐澳的報告，在國際引起很大的震撼，Le(a+b+) 的基因型及相關的基因到底是什麼？變成 1990 年代研究的重點。1995 年 Se 基因的 DNA 序列被訂出，而我們實驗室的余榮熾也在同年年底，在國際幾個著名的實驗室（包括瑞典

的 Karolinska Institute）的競賽中，首先成功的訂出 Se^w 基因的序列，我們發現了 Se^{w385} 基因（A385->T），引起 Se-transferase α 1,2 fucosyltransferase 在第 129 胺基酸位置的 isoleucine 被 phenylalanine 所取代，而造成弱功能的 Se-transferase，製造 Le^b 抗原的功能下降，很可能在與 Le 基因的產物 Le-transferase 在利用 substrate 競爭上因弱功能而佔下風，引起 Le 抗原量變少。Se^{w385} 廣泛的分布在亞洲及南太平洋地區，證明這是一個存在於亞洲的古老突變。[44,66,74]

我做台灣不同族群 Lewis 血型的測定，結果發現在 12 族原住民當中，除雅美族、卑南族及賽夏族外，都出現 Le(a+b-) 血型，而這血型在閩南人、客家人及外省人是看不到的。因 Le(a+b-) 是白種人的血型，有鑑於白種人曾經佔領過台灣，所以我們做 Le(a+b-) 血型相關的基因非分泌型 Se 基因的 DNA 序列研究，發現台灣原住民 se 基因為 se^{571}、se^{685}、se^{849}，和白種人的 se^{428} 不同。

se 基因是 Se 基因發生 DNA 序列上的定點突變，引起功能喪失，所以變成非分泌型。到 2002 年共發現 10 個 se 基因，其中在台灣原住民就看到三個 se 基因，se^{571} 首先在毛利人身上發現，除了廣泛的出現在台灣原住民，也在日本人、菲律賓人出現。se^{685} 只有在三族台灣原住民（排灣族、阿美族、卑南族）看到。se^{849} 也是廣泛的出現在台灣原住民身上，且也在菲律賓人出現。Le(a+b+) 血型的 Le^b 抗原，因抗原量少反應弱，所以在經驗不足的血庫常誤判為陰性，成 Le(a+b-) 血型，導致 Se 基因與 Lewis 血型間關係的混亂。我詳細做台灣各族群的 Lewis phenotyping 和 Se 間關係的研究，結果發現完全符合國際上公認的關係。[86,97]

Le 基因（FUT3）突變引起 Le(a-b-) 血型的相關基因共有 10

個，台灣不同族群的 Le(a-b-) 血型的相關 *Le* 基因，尚待將來的研究。

台灣人 Lewis 血型的發展過程：白種人的 Lewis 血型，從出生到成年有連續的改變，因台灣人有不見於白種人的 Le(a+b+) 血型，所以我測試台灣人不同年齡 Lewis 血型出現的情形及期間的改變，得到的結果是：台灣人在臍帶血的 Lewis 血型為 Le(a-b+) 或 Le(a-b-)，前者雖經過嬰兒期的 Le(a+b+) 型，但最後還是變回原來的 Le(a-b+) 血型。Le(a-b-) 型大部分經過嬰兒期的 Le(a+b+) 型，後變成成人的 Le(a+b+) 及 Le(a-b+) 血型，只有一小部分還是保持原來的 Le(a-b-) 血型沒改變到成人。[61]

Lewis 血型，特別是 Le(a+b+) 型，在生理上的意義及在疾病上的關係，尚待有志之士的投入研究。

F. K$_{null}$ 稀有血型的相對抗體 anti-Ku 引起的致死性溶血性輸血反應 [107] 及相關 *KEL* 基因 [99] 的研究

Kell 血型系統的抗原，在血球表面呈低密度的分布。這些抗原是在單一的 K 蛋白上由單一基因控制。1946 年在 K 抗體引起的新生兒溶血症發現 Kell (K) 抗原。白種人有 9% 帶 K 抗原，黑種人 2%，但黃種人包括中國人、日本人、韓國人，很少帶 K 抗原。約 3,000 個華人（香港、澳門及美國華僑）、3,000 個台灣人及 1,500 個台灣原住民中，只發現一個人帶 K 抗原，這個案雖無詳細家族資料，但很可能是白種人的後代。1994 年香港每 1,700 人有一個 Kk 血型（即 0.06%）。K 的對偶基因為 *k*，*k* 基因的抗原 k (Cellano)，白種人 99.8% 陽性，台灣人 100% 陽性，血液基金會

到 2020 年共收集到四袋 k 陰性的血。K 的抗原性強,所以輸血過的白種人,常見 anti-K,anti-K 不易經 manual Polybrene (MP) 法測出,須要加做 AHG phase(抗球蛋白試驗),anti-K 在白種人常引起輸血反應,為白種人最重要的抗體,其重要性與 Rh 血型的抗體並列。台灣沒 K 抗原,所以沒發現過 anti-K。

屬於這血型系統的,還有 Kp^a、Kp^b;Js^a、Js^b。Kp^a、Kp^b;Js^a、Js^b 為對偶基因,這些抗原和 K、k 抗原做相關連的遺傳。

K_{null} 血型:是稀有血型 K-、k-、Kp^a-、Kp^b-、Js^a-、Js^b-,缺少 K 系統所有的抗原,所以和 Rh_{null} 相似,亦稱 Ko。1957 年,在新生兒溶血症的個案,找到第一例 K_{null} 血型,為波蘭人,後來日本也發現另一個 K_{null} 血型。北京血液中心在篩檢 50 個 O 型捐血人時,發現一個 K_{null} 血型,為北方漢人,經家族的篩檢,發現兄弟姊妹中還有 2 個 K_{null} 血型。馬偕醫院在 2001 年從花蓮送過來的檢體中,發現台灣第一個 K_{null} 血型,病人為榮民,本籍雲南,從罕見的姓名研判,為雲南的少數民族。

病人因腎結石併發細菌感染開刀,住院 44 天中,共輸 34 單位的紅血球濃厚液。Hb(血紅素)在開始住院輸血有預期的上升,後來越輸血 Hb 越低,最後病人併發腎衰竭及敗血病死亡。我們在病人過世前的血清檢體中找到 anti-Ku,這抗體是在 K_{null} 血型發生,這抗體對抗所有 K 系統的抗原,所以和所有輸入的血球反應,因此病人的腎衰竭,是因 anti-Ku 引起的溶血性輸血反應的結果。在台灣,標準的交叉作業是 manual Polybrene 法,這方法對偵測 K 血型系統的抗體敏感度本來就不夠,所以 anti-Ku 在花蓮一直沒被注意到。這 anti-Ku 是近 20 年來,在台灣發現的唯一屬於 K 血型系統的抗體。我們篩檢約 3,000 個台灣人及原住民,

沒找到 K_{null} 血型。基因的研究發現，*K* 基因在 intron 3 (5' splice site) 發生 G>C 的變異，致使 *KEL* 基因成無功能基因 [99]。

G. Jk(a-b-) 血型

　　為稀有的血型，這種血型最先在菲律賓發現，是在帶菲律賓及西班牙血統的華裔身上發現，後來在巴西印地安人及紐澳地區的原住民也發現，其中紐西蘭原住民毛利人的頻率高達 0.9%，因而這血型被認為是波里尼西亞人的特徵之一。我們做台灣原住民血型分布的研究，測試近 1,500 個原住民的血液檢體，在排灣族的 165 個檢體中發現一個 Jk(a-b-) 血型，然後在其兄弟姊妹中找到另一個 Jk(a-b-) 血型，我們在魯凱族中也找到一個這血型，可見台灣南部的原住民和毛利人有關。日本已發現十幾個家族。馬偕醫院在 1987 年自高雄長庚醫院送來的檢體中發現 Jk(a-b-) 血型，血清因含 anti-Jk3（即 anti-Jk^{a}Jk^b），所以交叉試驗找不到合適的血。病人為 69 歲男，沒有族群資料。我們在 1992 年自亞東醫院送來新生兒黃疸症的檢體中發現 anti-Jk3，母親是 Jk(a-b-) 血型，女嬰的雙親都是閩南人。

　　Jk(a-b-) 的遺傳，主要是由不表現 Jk 抗原的隱性基因 *Jk* 引起的，因此在親子鑑定上，Jk(a+b-) 及 Jk(a-b+) 的雙親可以有 Jk(a+b-)、Jk(a+b-) 及 Jk(a-b+) 的小孩，在白種人如出現後兩者血型的小孩，即可否定親子關係，但在台灣因有 *Jk* 基因的可能，無法否定親子關係。Jk(a-b-) 血型的簡易測試方法，是將紅血球放在 2M Urea 中 15 分鐘，如為 Jk(a-b-) 血型，將不見溶血，須延遲到 15-30 分鐘才見溶血，如為一般血型，在 5 分鐘內就可以看到近全

部紅血球的溶血。

　　另外有部分 Jk(a-b-) 血型的遺傳是由顯性基因引起的，這基因稱 *In(Jk)*。日本曾發現母親 Jk(a+b+)，但兩個女兒及幾個外孫都是 Jk(a-b-) 血型。

H. Diego 血型系統

　　1956 年在委內瑞拉新生兒溶血症的母親血液中，找到對抗低頻率抗原的抗體，後來用該家族的名字，稱抗原為 Diego (Di)，抗體稱為 anti-Di^a，做了 Diego 家族的研究，發現有 30% 的家族屬 Di(a+)，這些帶 Di^a 抗原者，在體型上有印地安人的特徵。後來發現的幾例 anti-Di^a 引起的新生兒溶血症，都找到和黃種人的血緣關係。因美洲印地安人一直被認為和 Mongoloid（亞洲蒙古種族）有關，所以測試不同地區印地安人、美洲的日本人及中國人，結果發現 Di^a 頻率最高在美洲巴西印地安人，頻率近 46%，印地安人既然被認為屬於 Mongoloid，所以 Di^a 抗原被認為是屬於 Mongoloid 的標誌。在 1956 年測 156 個愛斯基摩人，意外發現愛斯基摩人並沒人帶 Di^a，測更多的愛斯基摩人，也一樣罕見帶 Di^a 抗原（2/1477），測美國阿拉斯加印地安人，也發現頻率低，加拿大的印地安人，也從較南方的 Alberta 的 3%，向北到近北極的 0%。北方的日本人 3-4%，南方的日本人 5-7%。1967-1970 年間，測試 1,374 個澳洲原住民及 1,741 個新幾內亞原住民，未發現 Di(a+) 者。

　　台灣閩南人 Di(a+) 的頻率為 3.2%，客家人 7%（篩檢 1,000 人的結果，我們測試許多血型系統，發現這是閩客唯一有明顯差別

的地方），南方外省人和閩南人相同3.2%，北方外省人10.3%。最近我們測了九族高山原住民及兩族平埔族（巴宰及邵族），共1,357個人的 Di^a 出現情形，結果發現只有5人爲 Di(a+) 血型，所以我們原住民不像是屬於蒙古族。Anti-Di^a 在台灣罕見，可能的原因是因過去所用的抗體篩檢細胞，並沒有刻意去含 Di^a 抗原。1995年台北榮總診斷出台灣第一例因anti-Di^{a}引起的新生溶血症，男嬰在出生後第三天被發現有黃疸而即刻換血，一星期後出院。

Di(a+b-) 爲稀有血型，anti-Di^b 爲罕見的抗體。馬偕醫院在1993年發現了台灣第一例、在國際上也罕見的，由 anti-Di^b 引起的新生兒溶血症，母親懷孕四次，第一胎正常，第二胎嬰兒發生黃疸現象且需要照光治療，這第四胎爲女嬰，女嬰出生時亦有黃疸，產後五天內 bilirubin（膽紅素）一直介於 14-15mg/dl 之間，因爲找不到合適的血換血，只有照光治療，幸好療效不錯。實驗結果，母親的血清和100袋捐血中心的紅血球及24個馬偕醫院血庫保存的稀有血型的血球全部反應。後來檢查母親的紅血球，發現爲 Di(a+b-) 血型，這母親很可能因前幾胎的懷孕，被胎兒的 Di^b 陽性血球敏感產生 Di^b 抗體，造成新生兒黃疸症，這母親的妹妹亦被測爲 Di(a+b-)，此個案經英國醫學研究委員會（MRC）的 Daniels 證實。根據文獻報告，在美洲印地安人因 Diego 血型抗體引起的新生兒溶血症，主要由母親的 Di^a 抗體引起，日本的新生兒溶血症也有由 Di^a 抗體引起的，但臨床上以 Di^b 抗體引起的較爲嚴重。在東方民族，因母親 Di^b 抗體引起的新生兒溶血症，可能比 Di^a 抗體引起的較爲嚴重。

我們在1995年接到自中國醫學科學院輸血研究所寄來的檢體，經我們實驗室測試，找到 anti-Di^b+E+Jk^a，病人爲20歲男

性，B血型，診斷為門脈高壓症，因做脾臟的切除術，輸入B型血1580ml，手術後兩天出現醬油色尿（溶血性輸血反應），發燒40度，黃疸，Hb（血紅素）自7gm/dl下降至3.9gm/dl，因找不到適合的血輸，後來病人死亡。Di(b+)的頻率，在台灣是超過99.9%，猜測在中國也同樣，所以很難找到Di(b-)的血來輸血。

I. 努力七年證明「只和新鮮血小板」反應的抗體，解決國際長久以來無法證明存在的血小板抗體 [69,129]

1986年，我們血庫紅血球的研究發現了幾個重要的血型，如米田堡血型和亞孟買血型，當時衛生署回應輸血學會的要求，提供公費，給四位血庫工作人員到國外受訓，當時只有馬偕醫院派了血庫的鮑博瑞先生，到英國的Bristol向Anstee教授學習製做anti-A及anti-B單株抗體的方法，隨後他到美國Community Blood Center of Greater Kansas City，跟Dr. Fred Plapp學習測試血小板抗體的方法，Dr. Plapp很慷慨的將要專利化的篩檢血小板抗體法SPRCA (Solid phase red cell adherence)法的試劑做法及檢驗的操作，教導鮑先生，於是鮑博瑞先生把SPRCA方法帶回台灣，從1988年做到現在（2025年），將近40年期間，我們用這個方法在馬偕醫院從事許多血小板的研究，也教導別的醫院，將這個方法發揚光大。

在白種人的國家，大部分新生嬰兒因母親的血小板抗體引起的新生兒血小板缺乏症（NAITP），最多的原因是anti-HPA-1a，因為白種人的國家有2%的人是HPA-1a陰性，這些陰性的媽媽可以經過懷孕或輸血被免疫而產生anti-HPA-1a血小板抗體，抗體

可以通過胎盤，破壞 HPA-1a 陽性胎兒的血小板（與 Rh 陰性的媽媽懷陽性胎兒的情況相同），引起胎兒的血小板破壞而成血小板缺乏症，所以在生產的過程中，胎兒通過產道，常因血小板數量太低而引起胎兒顱內出血（另外皮膚出現紫斑）。台灣人（可說全亞洲人）全部是 HPA-1a 陽性，但是像 98% 的白種人 HPA-1a 的陽性媽媽，也會發生新生兒血小板缺乏症，在一項研究 204 個白種人 HPA-1a 的陽性母親血小板抗體引起的新生兒血小板缺乏症的個案中，只有 11 例個案找到抗體的特異性，可見血小板的抗體特異性，除了 anti-HPA-1a 的鑑定，其他的抗體是非常困難鑑定的。

　　台灣的情形就是這個樣子，馬偕醫院篩檢過 1,000 個捐血人及 100 個員工，全部 HPA-1a 陽性，因為我們沒有 HPA-1a 陰性的人，大家都是陽性，也就不可能有對抗 HPA-1a 的抗體的發生，但是母親的血小板抗體引起的新生兒血小板缺乏症，還是在發生，因為血小板的抗原系統是相當龐大跟複雜，我們經常沒有辦法把血小板的特異型，清楚的鑑定出來。我們在 1995 年，經過七年的努力，從 1988 年測試一個母親生出兩個血小板缺乏症的嬰兒，其中一個嬰兒甚至發生顱內出血，這個母親經我們使用從美國學來的 SPRCA 法，證明有血小板的抗體，但是當我們準備寫報告，發現用幾種傳統的血小板研究方法，如 MAIPA、IF 等，都做不出有抗體。經多方的求證，終於證明這個母親所帶的血小板抗體是對抗 HPA-3a 抗原的不穩定部分，血小板經過一天以上的儲存或經過固定，造成抗原不穩定部分的破壞，因 MAIPA、IF 兩種方法都是用固定過的血小板，所以做不出來，而 SPRCA 是使用新鮮血小板，才有反應，有結果。論文在國際輸血學會會刊

發表以後，終於使國際了解到血小板抗原有不穩定的成分，經過固定（如 MAIPA、IF）以後，就失去了抗原性。這個可以說是一個大發現，變成研究血小板的一個里程碑 [69]，許多重要的血小板抗體研究，都會提到我們的這篇文章。

新生兒血小板缺乏症的發生頻率，台灣人（馬偕醫院）約每 6,600 個新生兒發生一個 NAITP。馬偕醫院從 1988 年開始以 SPRCA 做血小板抗體的篩檢，到 2018 年，30 年間，一共鑑定了 6 個 NAITP 的個案，抗體特異性：各 2 例 anti-HPA-3a、anti-HPA-5a、anti-CD36。

2019 年到 2024 年的五年間，共篩檢了 2,037 例的血小板抗體，這段時間，我們加入 EIA 血小板抗體篩檢法一起篩檢，共找到 8 例血小板特異抗體：6 例 anti-CD36 及各 1 例 anti-HPA-5a 和 anti-HPA-5b。臨床上，其中 5 例 anti-CD36 為血小板輸注無效的病例；各一例 anti-CD36 及 anti-HPA-5b 為 NAITP 的病例；及 1 例 anti-HPA-5a 為 ITP 的病人。顯然的，anti-CD36 因為 EIA 檢查的加入而有明顯的增加，同時證明這個抗體在台灣是最重要的血小板抗體。在臨床上，如果遇到血小板輸注無效，輸入 HLA 配合的血小板也沒有改善的話，必須要考慮有 CD36 抗體出現的可能，需要做病人血清的血小板抗體的篩檢。

J. HLA-class I 與 2003 年 SARS 冠狀病毒感染的關係 [106]

2003 年 5 月，我對 37 個疑似 SARS 病人、被排除的發燒病人、曾暴露的醫護人員、及健康對照組血液檢體做 HLA class I 及 class II 的篩檢。結果 HLA-B*4601 在嚴重或死亡的個案，有意義

的增加，Pc=0.0279。HLA-B46 是亞洲南方的血緣，在白種人、台灣原住民、亞洲北方人少見或沒有，2003 年 SARS 的傳播途徑，和古代越族的分布相似 [106]。本篇刊登後，經國際各大報報導，**變成國際醫藥的大新聞** [附件 5]。比較遺憾的是，本篇報告在台灣被抵制，以致只有少數國人知道這項重要的發現。

二、談台灣的血緣

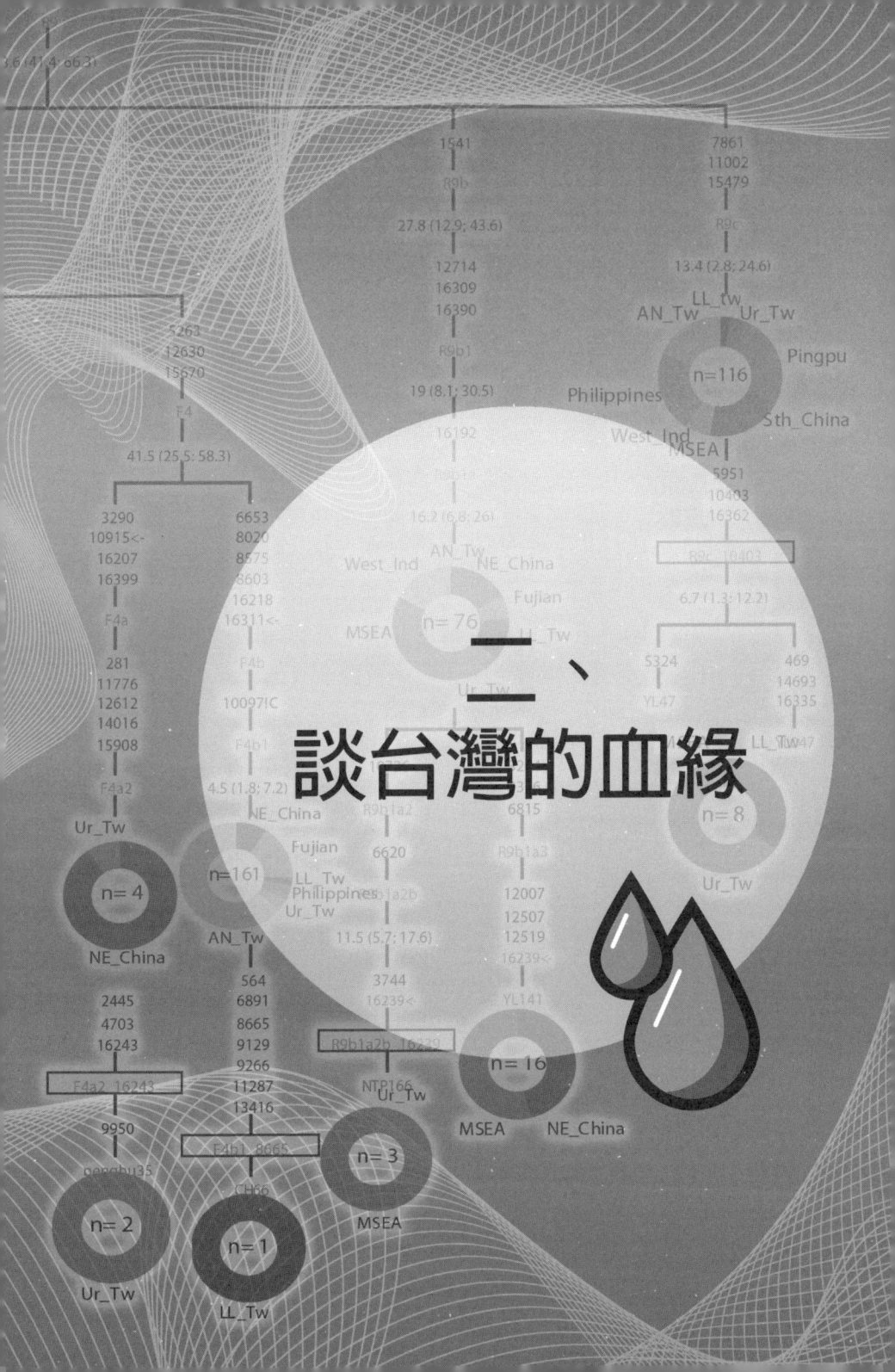

緣起：1990年代組織抗原（HLA）的研究，開始踏入分子人類學的領域

　　1993年在台北舉辦的HLA研討會，我又遇到前東京大學教授日本紅十字會東京血液中心的主任十字教授（Dr. Juji）。1990年代，所有HLA抗原的測驗是用血清學方法測的，台灣是用進口的HLA測定盤。事實上，正確的抗原測定方法，是要使用當地的血清（因含適合測當地居民的HLA抗原的抗體）做成的測定盤。十字教授跟我說，台灣政府花了很多經費，委託幾個實驗室做，結果沒有成功。他接著說，他願意用日本紅十字會做我的後盾，幫忙我，鼓勵我在馬偕醫院把台灣的HLA測定盤做出來。於是他派了紅十字會專家赤座達也醫師及助手來台，協助我建立一流的HLA實驗室。我在七年中，共收集了近20,000個馬偕醫院產房的胎盤，個個分離出血清，再分別和已知HLA抗原的台灣人的淋巴球反應，訂出血清中所含的HLA抗體，再做成測定盤。

　　當我們在2000年把HLA血清測定盤做出來的時候，HLA用DNA測定的方法，剛剛出來而且上市，這樣看來好像我們浪費七年，白忙一場。其實不然，我們因為要做台灣地區的測定盤，

因此我們收集台灣所有族群的淋巴球來測試，七年當中，我們上山下海收集到所有原住民、非原住民台灣人的淋巴球，我們將所得到的結果，參與日本紅十字會一年一度的全國 HLA 大會工作研討會，一起訂出台灣居民 HLA 的正確型別，再做成 HLA-A, B, DRB1 基因（血緣）關係樹，意外的發現，台灣人跟台灣高山原住民之間有很大的基因距離（見彩圖 8），這讓我非常的驚訝和興奮，從此我們就踏入人類學的範疇。

　　我查了許多資料才知道，地球在 20,000 年前開始暖化，以致冰河溶解，溶化的水流到海裡，讓海水上升，台灣海峽本來是乾的低地，將台灣連到歐亞大陸，但是在 10,000 年前海水開始上升，淹沒台灣海峽，台灣海峽的海水，在 7,000 年前上升到現在的海平面。原住民的祖先，很可能在台灣海峽陸連消失之前後時間，移民到台灣，而且因為台灣原住民和南北亞洲的族群都有血緣關係，顯示史前舊石器時代，人類可能沿著亞洲邊緣的低地，包括台灣海峽，從南到北的遷移。台灣原住民經過長期的隔離，變成現在基因（不多樣）的所謂純種的原住民族群，因而在基因關係樹上，與亞洲的族群，形成很大的基因距離（見彩圖 8）。

1. 台灣南島語族（高山原住民）的研究(1994-2014年)

A. 南島語族母系血緣（mtDNA）B4a1a 遷移的研究，顯示台灣很可能是南島語族的故鄉

B4a1a 血緣，在台灣原住民主要在阿美族看到（也在鄒族及雅美族看到），發生的年代約 10,000 年前。比 B4a1a 多一個突變（在第 14022 鹼基發生突變）稱為 B4a1a1，B4a1a1 血緣在新幾內亞找到，發生的年代約 6,000 年前。比 B4a1a1 多一個突變（發生在第 16247 鹼基）稱為 B4a1a1a 血緣，這血緣大量的在波里尼西亞人出現（>90% 波里尼西亞人屬這血緣），稱為波里尼西亞人的特徵（Polynesian motif），發生的年代約 6,000 年前。後來我們在菲律賓人及印尼人也找到 B4a1a 血緣，但頻率較阿美族低很多。B4a1a 血緣的前身 B4a1，在亞洲大陸（越南、中國及日本等）找到，發生的年代為 20,000 多年前，與 B4a1a 血緣相距 10,000 多年，所以 B4a1a 應發源在台灣或東南亞島嶼，從頻率來看，台灣是最有可能的發源地，而 B4a1a 與亞洲大陸的 B4a1 很可能早在冰河時期結束之前就已經分開。

從 B4a1a 血緣的演化，我們可以推測屬於母系社會 B4a1a 血緣的台灣原住民祖先，很可能是阿美族的祖先，在 4,000-5,000 年前，從台灣乘船出發，經過菲律賓、印尼東邊島嶼，到達新幾內亞，母系血緣突變成 B4a1a1 血緣，因為遷移的族群屬於母系社會，在這遷移過程，女人受到保護，男人找食物，男人大概在不友善的環境下被取代了，所以菲律賓、印尼及新幾內亞的父系血緣，取代了台灣原住民的父系血緣，成波里尼西亞人的父系血緣，所以波里尼西亞人是由不同來源的父母系血緣結合成的，母系與台灣原住民有共同的祖先，父系跟印尼及新幾內亞有共同的祖先。這些移民到新幾內亞後，經數千年的擴充，然後再擴散到太平洋變成波里尼西亞人（B4a1a1a 血緣），在這後段的擴散，母系社會變成父系社會（見彩圖 9）。

　　總結：2005 年我發表台灣九族南島語族（高山原住民）640 人母系血緣研究的結果，發現南島語族和非南島語族台灣人的母系血緣差異很大，南島語族有不少古老的血緣 [137]，其中 B4a1a 血緣主要出現在阿美族（45%）。這個血緣在菲律賓、印尼、新幾內亞也出現，因為在中國找不到，推測 B4a1a 遷移是從台灣出發，經菲律賓、印尼、新幾內亞，過程中，加上 14022 的變異，成 B4a1a1 血緣，到新幾內亞再增加 16247 變異，成波里尼西亞人的特徵血緣 B4a1a1a，這特徵血緣佔波里尼西亞人 80% 的母系血緣。2005 年文章刊登後，在 Yahoo 網站上出現 605 個評論，《經濟學人》（*The Economist*, 7/9/2005, Anthropology）評論「Taiwan, twinned with Hawaii」[附件 6]，結論是「台灣是南島語族的故鄉」。2011 年我們和英國的 Richards 等合作，繼續做 B4a1a 血緣的研究，發現台灣沒有 B4a1a1 血緣，菲律賓少，B4a1a1 主要在

印尼及新幾內亞出現 [178]，所以「台灣是南島語族的故鄉」好像有一點問題。然而，Richards 團隊用的方法，是採用固定式粒線體 DNA 的突變率去算每個粒線體 DNA 基因型的分布年紀，有其科學論證的缺失，若佐以古代 DNA 的結果（有考古年紀及粒線體 DNA 的定序資料），結果可能大大不同。事實上，我們的論點再經過 Reich 團隊分別以全基因體鹼基多樣性（SNP）資料及波里尼西亞人古代 DNA 的資料證實，證明台灣是南島語族的故鄉假說（*Nat Commun.* 5: 4689, 2014; *Current Biology* 30: 4846, 2020）。

B. 台灣南島語族群和南北亞洲的族群共有相同的 HLA haplotypes [89]

HLA haplotypes（組織抗原單倍型）是由幾個基因的組合而成的，如 HLA-A24-B48 haplotype，相同的組織抗原單倍型在不同族群出現，被認為是有共同的祖先，有血緣的關連，而組織抗原比父母系血緣顯示更古老的血緣關係。

大部分台灣高山原住民都具有高頻率的單倍型 A24-B48 及 A24-B61 haplotypes，這些單倍型也出現在東北亞的族群，包括愛斯基摩人（Inuit）、鄂倫春人及日本人。其中 A24-B48 被認為是東北亞族群特徵的血緣，所以台灣高山原住民與東北亞的族群共有 A24-B48 haplotype，是顯示古老的血緣關係、共有祖先，很可能顯示幾萬年前古代人類沿著亞洲大陸東邊東亞大陸棚（現已在海底）遷移的痕跡。從這裡，我們看到古代人類南北遷移留下的痕跡（見彩圖10）。

另外，由組織抗原的基因，可看到阿美族與澳洲原住民及

新幾內亞高地人的關係：尚令人不解的是，A34-B56 haplotype 在阿美族（18.6%）、新幾內亞高地人（10.6%）及澳洲原住民（4.1%）出現，顯示這些族群間具有很古老的關係，可能是五萬年前，當澳洲與新幾內亞還連在一起，屬於莎湖大陸，人類尚未遷移到台灣時，A34-B56 顯然是阿美族、澳洲原住民及新幾內亞高地人共同的祖先所帶有的 haplotypes（血緣），而這血緣一直保存到現在，因此阿美族與澳洲原住民及新幾內亞高地人應有共同的祖先，有古老的血緣關係，尚待將來的研究。

台灣南島語族群不少 HLA haplotypes 是和南北亞洲的族群共有，包含 Māori（毛利人）、Highlanders（新幾內亞高地人）、Archons（鄂倫春人）、Mongolians（蒙古人）、Inuit（愛斯基摩人）、Japanese（日本人）、滿族、Buryat（布里亞特人）、American Indian-Tlingit（特林吉特人，北美洲太平洋西北海岸原住民），表示這些族群和台灣的南島語族群有古老的血緣關係，顯示可能在萬年前舊石器時代的後期（冰河時期），當時台灣海峽是陸地，台灣陸連到歐亞大陸，人類的遷徙可能是從南亞到北亞（可能雙向），沿著歐亞大陸東邊沿海的東亞大陸棚遷徙（當時也是沿海陸地），台灣古代剛好位於遷移路線的中間，以致於台灣南島語族帶有南北亞洲的血緣[89]。

2. 台灣非南島語族（台灣人）的研究 (2000-2023 年)

　　非南島語的台灣人，就是非台灣高山原住民的台灣人，也是所謂的「台灣人」或稱為台灣漢人，包含閩南人、客家人。

　　我在 1980-1990 年代從事血型的研究，發現了台灣許多的新血型，其中有些血型是屬於東南亞特有的血型，如稀有血型的分泌型亞孟買血型（para-Bombay phenotype）[30]、米田堡血型（Miltenberger blood group）[53]，從這些血型的發現，顯示台灣人更像是東南亞的族群，讓我懷疑「台灣人是北方純種漢人的後代」的真實性。

A. 2001 年 HLA 基因的研究 [94]

　　我以閩南人、客家人 HLA-A, B, C 的基因頻率，和國際上不同族群的資料比較，發現閩南人、客家人是屬於亞洲南方的族群，不是北方人，屬東南亞族群 [94]（圖 6），這結果印證了我在血型方面的發現。但我 2001 年當時錯誤的認為，HLA 基因上屬

圖 6 HLA 基因研究結果顯示，台灣人（閩南人及客家人）的基因和北方漢人分開

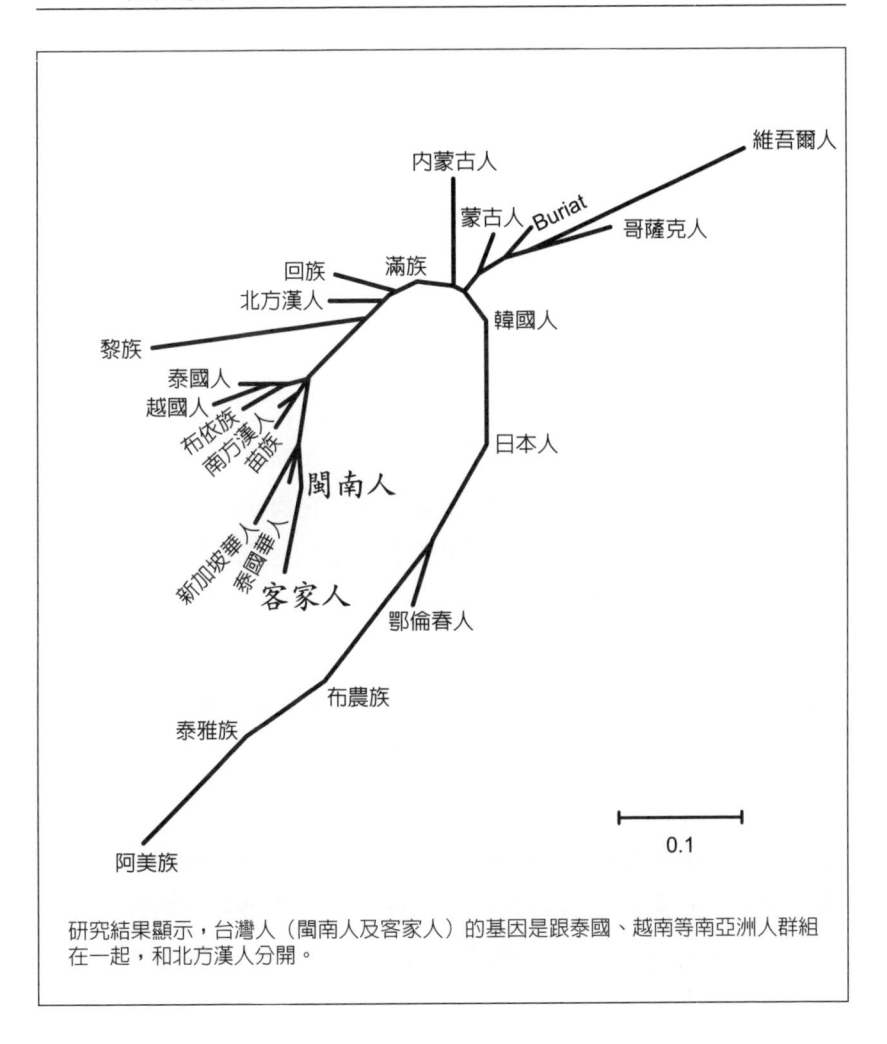

研究結果顯示，台灣人（閩南人及客家人）的基因是跟泰國、越南等南亞洲人群組在一起，和北方漢人分開。

東南亞的台灣人，是屬於百越族「唐山公」的後代，因為當時台灣看不到台灣近代史，只有社會的共識，就是台灣人是近 400 年

二、談台灣的血緣　95

來自中國福建、廣東移民「唐山公」的後代。這一篇「台灣人不是北方漢人」，曾引起一陣譁然，中國強烈反對。實際上，後來從台灣近代史（清朝康熙時期的記錄）漸漸發現，台灣人大部分應該是平埔族的後代。另外，根據荷蘭人《熱遮城日誌》的記載，1624年當荷蘭人到達台灣時，台灣沿海已居住許多平地的原住民「平埔族」。因平埔族在血緣上主要也是屬南方的亞洲人，平埔族基因資料和唐山公發生部分重疊，在血緣關係樹上分不出來，所以我在2001年誤認為血緣樹上的閩南人、客家人是唐山公的後代。近年來，台灣才逐漸有台灣近代史，明顯看到「平埔族」。

「平埔族」（Pinpu）是用來稱呼唐山公尚未來台之前，就已居住在台灣平地的居民，根據荷蘭時期（1624-1661）的記錄，有上百個平埔社分布在台灣的西部及北部平原，顯示在荷蘭時期，唐山公還沒到台灣之前，台灣西部、北部平原原本就有許多的居民（平埔社的居民平埔族），而且平埔族是當時台灣主要居民。1661年鄭成功打敗荷蘭，鄭成功父子一共帶進台灣36,000名中國人，1683年清朝打敗鄭成功，1683-1688年間，約有42,000名鄭成功的軍隊、官兵、家屬，全數被遣送回中國（王先謙：《東華錄選輯》第二冊[清朝順治、康熙、雍正之三朝記錄]，台中：台灣省文獻委員會，1969年，280-281頁）。平埔族在清朝大量漢化，以致1943年自認為平埔族的人口，曾一度下降到零[見專書4：《圖解台灣血緣》60頁]。

台灣人口籍貫的更迭，可以從日治時代戶口登記的改變看到，有些台灣人的戶口，在早期日治時期，原來登記為熟（平埔族），後來改為福（台灣人），如圖7。我們在2007年因從事

圖7 台北市凱達格蘭族塔塔悠社頭目家族戶口名簿上種族的更迭
（自熟變福，「福」為福佬人，即「閩南人」），可窺見平埔族漢化的情形。圖像來源：台北市松山戶政事務所。取自彭凌，「從一份古婚約書開始──台北市凱達格蘭族塔塔悠社歷史重建調查研究報告」，2013年。

大正九年（1920）潘氏熟屬於熟番

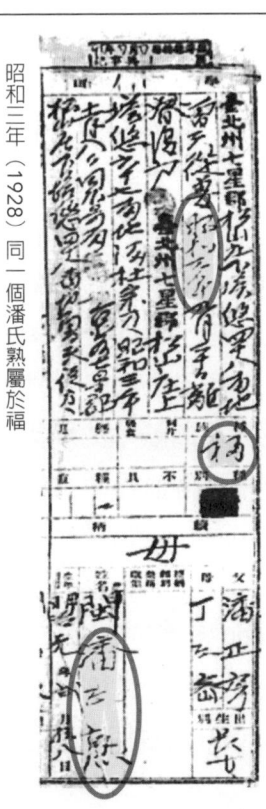

昭和三年（1928）同一個潘氏熟屬於福

平埔族的研究，又踩到政治紅線，而被製造（當時被媒體稱作）「噶瑪蘭口水事件」[見附錄3]。

二、談台灣的血緣　97

B. 2010 年代台灣母系血緣的研究 [見研討會摘要集 199、專書 4：《圖解台灣血緣》108 頁]

　　2000 年以後，我們的實驗室收集分析了共 7,000 人以上台灣不同族群及亞洲鄰國的父母系血緣，經過基因序列的比對，慢慢發現，有些台灣人的母系血緣是獨特的，只發現在台灣，屬於台灣人（及平埔族）特有的母系血緣，我們稱它為台灣特有的母系血緣或「TW 血緣」。TW 血緣在台灣以外的地方沒有，包括中國，表示 TW 血緣是台灣人的祖先到達台灣以後，才發展出來的血緣，也就是從移民到達台灣以後，母系血緣粒線體 DNA 發生的變異所形成台灣人特有的母系血緣。我們用粒線體 DNA 所新發生的鹼基的變異，來計算這些血緣可能發生的年代，以推測帶這個血緣的祖先到達台灣的時間。書前的彩圖 11 是台灣的 M10a1a 血緣系統，右邊黃色框的 M10a1a-9932 血緣，約 5,000 年前在亞洲發生，隨後增加 12786、152 兩個變異的血緣，約在 4,000 多年前到達台灣，在台灣發生相關的紅色框 M10a1a-12786 血緣，為台灣特有的血緣 M10a1aTW。黃色框中 4 人：2 人台灣人，2 人中國人。紅色框中 4 人：4 人皆為台灣人。

C. 2023 年台灣母系血緣的研究 [202,203]

　　我們從 2020 年開始整理在台灣西部及北部平原 16 處不同的沿海地區及城市（基隆、新北市、台北、宜蘭、苗栗、台中、彰化、嘉義、雲林、台南、屏東、高雄、澎湖、馬祖、小琉球、綠

島）收集到的622人DNA（父母親的祖先，至少三代以上都是住在同一個地方，沒有外來人口），加上145人（取自相近的地方）已發表在國際基因庫的台灣人全基因體序列，全部共767人做研究，這767人共帶有267個不同的血緣（haplotypes, lineages），其中有31個血緣為台灣特有的血緣（TW血緣），如表2、表3。

分析這些人母系血緣的來源，結果1/3來自東北亞（中國北方、西伯利亞、日本、韓國）；2/3來自東亞及東南亞（中國中南方、中南半島、印尼、菲律賓）。這些血緣有可能最早至5,000年前就來到台灣，最多移民到台的時間，是在約1,000到2,600年前，很可能是隨著古代南海、東海海上貿易網絡，移民到台灣。

我在這些血緣中，發現31個TW血緣（表3），帶這31個TW血緣的個案，在767人中有177人，佔23%，這些人應該是屬於古代台灣先民的後代，也許可被稱呼為廣義的平埔族的後代，在台灣現在的人口中，推測可能佔約1/4，真正的數目應該比這個大，因為大部分的檢體，實驗室只做部分序列的定序分析。剩下3/4的人，推測是近1,000年的移民。

31個TW血緣中，有10個TW血緣來源包含福建，佔TW血緣的32%，這10個血緣共有51人，佔767人的7%，發生的年代都不一樣，從1,300年到5,000年前之間，也就是唐山公不是只有近代200-300年來到台灣，而是因地緣的關係，在更久之前，在不同的時間已來到台灣。

亞洲大陸及東南亞島嶼的移民台灣，不只在現代台灣人的血緣研究上看到，也在實驗室的古代DNA研究上看到（ancient DNA, aDNA）。古代DNA是從古代遺骸萃取出的DNA，經定序與國際資料比對，再推測古代先民的遷移，我們的古代DNA的

表 2　參與研究的台灣人及引用的相關資料

人口	鄉鎮	代號	Groups	人數	語言	參考文獻
彰化	芳苑	CH	LL_Tw	71	漢語系	本研究
嘉義	布袋	CYI	LL_Tw	23	漢語系	本研究
綠島	綠島	GI	LL_Tw	25	漢語系	本研究
和平	和平島	HP	LL_Tw	10	漢語系	本研究
高雄	湖內	KH	LL_Tw	71	漢語系	本研究
苗栗	通霄	Miao	LL_Tw	18	漢語系	本研究
拍瀑拉	清水	Pa	LL_Tw	38	漢語系	本研究
澎湖	馬公	Penghu	LL_Tw	47	漢語系	本研究
屏東	萬丹	PT	LL_Tw	12	漢語系	本研究
台北(閩南跟客家)	五股、淡水	NTP	Ur_Tw	123	漢語系	本研究
小琉球	琉球	LC	LL_Tw	11	漢語系	本研究
宜蘭	宜蘭	IL	LL_Tw	24	漢語系	本研究
雲林	水林	YL	LL_Tw	149	漢語系	本研究
馬祖	南竿島	MS	East Coast of China	50	漢語系	24
馬卡道	萬巒	Mak	LL_Tw	50	漢語系	19
Hakka_Ko*	內埔	Hak	UR_Tw	45	漢語系	19
Minnan_Ko*	高雄市	Min	UR_Tw	50	漢語系	19
福建省(中國)	福建各處	Fj	East Coast of China	148	漢語系	25, 26
日本	東京、名古屋	Japan	Japan	664	日語系	32
中國東北	北京、河南、遼寧	NE_China	NE_China	257	漢語系	57, 58, 59
中國南方	詳見原始文獻	Sth_China	Sth_China	65	漢語系	57, 60
越南	詳見原始文獻	Vietnam	MSEA	603	南亞語系	28
泰國	詳見原始文獻	Thailand	MSEA	560	壯侗語系	30
馬來西亞	詳見原始文獻	Malaysia	MSEA	86	馬來-波里尼西亞語系	29
印尼(東)	詳見原始文獻	East_Ind	ISEA	72	馬來-波里尼西亞語系	61, 49, 62
印尼(西)	詳見原始文獻	West_Ind	ISEA	326	馬來-波里尼西亞語系	61, 49, 62
菲律賓	詳見原始文獻	Ph	ISEA	260	馬來-波里尼西亞語系	27
台灣南島語族	詳見原始文獻	AN_Tw	AN_Tw	426	南島語系	19, 60, 63-65

MSEA: Mainland Southeast Asia(東南亞); AN_Tw: Austronesian Taiwanese (台灣高山原住民);
ISEA: Island Southeast Asia(東南亞島嶼); Sth_China: South China(中國南方); NE_China(中國東北); LL_Tw: Lowland Taiwanese(平地台灣人); Ur_Tw: 都會台灣人(新北市、高雄市)。
* 我們在「閩南」及「客家」加入 * 在作者的名字「Ko」後面，以和我們的「台北」區別。

表3　台灣特有的母系血緣（TW 血緣）

	新血緣的暫時名稱	推測發生的年代 (kya, 千年前)	全基因體及部分基因定序的個案數	台灣主要居住地	可能的來源
1	A20_16148	1	9	彰化, 雲林	東北亞
2	B4a_16234	0.7	7	高雄	福建
3	B4c1b2b_16305	3.2	10	台灣郊區	東南亞、台灣原住民
4	B4c1b2c1_16280	2.6	3	彰化	東南亞、台灣原住民
5	B4c1b2c2_10250	na<8.84	4	高雄	福建、東南亞、東南亞島嶼
6	B4h1_10581	na<9	8	彰化	福建、東南亞
7	C7a_10310	8.8	9	台灣郊區	中國、東南亞
8	D4a3b_16294	7.8	5	台灣郊區	福建
9	D4b1b2_16380	3.2	7	台灣郊區、綠島	東北亞、日本
10	D4b2b2b_16274	4.3	3	雲林	東北亞、日本
11	D4b2b_10310	7.8	3	雲林	中國、日本
12	D5a2a1b1_16293	2.6	12	澎湖	東北亞、日本
13	D5b1b2_16249	2.6	3	雲林	中國、東南亞
14	F1a1_8589	2.6	5	拍瀑拉	中國東岸
15	F2_10313	2.2	7	彰化	福建、東南亞
16	F2_8264	4.6	11	宜蘭	福建、東南亞
17	F4a2_16243	6.7	3	澎湖	東北亞
18	F4b1_8665	4.5	2	彰化	福建、台灣原住民、東南亞島嶼
19	M7b1a1_11659	na<10.3	2	綠島	福建
20	M7b1a1a1b_16162	na<3.6	5	高雄	中國、東南亞
21	M7b1a1a_8406	1.9	4	高雄	中國、東南亞
22	M7b2a_8389	2.6	6	宜蘭	中國東岸、東南亞、東南亞島嶼
23	M7c1a3a_469	2.6	6	彰化, 宜蘭, 雲林	東北亞、日本
24	M7c1a3a_1664	na<5	2	馬祖	東北亞、日本
25	M7c1a3_3027	1.9	4	台灣郊區, 嘉義	東北亞、日本
26	M7c1a4a_16173	3.7	13	澎湖, 苗栗	中國、東南亞島嶼
27	M7c1a4b(16295<-)	5.2	7	郊區的台灣人	台灣原住民
28	M8a2_8503	1.3	4	雲林	中國
29	M8a2a1_8410	1.7	4	宜蘭	中國
30	N10_10586	1.3	3	嘉義	東南亞島嶼
31	Z4_16248	1.3	6	雲林	東北亞、福建

研究證明，花蓮嶺頂 3,000 年前的古代遺址中，四具遺骸的血緣（B4b, C4a2, N9a1, Z）是現今在台灣人及亞洲人常常看到的血緣，證明台灣人的祖先，早在 3,000 年前就從亞洲來到台灣 [194]。另一方面，考古學的研究發現，在 2,400 到 1,800 年前新石器時代晚期，在台灣許多沿海地區突然出現不同的成熟的文化 [203]。台灣古代花蓮的豐田玉，出現在南海沿岸的菲律賓、越南、泰國的 3,500 年前的古代遺址，表示在 3,500 年前，南海已經有很活躍的海上貿易網絡，台灣當時也是屬於這個網絡的一部分 [見專書 4：《圖解台灣血緣》80 頁]，台灣人祖先的來到台灣，可能是屬於這個海上活動的一環。

　　結論：歷史記載唐山公是在近代 400 年從中國東南沿海移民來台，但實際上，在近代移民之前，可能遠到 5,000 年前，台灣人的祖先就陸續從亞洲北部、中部、南部，主要從東南亞，在不同的時間來到台灣。

D. 談台灣的父系血緣：「平埔公」並沒有消失，而是意氣風發的生活著，「唐山公」的後代恐怕只佔部分的台灣男性人口 [188]

　　台灣主要的父系血緣，是屬於 Y 染色體 O-M175 血緣（Y-SNP 單倍群）的分枝 O1-M119 O1a1* 血緣及 O3-M122 的 O3a1c1 及 O3a2c1a 血緣（見表 4）。

表 4　台灣的主要父系血緣分布及這些血緣在福建、中南半島、菲律賓及印尼的分布情形（%）

O-M175血緣[1]		台灣人	平埔族	高山原住民	福建	中南半島	菲律賓	印尼
O1-M119	O1a1*	14	34	60	22	1	16	14
O3-M122	O3a1c1	12	7	0	20	2	5	2
	O3a2c1a	23	8	0	13	11	2	2
人數		1218	286	355	55	153	139	246

[1] Y染色體單倍群（Y-SNP）

　　O血緣（Y染色體O單倍群）的起源，可以追溯到3.5萬年到3萬年前，起源於亞洲的南方，主要分布在東亞及東南亞。O血緣的分枝O1-M119血緣（O1a1*血緣），主要分布在南島語族（台灣原住民、東南亞島嶼族群）及傣語族群（百越族），O1-M119血緣在18,000-16,000年前可能起源於台灣或亞洲西南方，然後再向南擴散到東南亞島嶼 [188]。在台灣，父系血緣的分布如表4所示：台灣人（14%）、平埔族（34%）、高山原住民（60%）及福建（22%）。台灣人的O1a1*和高山原住民的O1a1*，大部分可以經由Y-STR分開，平埔族的O1a1*分布在台灣人，同時也分布在原住民中。

　　比較意外的是，我們福建的檢體有22%的O1a1*，因為照Wen B.等2004年的研究報告（*Nature* 431: 302-305），O1a1*在福建是0%，是照2003年研究福建古代客家人的移民中心古鎮長汀，148個互相沒血緣關係男性的檢體檢驗研究結果，發現沒有O1-M119血緣（O1a1*），只有O3-M122血緣，該文章資料是用Li H.等2003年的報告（遺傳學報30: 873-880），但是Li的報告中，148人當中仍然可見有3人（2%）H9，很可能是屬於

二、談台灣的血緣　103

O1a1*，所以在客家移民中心的古鎮，還是可能可以找到百越族的基因（O1a1*）。這個可以配合我們馬偕醫院分子人類學研究室55個福建男性的檢體中，看到12人（22%）屬於O1a1*（表4）。所以古代的百越族，並沒有因為漢武帝的南征，而從福建、廣東消失，所謂的「百越族的男性全部被消滅，且被漢人的O3-M122血緣所取代」的傳說，看起來是有問題的。真實的情況可能是，百越族的父系血緣，應該還是存在中國東南沿海地區。

台灣人的O1a1*血緣，最有可能是台灣原本擁有的血緣，萬年前從O1-M175演化出來的分枝O1-M119的O1a1*血緣，所以大部分的「平埔公」應該是帶有台灣原有的台灣先民的O1a1*血緣。另外，台灣的O1a1*血緣的來源，尚有400年來，自中國東南沿海移民的O1a1*血緣的「唐山公」，還須要考慮來自東南亞島嶼國家菲律賓及印尼的O1a1*血緣，這兩個東南亞島嶼國家和台灣一樣，有高頻率的O1a1*（14-16%）。

圖8，大圓圈中的左邊括弧12人的第4人AD179，是高雄湖內人，被家中長輩告知（也看到族譜），他的祖先是跟隨鄭成功400年前從福建遷移來台，自認是唐山公的後代，但血緣演化關係圖顯示，他的祖先可能早在距今約700年前，因演化而與第5人（AD612）及第6人（KH24）的祖先分開（小圓圈），演化而分開時間約為700年前（利用星號點的時間約3,200年，推測小圓點的時間為700年左右），約比鄭成功來台的時間提早300年，所以AD179照理說應該是「平埔公」的後代。因此，從這個案看到，當人們自稱為唐山公的後代時，不一定是真實的，因為可能是平埔公的後代，許多問題尚待解決。

圖8　O1a1*血緣的演化關係圖

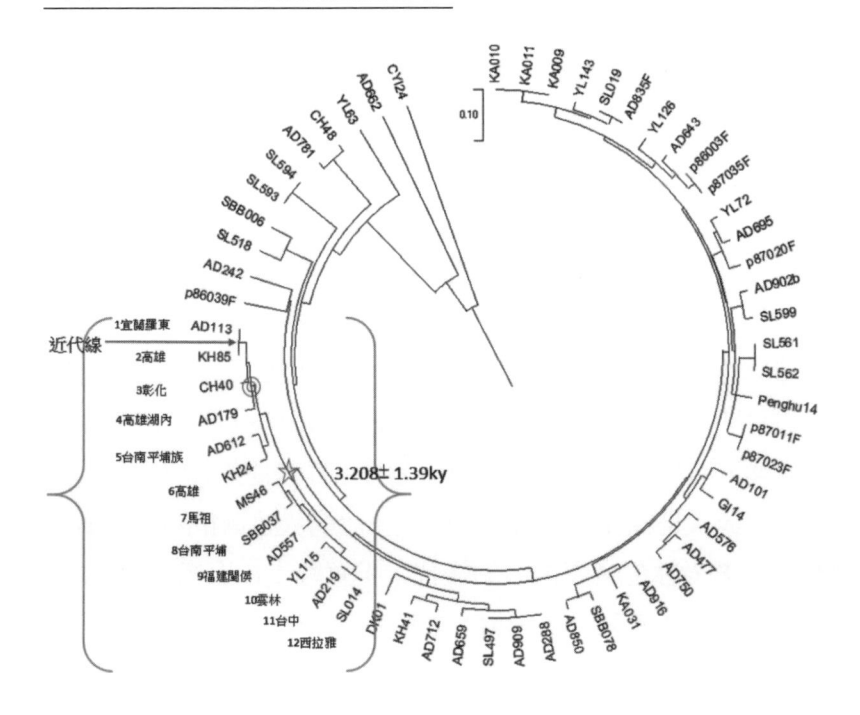

講到台灣人的父系血緣，大部分的人都會說他們的祖先是跟隨鄭成功來台的。事實上，根據沈建德先生的研究，荷蘭時代的記錄（1624-1661年），平埔族是台灣主要居民，推測當時台灣平埔族約有300,000人，高山原住民約有200,000人，中國人數非常有限。1661年鄭成功據台後，鄭成功父子一共帶36,000中國人進入台灣。1683年鄭氏王朝被清朝打敗，在1683-1688年間，約有42,000軍民、文武官員及家眷等，全部從台灣遣送回中國。（王先謙：《東華錄選輯》第二冊［清朝順治、康熙、雍正之三朝記錄］，280-281頁）

二、談台灣的血緣　105

我們研究 Y 血緣的另外一個基因系統 Y-STR 血緣：用每個人在不同基因位點 Y-STR 長度的不同，比較分析，來研究在台灣及周圍地區男性染色體血緣的演化遷移情形，經把測得的 Y-STR 資料演算成血緣的演化關係圖，可得到其中一群血緣的起點，如圖 8 的星號點，時間約為 3,000 年前（Zhivotovsky LA. *Am J Hum Genet*. 74: 50-61, 2004）。

O1-M119 血緣 O1a1* 在福建的出現：在客家移民的中國古鎮長汀 2% 很可能是 O1-M119 血緣，及馬偕醫院分子人類學研究室的福建男性檢體 22% 是 O1a1* 血緣，是很重要的事實，因為這樣子可以證明，從福建、廣東移民到台灣的唐山公，不一定全部都是北方漢人 O3-M122 的後代，也就是可以打破長久以來台灣人的迷思：台灣人是純種北方漢人的後代。台灣人普遍錯誤地認為，所有的台灣男性都是唐山公的後代。但實際上，台灣人 14% 的 O1a1* 血緣，應有大部分 O1a1* 血緣是原本在 18,000-16,000 年前起源於台灣的「平埔公」的後代。

O3-M122 是台灣人的主要父系血緣，起源於亞洲大陸南方，在 6,000-5,000 年前開始遷移到台灣，變成非南島語系（即台灣人）的父系血緣，佔台灣人父系血緣的 54%，共有 18 個單倍群，其中兩個主要的單倍群是 O3a1c1 及 O3a2c1a（表 4），佔台灣父系血緣的 12% 及 23%。O3a2c1a 父系血緣在福建是 13%，在中南半島包括泰國、越南、緬甸約 10%，可見是屬於東南亞大陸重要的父系血緣，但東南亞島嶼國家菲律賓及印尼的 O3a2c1a 頻率就偏低，約 2%。

O3-M122 血緣主要分布在台灣全島非原住民台灣人及少數的平埔族中，O3-M122 血緣高頻率、廣泛的在台灣出現，這些屬於

O3血緣的O3a2c1a、O3a1c1血緣，也可能大部分是古代台灣先民的後代，也就是「平埔公」的後代，也有可能是古代來自中南半島移民的後代。部分O3-M122的台灣男性，應該是近400年唐山公移民的後代。

　　台灣的父系血緣除了O-M175血緣外，尚有3-4% C血緣、N血緣，少數的R血緣，及少數古老的P血緣、Q血緣，台灣可能沒有古老的D-M174血緣[見附錄4]。

3. 古代 DNA（Ancient DNA, aDNA）的研究 [1] [194]

　　台灣島位於歐亞大陸東邊沿岸島鏈的中央，自古就在人類遷徙的途徑上，可以解釋為何島上發現超過 2,800 處史前遺址。古代 DNA 研究，是通過萃取考古遺址發掘的遺骸 DNA，探索古代先民的遷徙歷程。在冰河時期，台灣曾多次與亞洲大陸相連，當兩地相連時，大陸的古代人群與生物可以遷徙至台灣。考古發現顯示，台灣早在舊石器時代晚期（約 50,000 至 10,000 年前）便有人類居住，長濱文化與八仙洞遺址證明了這一點。

　　若要了解台灣人祖先的來源，除了生物統計分析外，透過古代 DNA 的研究，可以直接追溯當時先民的血緣擴散。2005 至 2008 年，我們參與了國科會人文處的跨領域研究計畫，專注於研究南島民族的分類與擴散，並在馬偕醫院建立了專門的古代 DNA 的實驗室，為台灣第一個古代 DNA 實驗室。實驗室成功從約 4,500 年前的牙齒中萃取 DNA，並定義了粒線體 DNA 的單倍群。

　　研究發現，距今 4,500 年前的台南科學園區出土的古代

---

1 本篇由黃錦源執筆。

表5 馬偕醫院古代DNA研究的初步分析結果

遺址地點	距今時間	粒線體DNA型別	可能母系血緣來源	檢體來源
南部科學園區（台南）	4200-4800	M7c D4	SEA, ISEA, Taiwan Aborigine NEA	臧振華
嶺頂（花蓮）	2950-3160	C4a B4c1b2a N9a1(extinct) Z B4b	NEA(including Sibera) SEA, ISEA, Taiwan Aborigine EA, NEA EA SEA, ISEA	胡正恆
南部科學園區（台南）	4000	A	EA	朱正宜
西寮（台南）	1500	A	EA	劉益昌
清水（台中）	1000	F2 M R9	SEA EA SEA	劉益昌
南部科學園區（台南）	500	M33	SEA	朱正宜
燕巢（高雄）	>400	F2	SEA	簡炯仁

DNA，顯示當時台灣已有來自東南亞大陸的血緣，這挑戰了以往認為台灣人祖先只有在距今400年才開始來台居住的共識。隨後，研究團隊也分析了來自台灣其他考古遺址的DNA樣本，發現各時期的台灣遺址中，台灣原住民與東亞大陸血緣混居的現象普遍存在（表5）。

例如，嶺頂遺址出土的遺骸，經碳14定年，確定為3,000年

前的新石器時代晚期,萃取出的 DNA 揭示了五個不同的母系血緣型別(單倍群),包括 C4a2、N9a1、B4c1b2a、Z 和 B4b1,這些血緣常見於今日亞洲大陸及台灣人當中。其中,B4c1b2a 血緣與台灣中部高山原住民有關,C4a2 和 Z 血緣與東北亞人群相關,B4b1 血緣屬於東南亞大陸血緣,N9a1 血緣則屬於東北亞和東亞的血緣(見彩圖 12)。

綜合這些研究結果,我們可以證明,在新石器時代晚期,來自東北亞、東亞大陸、東南亞大陸和東南亞島嶼的血緣已經進入台灣,並與台灣原住民共居。這些發現顯示,台灣的先民在 3,000 多年前,已經有來自不同的地區的混合及混居,也可能代表當時社會階級的存在。此外,某些墓葬的特殊結構(如石板棺),表明當時可能已經存在社會分層。這項研究不僅揭示了台灣過去人群的遷移史,還提供了關於台灣原住民及其與鄰近地區的血緣關係的寶貴資訊。

參考資料（請參閱林媽利醫師期刊論文集）

[17] **Lin-Chu M***. Experience with the manual Polybrene method in Taiwan (letter). *Transfusion*, 1984; 24: 543.

[22] **Lin-Chu M***. Broadberry RE, Yen LS. An appraisal of Rh(D) typing in Chinese. *J Formosan Med Assoc*, 1986; 85: 196-198.

[27] **Lin-Chu M***. Broadberry RE, Chiou FW. The B$_3$ phenotype in Chinese. *Transfusion*, 1986; 26: 428-430.

[30] **Lin-Chu M***. The para-Bombay phenotype in Chinese persons. *Transfusion*, 1987; 27: 388-390.

[33] **Lin-Chu M***. Inspection and continuing education on blood banking in Taiwan. *Excerpta Medica, Current Clinical Practice Series*, 1988; 47: 249-253.

[40] **Lin-Chu M***, Broadberry RE. Blood transfusion in the para-Bombay phenotype. *Brit J Hemat*, 1990; 75: 568-572.

[44] Brodberry RE, **Lin-Chu M***. The Lewis blood group system among Chinese in Taiwan. *Human Heredity*, 1991; 41: 290-294.

[47] **Lin-Chu M**, Broadberry RE, Tanaka M, Okubo Y. The i phenotype and congenital cataracts among Chinese in Taiwan. *Transfusion*, 1991; 31: 676-677.

[51] **Lin M***. Shien SH, Yang TF. Frequency of platelet-specific antigens among Chinese in Taiwan. *Transfusion*, 1993; 33: 155-157.

[53] Broadberry RE, **Lin M***. The incidence and significance of anti-"Mi^a" in Taiwan. *Transfusion*, 1994; 34: 349-352.

[54] **Lin M**. The national blood program of Taiwan, ROC (letter). *Vox Sang*, 1994; 66: 299.

[55] **Lin M***, Broadberry RE. The modification of standard Western pretransfusion testing procedures for Taiwan. *Vox Sang*, 1994; 67: 199-202.

[57] **Lin M***, Broadberry RE. The clinical significance of anti-'Mi^a' (letter). *Transfusion*, 1994; 34: 1013-1014.

[58] **Lin M***, Broadberry RE. Elimination of Rh(D) typing and the antiglobulin test in pretransfusion compatibility tests for Taiwanese. *Vox Sang*,1994; 67: 28-29.

[61] **Lin M***, Shieh SH. Postnatal development of red cell Lea and Leb antigens in Chinese infants. *Vox Sang*, 1994; 66: 137-140.

[66] **Lin M***. Broadberry RE. The Lewis phenotype in Orientals (letter). *Vox Sang*, 1995; 68: 68-9.

[69] **Lin M***, Shieh SH, Liang DC, Yang TF, Shibata Y. Neonatal alloimmune thrombocytopenia in Taiwan due to an antibody against a labile component of HPA-3a(Bak[a]). *Vox Sang*, 1995; 69: 336-340.

[73] Broadberry RE, **Lin M***. The distribution of the MilII (Gp.Mur) phenotype among the population of Taiwan. *Transfusion medicine*, 1996; 6: 145-148.

[74] Broadberry RE, **Lin M***. Comparison of the Lewis phenotypes among the different population groups of Taiwan. *Transfusion Medicine*, 1996; 6: 255-260.

[81] Yu LC, Yang YH, Broadberry RE, Chen YH, **Lin M***. Heterogeneity of the human H blood group alpha (1,2) fucosyltransferase gene among para-Bombay individuals. *Vox Sang*, 1997; 72: 36-40.

[83] **Lin M**, Broadberry RE. Immunohematology in Taiwan. *Transfusion Medicine Review*, 1998; 12: 56-72.

[86] Yu LC, Lee HL, Chu CC, Broadberry RE, **Lin M***. A new identified nonsecretor allele of the human histo-blood group alpha (1,2) fucosyltransferase gene (FUT2). *Vox Sang*, 1999; 76: 115-119.

[89] **Lin M**, Chu CC, Lee HL, Chang SL, Ohashi J, Tokunaga K, Akaza T, Juji T. Heterogeneity of Taiwan's indigenous population: possible relation to prehistoric Mongoloid dispersals. *Tissue Antigens*, 2000; 55: 1-9.

[92] Chu CC, **Lin M***, Nakajima F, Lee HL, Chang SL, Tokunaga K, Juji T. Diversity of HLA among Taiwan's indigenous tribes and the Ivatans in the Philippines. *Tissue Antigens*, 2001; 58: 9-18.

[94] **Lin M**, Chu CC, Chang SL, Lee HL, Loo JH, Akaza T, Juji T, Ohashi J, Tokunaga K. The origin of Minnan and Hakka, the so-called "Taiwanese", inferred by HLA study. *Tissue Antigens*, 2001; 57: 192-199.

[97] Yu LC, Chu CC, Chan YS, Chang CY, Twu YC, Lee HL, **Lin M***. Polymorphism and distribution of the Secretor α (1,2)-fucosyltransferase gene in various Taiwanese populations. *Transfusion*, 2001; 41: 1279-1284.

[98] Yu LC, Twu YC, Chang CY, **Lin M***. Molecular basis of the adult i phenotype and the gene responsible for the expression of the human blood group I antigen. *Blood*, 2001; 98: 3840-3845.

[99] Yu LC, Twu YC, Chang CY, and **Lin M***. Molecular basis of the Kell-null phenotype: a mutation at the splice site of human *KEL* gene abolishes the expression of Kell blood group antigens. *J Bio Chem*, 2001; 276: 10247-10252.

[105] Yu LC, Twu YC, Chou ML, Chang CY, Wu CY, **Lin M***. Molecular genetic analysis for the B^3 allele. *Blood*, 2002; 100: 1490-1492.

[106] **Lin M**, Tseng HK, Trejaut JA, Lee H L, Loo JH, Chu CC, Chen PJ, Su YW, Lim KH, Tsai ZU, Lin RY, Lin RS, Huang CH. Association of HLA class I with severe acute respiratory syndrome coronavirus infection. *BMC Medical Genetics*, 2003; 4: 9.

[107] **Lin M***. Wang CL, Chen FS, Ho LH. Fatal hemolytic transfusion reaction due to a anti-Ku in a K_{null} patient. *Immunohematology*, 2003; 19: 19-21.

[109] Yu LC, Twu YC, Chou ML, Chang CY, Reid ME, Gray AR, Moulds JM, **Lin M***. The molecular genetics of the human I locus and molecular background explaining the partial association of the adult i phenotype with congenital cataracts (Plenary paper). *Blood,* 2003; 101: 2081-2088.

[129] Kataoka S, Kobayashi H, Chiba K, Nakamura M, Shinada, Moritas, **Lin M**, Shibata Y. Neonatal alloimmune thrombocytopenia due to an antibody against a labile component of human platelet antigen-3b (Bak[b]). *Transfu Med*, 2004; 14: 419-423.

[137] Trejaut JA, Kivisild T, Loo JH, Lee CL, He CL, Hsu CJ, Li ZY, **Lin M***. Traces of archaic mitochondrial lineages persist in Austronesian-speaking Formosan populations. *PLoS Biology,* 2005; 3: e247.

[142] **Lin M***. Taiwan experience suggests that RhD typing for blood transfusion is unnecessary in southeast Asian populations. *Transfusion,* 2006; 46: 95-98.

[178] Soares P, Rito T, Trejaut J, Mormina M, Hill C, Tinkler-Hundal E, Braid M, Clarke DJ, Loo JH, Thomson N, Denham T, Donohue M, Macaulay V, **Lin M**, Oppenheimer S, Richards MB. Ancient Voyaging and Polynesian Origins. *Am J Hum Genet*, 2011; 88: 239-247.

[182] Yu LC, **Lin M***. Molecular genetics of the blood group I system and the regulation of I antigen expression during erythropoiesis and granulopoiesis. *Curr Opin Hematol*, 2011; 18: 421-426.

[188] Trejaut JA, Poloni ES, Yen JC, Lai YH, Loo JH, Lee CL, He CL, **Lin M***. Taiwan Y-chromosomal DNA variation and its relationship with Island Southeast Asia. *BMC Genet*, 2014; 15: 77.

[194] Huang JY, Trejaut JA, Lee CL, Wang TY, Loo JH, Chen ZS, Chen LR, Liu KH, Liu YC, Hu CH, **Lin M***. Mitochondrial DNA Sequencing of Middle Neolithic Human Remains of Ling-Ding Site Implication for the Social Structure and the Origin of Northeast Coast Taiwanese. *Journal of Phylogenetics & Evolutionary Biology*, 2018; 6: 6.

[200] **Lin M**. Elimination of pretransfusion RhD typing at Mackay Memorial Hospital, Taiwan-30-year experience (1988-2017). *Vox Sang*, 2021; 116: 234-238.

[202] **Lin M**, Trejaut JA. Diversity and distribution of mitochondrial DNA in non-Austronesian-speaking Taiwanese individuals. *Hum Genome Var*, 2023; 10: 2.

[203] 林媽利. 台灣人的來源— DNA 的探索. *台灣醫界*, 2023. 66: 261-266.

[研討會摘要集 199] **Lin M**, Lee CL, Loo JH, Yen JC, Chu CC, Lee HL, Trejaut JA. More genetic sharing among the populations of Taiwan than expected: a plain tribe (Pinpu) perspective. PNC 2009 Annual Conference, Taipei, Taiwan.

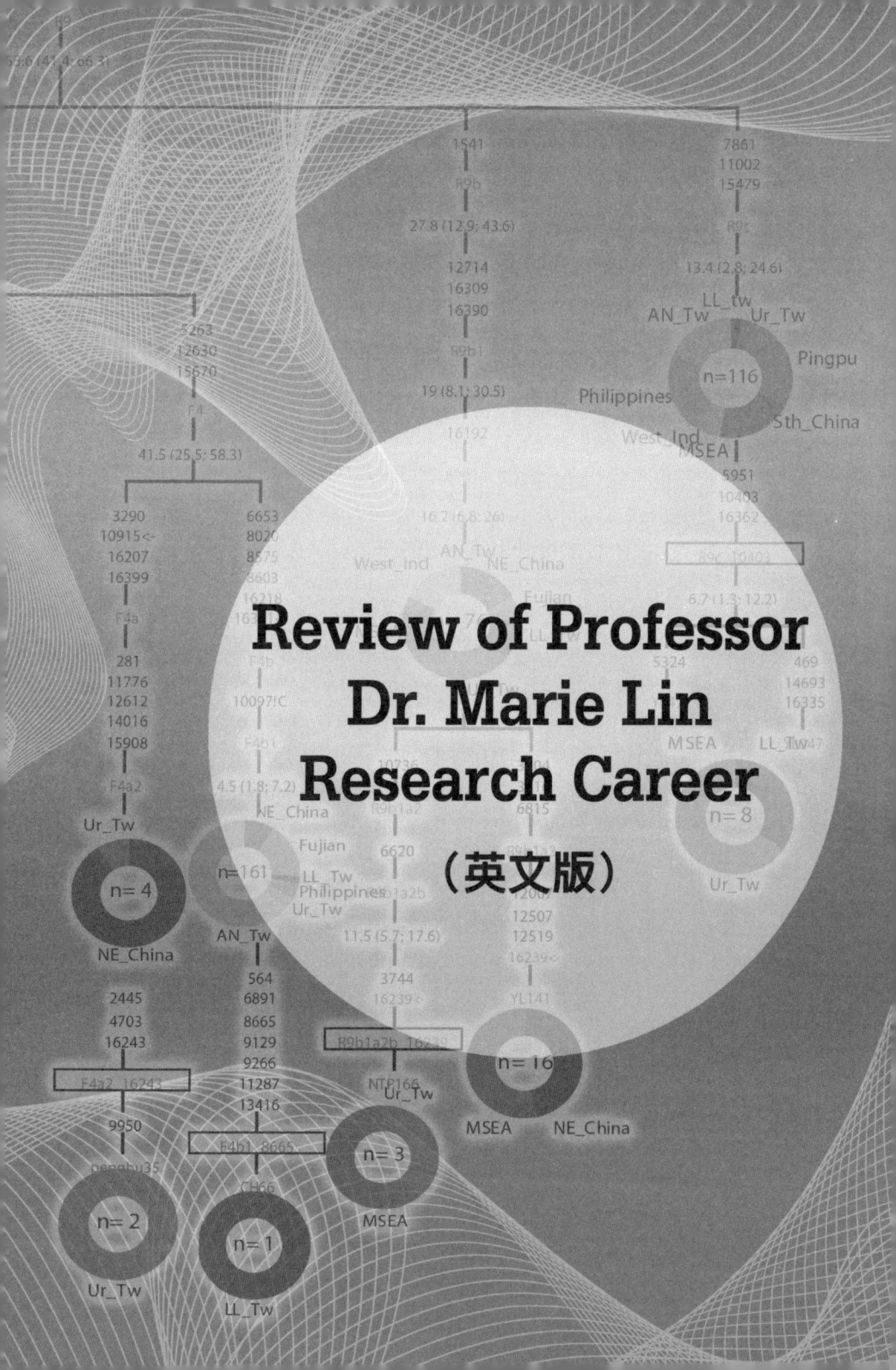

Review of Professor Dr. Marie Lin Research Career
（英文版）

Foreword

In 1981, after completing four years of pathology specialist training at the University of Texas in the United States and obtaining my American Board of Pathology certification, I returned to Taiwan. On October 1st, I arrived at Mackay Memorial Hospital (MMH), carrying the prestige of being both an Associate Professor at the Institute of Pathology at National Taiwan University (NTU) and an American Board-certified pathologist. However, I quickly discovered that I was unable to continue practicing anatomical pathology (which I had been engaged in for 16 years at NTU). Instead, my work at MMH's Clinical Laboratory was confined solely to the blood bank.

At that time, immunohematology (the study of blood banking and transfusion medicine) was still a new and relatively unfamiliar field in Taiwan. Since my four years of training in the U.S. had mainly focused on blood banking, I reluctantly accepted this role. Like most hospitals, the blood bank at MMH was only about 6 to 10 square meters in size. It contained a refrigerator, a centrifuge, a table, and one medical technologist. My colleagues from NTU, upon seeing the limited setup, couldn't help but ask, "What are you doing in such a small blood bank?"

Engaging in Blood Policy and Blood Group Research

Every day at work, I watched the medical technologist busy drawing blood from paid donors (often referred to as "blood cows"). At that time, voluntary blood donation was scarce, and the hospital could only supply a small portion of the patients' transfusion needs. I started by teaching the medical technologist the most basic cross-matching techniques, showing her how to shake test tubes and interpret the results.

I also realized that Taiwan had very limited blood group data—aside from ABO and Rh, there were only a few scattered records on the MN blood group. Everything had to start from scratch!

During that period, Taiwan was deeply concerned about the high prevalence of hepatitis B carriers. In my spare time, I frequently visited the Department of Health, as I had been invited by Dr. Hsu Tzu-Chiu, the Minister of Health, to participate in the formulation of Taiwan's national blood policy [see Attachment 1].

In the early 1980s, Taiwan's blood donation and transfusion systems were chaotic. Alongside fellow transfusion medicine experts—including Dr. Sun Chien-Feng, Dr. Lee Cheng-Hua, and Dr. Kao Yuan-Hsiang from the U.S.—as well as Department of Health officials such as Dr. Yeh Chin-Chuan, MS. Tsai Su-Ling, and assistant Ms. Shih Mei-Chun, we conducted nationwide evaluations and inspections of blood donation institutions and hospital transfusion units (blood banks). Based on these assessments, we established standards and regulations for blood banking.

Between 1984 and 1992, over the span of eight years, we transformed Taiwan's blood donation and transfusion system. By 1992, the country's blood supply was sufficient to meet the needs of all hospitals, and paid blood donations (blood cows) were completely abolished. Taiwan became one of the few countries in the world to transition from a commercial blood trade system to an entirely voluntary donation-based system in just eight years—a feat that most likely was unprecedented globally.

Discovering and Researching Blood Groups

In 1983, British blood bank expert and missionary Richard E. Broadberry (FIMLS) arrived at Mackay Memorial Hospital, responding to a divine calling. He became my closest research partner, and together we embarked on two decades of groundbreaking blood group research in Taiwan.

Later, Dr. Yu Lung-Chih joined our team as a young researcher, further advancing genetic studies on blood groups. Through our work, numerous previously unknown blood groups specific to Asia—particularly Southeast Asia—were identified.

To the surprise of many, blood group distributions not only differed between Caucasians and Asians, but also between Northeast Asia (e.g., Japan) and Southeast Asia (e.g., Taiwan). At the time, China had not yet conducted blood group research, so there was no available comparative data.

Our discoveries in Taiwan drew global attention. Between the 1980s and 1990s, Taiwan became a hot topic in international transfusion medicine. Each year, we exchanged around 100 letters with international experts, discussing our findings, corresponding with researchers worldwide, and even exchanging rare blood type samples [see Appendix 6]. This global recognition also paved the way for younger Taiwanese scientists to establish themselves in the international transfusion medicine community.

Key Blood Group Discoveries

One of our most famous discoveries was the secretor of the para-Bombay phenotype. This blood group can create discrepancies in ABO compatibility between parents and children.

For example, in 1985, a newborn boy in MMH's nursery caused a family dispute—both parents were groups O, yet their child was group B. We quickly identified the father as a para-Bombay individual carrying a latent *B* gene, which was passed on to the child and expressed due to the mother's *H* gene. This case illustrated the complex genetic interplay required for ABO expression (see Figure 1 on Page 66).

Additionally, our research revealed that the para-Bombay blood group in Taiwan differs from that in Caucasians. Unlike Western para-Bombay individuals—who must receive Bombay group blood for transfusions—Taiwanese para-Bombay individuals can safely receive regular ABO-matched blood. We confirmed this finding through human trials.

Another major discovery was the Le(a+b+) blood group, previously unseen outside of Asia. Initially, Western scientists doubted our results, believing we had made an error. However, through extensive blood sample exchanges and reagent testing, we successfully convinced the global scientific community of its existence. Notably, we identified the Se^w gene—a key gene associated with this blood group—one year ahead of Sweden's prestigious Karolinska Institute.

In 2003, during the SARS outbreak, we identified that HLA-B*4601 (a genetic marker common in Southeast Asian populations) increased susceptibility to severe SARS infections. We quickly collected 166 blood samples from individuals exposed to SARS and conducted research in a biosafety-controlled lab. In just one and a half months, we completed the study, wrote the report, and submitted them to an international journal, where they were published within three months.

Our discovery became a major international medical news story and was reported by *The Wall Street Journal,* Reuters, and *Asahi Shimbun* [see Attachment 5]. Yet, strangely, Taiwanese media only covered it briefly before going silent. I never understood the reasons behind this, but I do know that when the Minister of Health presented a report to the Legislative Yuan, he dismissed our findings as "statistically insignificant"—even though international experts believed our sample size was sufficient.

Taiwan's Leadership in Transfusion Medicine

Many wonder why Taiwan became a leader in transfusion medicine in Asia. The reason is that, apart from Japan in Northeast Asia, most Southeast Asian nations were still developing their healthcare systems. Transfusion medicine requires both advanced healthcare infrastructure and experts in immunohematology—which Taiwan uniquely possessed.

Our genetic research on blood groups officially began in 1993, when Dr. Yu Lung-Chih joined our team after completing his PhD at NTU's Institute of Biochemistry. Over the next nine years, he dedicated himself to blood group genetics, publishing numerous high-impact papers.

In just a decade, Taiwan caught up with Western countries in transfusion medicine, thanks to the dedication of our team at Mackay Memorial Hospital. Our discoveries not only contributed to global medical knowledge but also provided invaluable reference data for Southeast Asian countries.

Developing a Domestic HLA Typing Tray

In 1993, at the HLA Symposium in Taipei, we invited Dr. Takeo Juji, the Director of the Tokyo Red Cross Blood Center, to deliver a lecture. As fellow members of the International Society of Blood Transfusion (ISBT), we had met frequently at conferences and were well-acquainted.

After the symposium, Dr. Juji expressed his bewilderment over why Taiwan's government had spent significant funding on research institutions for HLA typing tray development for years but had not produced any results. He encouraged me to take on the task and offered the full support of Japan's national HLA team under the Red Cross. With his backing, I was able to establish an HLA laboratory at Mackay Memorial Hospital and begin developing a domestic typing tray.

Without official funding, I immediately requested the hospital's obstetrics and gynecology department to preserve placentas that were originally meant for disposal, allowing me to collect serum from placental blood to develop the typing tray.

Accurate HLA typing is crucial for disease diagnosis, treatment (including bone marrow transplantation), and transplantation medicine. During the 1960s to 1990s, global HLA typing relied on serological methods. However, to ensure precise results, the typing tray must be developed using local serum antibodies, as different populations exhibit unique antigenic variations. Thus, advanced nations strived to tailor their HLA typing trays using antibodies derived from local sera.

In August 1994, Dr. Tatsuya Akaza from the Tokyo Red Cross Blood Center arrived in Taiwan with an assistant, reagents, and Japanese HLA typing trays. Over the course of one month, they helped us establish Taiwan's most advanced HLA laboratory.

Pioneering Research on Taiwan's Indigenous Populations

Following this, we published several groundbreaking papers, including:
- "Heterogeneity of Taiwan's indigenous population: possible relation to prehistoric Mongoloid dispersals" (2000) [89]
- "Diversity of HLA among Taiwan's indigenous tribes and the Ivatans in the Philippines"(2001) [92]

One particular illustration of Taiwan's indigenous genetic makeup (Figure 9, also referenced as "Color Figure 8" in the book) astonished me. It revealed a significant genetic gap between Taiwanese people and Taiwan's indigenous Austronesian tribes.

Perplexed by this finding, I turned to historical records on Taiwan's ancient geography and climate changes. I learned that during the Late Paleolithic period (~10,000 years ago), Taiwan was still connected to the Eurasian continent. Early human populations likely migrated along coastal lowlands. However, as global warming melted glaciers, rising sea levels submerged these lowlands, isolating ancient settlers on Taiwan. Prolonged genetic isolation over millennia widened the genetic divergence between Taiwan and the Eurasian mainland.

This realization gradually shifted my research focus toward anthropology. In 2001, we published "The origin of Minnan and Hakka, the so-called 'Taiwanese', inferred by HLA study" [94], concluding that Taiwanese Minnan (Hoklo) and Hakka people belong to southern Asian populations, not northern Han Chinese.

While this delighted many in Taiwan, it also sparked controversy, criticisms, and even an official condemnation from China's State Council, which called our study "shameful and politically motivated." Due to political sensitivities, the journal's editorial board—where Chinese representatives were present—delayed publication for a year before it was finally approved by other board members and published.

Transitioning into Taiwanese Population Genetics

To develop a localized HLA typing tray, we needed comprehensive data on Taiwan's ethnic groups' HLA distribution. This gradually led us to population genetics research on Taiwanese ethnic groups, eventually expanding into Taiwanese DNA studies.

On March 5, 2024, I returned to Tokyo to personally thank Dr. Juji for his unwavering support 30 years ago, which enabled us to establish our HLA laboratory (see Color Figure 14). This laboratory provided me with the opportunity to study Taiwanese genetics, and our team's research has had a profound impact on Taiwan's identity.

In the early 1990s, only 20% of Taiwanese identified primarily as Taiwanese. When I began HLA research in 1994 and published our 2001 findings, I faced significant backlash. However, Taiwanese identity gradually rose to around 40%.

From 2003 to 2005, while editing and revising the third edition of my textbook, *Transfusion Medicine*, I included all of Taiwan's newly discovered blood groups. By this time, Taiwan's transfusion medicine had flourished, and blood bank operations and research capabilities had significantly improved.

Recognizing that Taiwan's blood banking system was now well-established, I felt that my mission in transfusion medicine was complete. This allowed me to fully commit to researching Taiwanese genetics. I distributed the 14-chapter third edition of *Transfusion Medicine* to 14 leading experts in Taiwan's transfusion medicine field, urging them to contribute to the future fourth edition, as I could no longer afford to divide my time.

Unraveling the Genetic Origins of Taiwan's Populations

Taiwan's genetic research has primarily focused on indigenous Austronesian groups. Internationally, the Austronesian migration is considered one of the most significant events in human history, making it a highly studied topic. Moreover, research on Taiwan's indigenous peoples is less politically sensitive, making it easier to secure funding.

Like many scholars, we initially studied Taiwan's indigenous Austronesians. In 2005, we participated in Academia Sinica's large-scale research project on indigenous peoples. However, by the time we received funding, the cost of DNA sequencing had halved, leaving us with excess funds. We decided to use this funding to study the remaining 98% of Taiwan's population—Taiwanese (non-Austronesian groups).

Discovering Unique Taiwanese Genetic Lineages

In the 2010s, we studied the paternal and maternal genetic lineages of Taiwan's population and compared them with surrounding regional groups.

Our research revealed that many of the maternal lineages among Taiwanese are unique to Taiwan—they are absent in neighboring China. This suggests that these lineages originated in Taiwan and developed in isolation after early ancestors arrived.

By 2023, we had collected and analyzed DNA from over 7,000 individuals to trace Taiwanese ancestry. We also studied 767 unrelated individuals with at least three generations of Taiwanese ancestry, analyzing their maternal lineage.

Our findings indicate that Taiwan's ancestors partially originated from Northeast Asia, but the majority came from East Asia and Southeast Asia, including the Island Southeast Asia. Furthermore, most of Taiwan's population descended are from immigrants who arrived within the past 1,000 years, with some lineages tracing back over 5,000 years—corresponding to the Late Neolithic period in archaeology.

Our study, published in *Nature*'s *Human Genome Variation* journal, confirmed that Taiwanese settlement and expansion occurred long before the Ming and Qing-era migration from China.

Our Current Dilemma

Taiwan is a multi-ethnic island, composed of Austronesian (indigenous) and non-Austronesian (Taiwanese) groups.

Since the 1990s, Mackay Memorial Hospital's Molecular Anthropology Laboratory has focused on Taiwanese genetic research, particularly the question: *Are all Taiwanese men descendants of Chinese immigrants (Tangshan Gong, or Tangshan men)?*

However, as a Christian hospital, MMH primarily serves the general public and lacks funding for high-tech DNA research—especially ancient DNA (aDNA) studies. The COVID-19 pandemic further strained hospital finances, leading to staff reductions.

In contrast, China has heavily invested in molecular anthropology and ancient DNA research over the past 20 years, establishing multiple internationally recognized research institutes.

Taiwan, meanwhile, has only two active teams in molecular anthropology research:

1. Mackay Memorial Hospital (4 researchers)

2. National Yang Ming Chiao Tung University (3 researchers)

I call upon the Taiwanese government to support our research efforts, as molecular anthropology and ancient DNA studies are crucial to Taiwan's sovereignty, historical narrative, and even national security.

Finally, I thank the people of Taiwan and God for allowing me to embark on this lifelong journey of discovering Taiwan's origins. May God bless Taiwan.

I.
About Blood Transfusion and Blood Groups

1. Assistance in Formulating Taiwan's National Blood Program [54, Attachment 1]

A. Development and Evolution of Taiwan Transfusion Medicine

Establishing National Standard for Pretransfusion Testing [54]: In the 1980s, blood bank testing before transfusion in Taiwanese hospitals relied mainly on the unsafe saline slide method, leading to operational chaos in blood banks across the country. Marie Lin and her team [referred to as ML, see Color Figure 1] discovered that manual Polybrene (MP) was the most suitable approach for the Taiwanese in 1984 [17]. ML introduced the manual Polybrene (MP) method without AHG phase for Taiwanese needs. Taiwan Blood Transfusion Society received ML's guidance for continuous training, making MP the standard pre-transfusion testing in the 1980s-90s. *Vox Sang* acknowledged ML's contribution and recommended Taiwan's approach as a reference for other country [57, Attachment 2]. In 1994, ML revolutionized Taiwan's transfusion practices and published "The modification of standard Western pretransfusion testing procedures for Taiwan" [55].

In 1988, ML established the "Taiwan Blood Bank Consultation Center" at Mackay Memorial Hospital (MMH) to provide free and prompt consultation on challenging transfusion cases, thereby enhancing the overall standards of blood banks nationwide.

Discovery of the Miltenberger Blood Group and Anti-'Mi^a' Antibody: The discovery of the Miltenberger blood group in the Taiwanese population marked a significant advancement in transfusion medicine. ML team (Richard Broadberry) and many blood group experts worked on identified this phenotype from 1983 to 1986, including Patricia Tippett of MRC, UK; Marcela Contreras of North London Blood Center; Dasnayanee Chandanayingyong of Siriraj Hospital, Thailand; Yasuto Okubo of Osaka Red Cross Blood Center and Makoto Uchikawa of Tokyo Red Cross Blood Center. This discovery turned out to be of most importance in Taiwan, akin to the ABO blood group, as the corresponding anti-'Mi^a' antibody was common (2% of patients) and posed risks of both intravascular hemolysis during transfusions reaction and hemolytic disease of newborns. Taiwan's blood banks began screening for anti-'Mi^a' antibodies in 1990. This issue was also found to be prevalent in the entire Southeast Asian region, leading to the Miltenberger also becoming a critical blood group in Southeast Asia. [53,59,71,73].

Suggestion to Eliminate RhD Pre-Transfusion Screening (Addressing RhD Negative Blood Transfusion Challenges in Taiwan) [Attachment 3]: RhD-negative (RhD–) patients often faced difficulties in finding RhD– blood for emergency transfusions due to the low frequency of RhD– individuals in Taiwan (0.3%). This scarcity led to RhD– patients in dangerous situation of lacking blood since general Taiwan population including medical personels were usually afraid of giving RhD+ blood to RhD– patient. Internationally, the consensus was that RhD– individuals without anti-D could safely receive RhD+ blood. Following the advice of international Rh experts Prof. P. L. Mollison, who proposed that Taiwan, unlike the West, may not need RhD pre-transfusion screening, Mackay Memorial Hospital eliminated RhD pre-transfusion screening in 1988 [22,58]. Despite initial concerns, reviewing 30 years of data in 2017 revealed that the frequency of anti-D complications remained unchanged, whether pre-transfusion screening was conducted or not [142,200]. This approach was intended to alleviate the increasing focus on Rh blood group and the anxiety surrounding RhD-negative status in society, allowing RhD-negative individuals without anti-D to confidently receive both RhD+ and RhD– blood.

This comprehensive effort led by Marie Lin and her team, spanning decades, revolutionized Taiwan's blood transfusion practices and laid the foundation for safe and efficient blood banking operations. Their discoveries and practices had a significant impact, not only on Taiwan but also across East Asia and beyond.

B. Enhancing the Blood Donation System [33,54]

The blood donation system was initially under the Ministry of the Interior and lacked supervision from the Department of Health. This absence of oversight led to improper practices by blood collection organizations. Moreover, without a plan for sourcing blood and a high prevalence of hepatitis B in the early days, the need for a robust blood donation system became imperative. ML, alongside members of the Transfusion Society and health officials, established standards and operational protocols through comprehensive evaluation and supervision of blood collection organizations and medical institutions' blood banks [33]. This effort led to the establishment of the Taiwan Blood Services Foundation in 1990, placing the blood donation system under the jurisdiction of the Department of Health (DH). Quality control and supervision by the DH ensured safe blood supply through donations, replacing the unsafe commercial blood trade. By 1992, Taiwan achieved self-sufficiency in blood supply, meeting nearly 100% of domestic hospital demand through donations. The successful elimination of the blood trade in 1992 garnered international recognition for Taiwan's achievements in blood donation policies, and was placed alongside 15 other developed nations as a "Developed Countries" (*Transfusion* 1996; 36: 1019-32) [Attachment 4].

2. Extensive Taiwanese Blood Groups Studies

Immunohematology Study in Taiwan [83]: ML conducted long-term (1980s-2000s) research on various blood groups in Taiwan, leading to the discovery of new blood groups and related genes unique to Taiwanese population as shown below. ML also investigated feasible strategies for transfusion involving rare blood groups [40]. All these work earned recognition from international scholars as a treasure trove of knowledge of blood transfusion.

The new blood groups, rare blood groups and related genes discovered by ML including A_2, A_3, A_{el}, A_m, A_x, B_{el}, B_m, B_x, D_{el}, Jk(a-b-), Lu(a-b-), Di(a+b-), D^{v1}, Dc-, St^a, Tj^a and Miltenberger of total 17 blood groups and following 5 blood groups: para-Bombay phenotype, B_3, Le(a+b+), i, K_{null}; and also the additional Tn, Cad polyagglutination. The discovery became essential references for Southeast Asian blood banks, benefiting countries like China, Vietnam, Myanmar, and India.

Para-Bombay Phenotype (H Antigen Deficient Secretor Type); O_h-Secretor; O_{Hm}: In 1985, ML discovered the first case of the para-Bombay phenotype in a Taiwanese at Mackay Memorial Hospital [30,81]. This blood group lacks the H antigen, making it unable to express the *A* or *B* genes, resulting in an O-type appearance. However, it can pass on the unexpressed *A* or *B* genes to their children, leading to ABO blood group incompatibility between parents and children. The expression of the para-Bombay phenotype differs in Caucasians, who lack secretor genes and require para-Bombay or Bombay phenotype for transfusion. Asians, on the other hand, likely have secretor genes associated with the para-Bombay phenotype, preventing the production of corresponding antibodies, allowing them to receive blood from regular donors [40].

Discovery of B_3 Blood Group (IVS3+5G>A Mutation): ML identified the first ABO sub-blood group in a blood donor in 1983 [27], with a genetic basis intron 3 mutation [105] leading to structural changes in B transferase.

Discovery of the Le(a+b+) Blood Group and the Related New *Se^w* Gene: In 1990, ML revealed that 25% of Taiwanese individuals possess the Le(a+b+) blood type, which is absent in Caucasians, while the common Le(a+b-) type is not prevalent among Taiwanese [44,66,74]. The ML team discovered new *Se^w* genes related to this blood group a year earlier than the Karolinska Institute in Sweden [72]. Additionally, three new non-secretor genes (se^{571}, se^{685}, se^{869}) were found in Taiwanese indigenous people with the Le(a+b-) blood group [74,86,97].

Demonstration of the *I* Blood Group Gene and Its Link to Congenital Cataracts: In 1991, ML found five individuals from three Taiwanese families who exhibited the rare i blood group along with congenital cataracts [47]. Molecular biology studies in 2001 and 2003 revealed that these conditions were caused by mutations in the *GCNT2* gene structure [98,109,182]. ML's 2003 paper [109] on this topic was recognized as a Plenary paper in the *Blood* Journal, and its significance was highlighted in a special editorial.

K$_{null}$ Blood Group Study and Lethal Anti-Ku Hemolytic Transfusion Reaction [107]: ML found a rare K$_{null}$ blood group case in 2003. Genetic analysis showed a nonfunctional *KEL* gene caused by a mutation [99].

Identification of Anti-HPA-3a, -3b Antibodies Reactive Only with Fresh Platelets [69,129]: ML's discovery in 1988 a maternal allo-anti-HPA-3a against newborn platelets could lead to neonatal thrombocytopenia (NAIT), and this anti-HPA-3a antibody was found exclusively reacting with fresh platelets. Anti-HPA-1a were not found in Asian populations since lacking HPA-1a negative individual [51]. The unique case of a mother giving birth to two NAIT infants due to anti-HPA-3a antibodies was reported, the incriminated anti-HPA-3a couldn't be detected by traditional methods of using fixed platelet like MPHIA, MAIPA, IF, Immunobloting, or EIA. This report become an important reference paper in platelet immunology. In 2004 a similar anti-HPA-3b NAIT was found in a Japanese baby (Citations 205 times in 2023).

HLA-Class I and its Relation to the 2003 SARS Coronavirus Infection [106]: In 2003, ML conducted HLA class I and class II screenings on blood samples from 37 suspected SARS patients, feverish patients, healthcare workers exposed to SARS, and general healthy Taiwanese individuals. The significant increase of HLA-B*4601 in severe or fatal cases (Pc=0.0279) was noted. HLA-B46 is mainly found in SEA descent and is almost absent in Caucasians, Taiwan indigenous populations, and rarely in other Asians. The distribution of the 2003 SARS outbreak correlated with the ancient distribution of the Yue ethnic group [106], leading to international attention and news coverage [Attachment 5] (Citations 366 times in 2023).

II.
Research on the Molecular Anthropology of Taiwan Ethnic Groups

1. Studies of the Austronesian Speakers in Taiwan (1994-2014)

A. Research on the Migration of Maternal Lineage (mtDNA) B4a1a among the Austronesian Speakers

Taiwan is likely the homeland of the Austronesian speakers. In 2005, ML published the results of maternal lineage research on 640 individuals from nine Austronesian speaking (highland indigenous) groups in Taiwan [137]. They found significant differences in maternal lineage between Austronesian speakers and non-Austronesian speaking Taiwanese individuals, with Austronesian speakers showing a presence of ancient lineages. Among these, the B4a1a lineage was prominent in the Amis tribe (45%). This lineage is also found in the Philippines, Indonesia, and New Guinea but not in China. It is hypothesized that the B4a1a migration originated from Taiwan, passed through the Philippines, Indonesia, and New Guinea, accumulating variations to form B4a1a1 and eventually developing into the characteristic B4a1a1a lineage found in Polynesians, constituting 80% of their maternal lineage. The publication in

2005 sparked significant discussion, with *The Economist* (7/9/2005 anthropology) stating, "Taiwan, twinned with Hawaii," [Attachment 6] and suggesting that Taiwan could be the homeland of the Austronesian speaker. In collaboration with researchers in the UK in 2011, ML continued their research on the B4a1a lineage and found that Taiwan had no B4a1a1 lineage, with fewer occurrences in the Philippines. B4a1a1 was primarily found in Indonesia and New Guinea, casting doubt on the theory that Taiwan was the sole homeland of the Austronesian speaker [178]. However, further studies by Reich et al of genome-wide single-nucleotide polymorphisms (SNPs) on Island Southeast Asian populations and ancient DNA studies in Vanuatu archaeological remains reconfirmed that Taiwan as the homeland of Austronesian speakers (*Nat Commun.* 5: 4689, 2014; *Current Biology* 30: 4846, 2020).

B. Shared HLA Haplotypes between Austronesian Language Family Groups in Taiwan and South/North Asian Populations [89]

Many Austronesian language family groups in Taiwan share HLA haplotypes with populations from South and North Asia, including Māori, Highlanders, Archons, Mongolians, Inuit, Japanese, Man, Buryat, and American Indian-Tlingit. This suggests a genetic relationship between these populations and Austronesian language family groups in Taiwan. It indicates that during the late Pleistocene era, specifically during the Ice Age, when Taiwan was connected to the Asian mainland due to lower sea levels, human migrations likely occurred from South Asia to North Asia (possibly in both directions) along the eastern coastal continental shelf of Eurasia. This could have been a route for early human migrations, and Taiwan, being located in the middle of this migration path, may have inherited genetic elements from both South and North Asia.

2. Studies of Non-Austronesian Speakers in Taiwan (2000-2023)

Non-Austronesian language family groups in Taiwan refer to individuals who are not part of Taiwan's highland indigenous population but include groups like the Minnan and Hakka people.

In the 1980s and 1990s, ML conducted research on blood groups in Taiwan, discovering several new blood types unique to Southeast Asia. This research raised questions about the idea that Taiwanese people are descendants of northern Han Chinese.

A. HLA Research in 2001 [94]

In 2001, ML compared the HLA gene frequencies of Minnan and Hakka people in Taiwan to international data on different populations. The results indicated that Minnan and Hakka people belong to the Asian southern group of populations, not northern Chinese. This finding supported the discoveries made in blood group research. At the time, ML mistakenly associated this result with the descendants of "Tangshan Gong," a term used to describe migrants from Fujian, China, who were believed to have come to Taiwan in the last 400 years. This assertion caused controversy, particularly with strong opposition from China. In reality, most Taiwanese are likely descendants of the Pinpu people, who were also of southern Asian origin. Recent historical records reveal that Taiwan had a significant population of Pinpu people even before the arrival of Tangshan Gong. According to records from the Dutch period (1624-1661), there were hundreds of Plains Indigenous (Pinpu) communities distributed in the western and northern plains of Taiwan. This indicates that even before the arrival of the Dutch in Taiwan, there were already many inhabitants in the western and northern plains (the residents of Plains Indigenous communities), and the Plains Indigenous people were the main residents of Taiwan at that time. In 1661, Koxinga defeated the Dutch, and he and his son brought a total of 36,000 Chinese settlers to Taiwan. In 1683, the Qing Dynasty defeated Koxinga, and between 1683 and 1688, approximately 42,000 of Koxinga's soldiers, officials, and their families were all repatriated to China. (王先謙：《東華錄選輯》第二冊 [清朝順治、康熙、雍正之三朝記錄], 台中: 台灣省文獻委員會, 1969年, 280-281頁) The Plains Indigenous people underwent significant Sinicization during the Qing Dynasty, to the extent that by 1943, the population of people identifying as Plains Indigenous had temporarily dropped to zero.

B. Research on Maternal Lineages in the 2010s

After 2000, Loo Junhun of ML team analyzed the maternal and paternal lineages especially the maternal lineages of over 7,000 individuals from various Taiwanese ethnic groups and neighboring Asian countries [see conference abstract collection 199]. By comparing genetic sequences, we identified unique maternal lineages, referred to as "TW lineages," which were not found outside of Taiwan, including China. These lineages are considered specific to the Taiwanese population, formed after the ancestors arrived in Taiwan, reflecting genetic variations in the maternal lineage (mtDNA) that occurred in Taiwan. Using newly discovered mtDNA variations, ML estimated the time when these ancestors arrived in Taiwan, could dating back as far as 5,000 years ago.

C. Research in 2023 [202,203] and Ancient DNA Study

ML analyzed DNA samples collected from different coastal regions and cities in western and northern Taiwan. These samples were obtained from individuals whose ancestors had lived in the same region for at least three generations without external immigration. In this group of 767 individuals, ML identified 267 different lineages. The analysis of maternal lineages revealed that one-third originated from Northeast Asia (Northern China, Siberia, Japan, Korea), while two-thirds came from East Asia and Southeast Asia (Central and Southern China, Indochina, Indonesia, the Philippines). These lineages may have arrived in Taiwan as early as 5,000 years ago, with the majority migrating between approximately 1,000 to 2,600 years ago. Among these lineages, ML identified 31 TW lineages, representing the descendants of ancient Taiwanese ancestors. These individuals may be considered broadly as descendants of Pinpu people, possibly accounting for approximately 25% of Taiwan's current population. However, the actual number is likely higher, as most DNA testing, laboratories only perform partial sequence analysis (15% of mtDNA), and the remaining 75% of the population is estimated to be recent 1,000 years immigrants. Among the 31 TW lineages, 10 have origins that include Fujian, with a total of 51 individuals. These lineages vary in terms of their time of occurrence, ranging from 1,300 to 5,000 years ago. This indicates that the arrival of individuals associated with Tangshan Gong was not limited to the last 200-300 years but likely occurred earlier in different periods.

Evidence from ancient DNA (aDNA) research, which involves the analysis of DNA extracted from ancient remains, further supports the presence of immigrants from the Asian mainland and Island Southeast Asia. The aDNA research demonstrated the presence of common lineages, which are frequently observed in current Taiwanese and Asian populations. The human remains found in Hualien's Ling-Ding archaeological site dating back 3,000 years. This provides strong evidence of active maritime trade networks in the South China Sea as early as 3,000 years ago, with Taiwan being a part of this network [194], and the settlement of Taiwan ancestors of non-Austronesian speakers from Asian continent and Southeast Asian islands occurred at least 3,000 years ago.

D. The Paternal Lineage in Taiwan: the "Pinpu Gong" (or Pinpu men) have not disappeared but continue to thrive, while descendants of "Tangshan Gong" likely constitute a portion of Taiwan's male population [188]

Taiwan's main paternal lineages belong to the Y-chromosome O-M175 lineage (Y-SNP haplogroup), specifically the O1-M119 O1a1* lineage, as well as the O3-M122 lineages, including O3a1c1 and O3a2c1a (see Table 1).

Table 1 Distribution of Paternal Lineages in Taiwan and Neighboring Regions (%)

O-M175 Paternal Lineages [1]		Taiwan Population	Pinpu	Tawan Aborigin	Fujian	Indochina	Philippines	Indonesia
O1-M119	O1a1*	14	34	60	22	1	16	14
O3-M122	O3a1c1	12	7	0	20	2	5	2
	O3a2c1a	23	8	0	13	11	2	2
Number of people		1218	286	355	55	153	139	246

[1] Y haplogroup (Y-SNP)

Haplogroup O (Y-DNA Haplogroup O) originated approximately 30,000 to 35,000 years ago in southern Asia and is primarily distributed in East and Southeast Asia. A sublineage, O1-M119 (O1a1*), is predominantly found among Austronesian-speaking populations (Taiwan Aborigins and Southeast Asian islanders) and the Tai-Kadai-speaking Bai-Yue people. This haplogroup likely originated in Taiwan or Continental Southwestern Asia around 16,000-18,000 years ago before spreading southward to Southeast Asian islands [188].

The haplogroups distribution in Taiwan is shown in Table 1: Taiwanese (14%), Pinpu tribes (34%), Taiwan Aborigins (Austronesian speakers) (60%), and Fujian (22%). The O1a1* lineage of Taiwanese and Taiwan Aborigins can largely be distinguished through Y-STR analysis. The O1a1* lineage of the Pinpu tribes is distributed among both the Taiwanese and the Taiwan Aborigins. Interestingly, 22% of MMH Fujian males samples are found to carry O1a1*, which contradicts the findings of Wen B. et al. (2004, *Nature* 431: 302-305), who reported 0% O1a1* in Fujian. This earlier study was based on samples from 148 unrelated Hakka males from Changting, an ancient Hakka migration center in Fujian. The results showed no O1-M119 haplogroup but exclusively O3-M122. The data used in that study referenced Li H. et al. (2003, *Journal of Genetics* 30: 873-880), which noted that 3 of the 148 samples (2%) were likely O1a1*. This aligns with findings from the Mackay Memorial Hospital Molecular Anthropology Laboratory, where 22% of 55 Fujian male samples were identified as O1a1* (see Table 1). These findings suggest that the Bai-Yue paternal lineage did not disappear from Fujian and Guangdong due to Emperor Wu of Han's southern conquests. The theory that Bai-Yue males were entirely replaced by Han Chinese O3-M122 is likely inaccurate. Instead, Bai-Yue paternal lineages, including O1a1*, continue to exist significantly in southeastern coastal China. The O1a1* haplogroup in Taiwan likely represents a lineage native to Taiwan, derived from the evolution of O1-M175 tens of thousands of years ago. Thus, part of the "Pinpu Gong" lineage can be traced back to this original O1a1*. Additionally, another source of Taiwan's O1a1* haplogroup comes from migrations over the past 400 years from southeast cost of China (Fujian and Guangdong), representing the "Tangshan Gong." Another potential contributor is the O1a1* haplogroup from Southeast Asian island nations like the Philippines and Indonesia, both of which have high frequencies of O1a1* (14-16%), similar to Taiwan.

Figure 1 Evolutionary Relationship Diagram of the O1a1* Lineage (Y-STR)

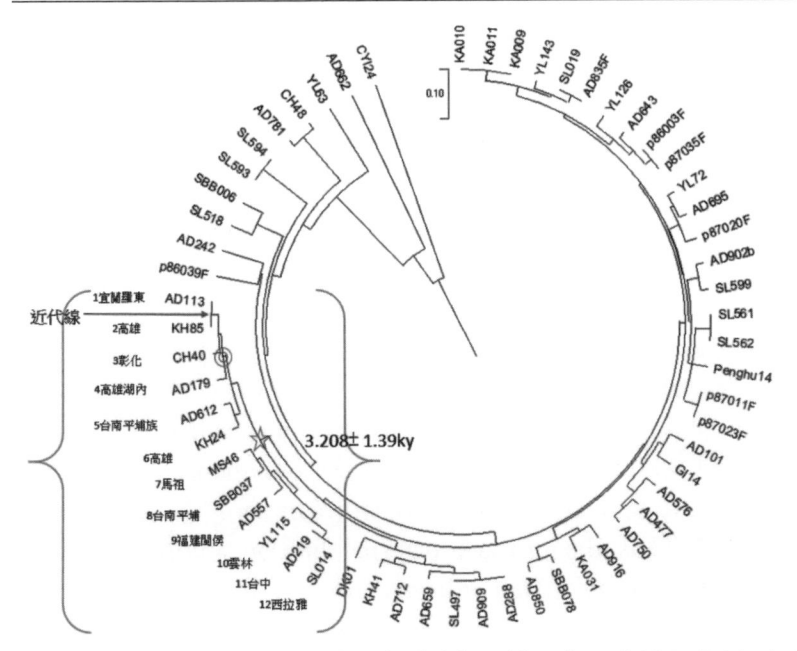

Figure 1, the 4th individual within the left-hand bracket of 12 individuals, labeled AD179, is a resident of Kaohsiung County. According to family elders and ancestral records, his ancestors migrated to Taiwan from Fujian with Koxinga 400 years ago. However, the evolutionary relationship diagram suggests that his ancestors may have diverged (marked with a double circles) from those of the Tainan Pinpu individual (5 AD612) and Kaohsiung Taiwanese (6 KH24) approximately 700 years ago. This divergence predates Koxinga's arrival in Taiwan 400 years ago by about 300 years. In this case AD179 is likely a descendant of the "Pinpu Gong." Therefore when people claims that they are the decendent of Tangshan Gong is not nessary to be real, since they could be the decendent of Pinpu Gong.

In our research, another genetic system, Y-STR lineage, was analyzed. By comparing variations in Y-STR lengths at different loci, we examined the evolutionary migration patterns of male Y-chromosome lineages in Taiwan and surrounding regions. Using the Y-STR data, an evolutionary relationship diagram was constructed, identifying one lineage cluster originating approximately 3,000 years ago (marked with a star in Figure 1). This estimation aligns with the methodology described in Zhivotovsky LA. (*Am J Hum Genet*. 74: 50-61, 2004).

The finding that 2% of individuals in the Hakka ancient town of Changting in China potentially belong to the O1-M119 lineage and that 22% of Fujian male samples from the Mackay Memorial Hospital Molecular Anthropology Laboratory exhibit the O1a1* lineage is significant. This evidence suggests that the migrants from Fujian and Guangdong to Taiwan, referred to as "Tangshan Gong" were not exclusively descendants of the northern Han lineage (O3-M122). This finding challenges the longstanding misconception among Taiwanese people that they are purely descendants of northern Han Chinese. Many Taiwanese mistakenly believe that all Taiwanese males are descendants of "Tangshan Gong." In reality, 14% of Taiwanese men belong to the O1a1* lineage, and a substantial portion of this lineage likely originates from the "Pinpu Gong" whose ancestry dates back to the emergence of O1a1* in Taiwan approximately 18,000 to 16,000 years ago.

O3-M122 is the primary paternal lineage among Taiwanese people. Originating in the southern regions of the Asian continent, it began migrating to Taiwan around 6,000-5,000 years ago. Over time, it became the dominant paternal lineage among non-Austronesian-speaking populations (i.e., modern Taiwanese), accounting for 54% of the paternal ancestry in Taiwan. This lineage consists of 18 haplogroups, with the two main subgroups being O3a1c1 and O3a2c1a (as shown in Table 1), comprising 12% and 23% of the Taiwanese paternal lineage, respectively. The O3a2c1a haplogroup accounts for 13% of paternal lineage in Fujian and approximately 10% in the Continental Southeast Asian, including regions such as Thailand, Vietnam, and Myanmar. This indicates its significance as a major paternal lineage in the Southeast Asian continent. Therefore its frequency in Southeast Asian island nations, such as the Philippines and Indonesia, is much lower, at around 2% [188].

In Taiwan, the O3-M122 lineage is predominantly distributed

among non-indigenous Taiwanese populations, with smaller representations among certain Pinpu tribes. Its high frequency and widespread presence across Taiwan suggest that O3a2c1a and O3a1c1, both subgroups of the O3 lineage, largely descend from ancient migrants, who are also considered ancestors of the "Pinpu Gong." Additionally, some Taiwanese men with the O3-M122 lineage may trace their ancestry to the "Tangshan Gong" immigrants from China within the past 400 years, or to ancient migrants from the Continental Southeast Asian.

In addition to the O-M175 lineage, Taiwan's paternal lineages also include 3-4% of C and N lineages, a small proportion of R lineage, and traces of ancient P and Q lineages. It is likely that the ancient D-M174 lineage is absent in Taiwan. [refer to *Liberty Times*, July 30, 2024, Free Forum section, Appendix 4]

References
(Please refer to Dr. Lin Marie's journal article collection)

[17] **Lin-Chu M***. Experience with the manual Polybrene method in Taiwan (letter). *Transfusion*, 1984; 24: 543.

[22] **Lin-Chu M***. Broadberry RE, Yen LS. An appraisal of Rh(D) typing in Chinese. *J Formosan Med Assoc*, 1986; 85: 196-198.

[27] **Lin-Chu M***. Broadberry RE, Chiou FW. The B_3 phenotype in Chinese. *Transfusion*, 1986; 26: 428-430.

[30] **Lin-Chu M***. The para-Bombay phenotype in Chinese persons. *Transfusion*, 1987; 27: 388-390.

[33] **Lin-Chu M***. Inspection and continuing education on blood banking in Taiwan. *Excerpta Medica, Current Clinical Practice Series*, 1988; 47: 249-253.

[40] **Lin-Chu M***, Broadberry RE. Blood transfusion in the para-Bombay phenotype. *Brit J Hemat*, 1990; 75: 568-572.

[44] Brodberry RE, **Lin-Chu M***. The Lewis blood group system among Chinese in Taiwan. *Human Heredity*, 1991; 41: 290-294.

[47] **Lin-Chu M**, Broadberry RE, Tanaka M, Okubo Y. The i phenotype and congenital cataracts among Chinese in Taiwan. *Transfusion*, 1991; 31: 676-677.

[51] **Lin M***. Shien SH, Yang TF. Frequency of platelet-specific antigens among Chinese in Taiwan. *Transfusion*, 1993; 33: 155-157.

[53] Broadberry RE, **Lin M***. The incidence and significance of anti-"Mi[a]" in Taiwan. *Transfusion*, 1994; 34: 349-352.

[54] **Lin M**. The national blood program of Taiwan, ROC (letter). *Vox Sang*, 1994; 66: 299.

[55] **Lin M***, Broadberry RE. The modification of standard Western pretransfusion testing procedures for Taiwan. *Vox Sang*, 1994; 67: 199-202.

[57] **Lin M***, Broadberry RE. The clinical significance of anti-'Mi[a]' (letter). *Transfusion*, 1994; 34: 1013-1014.

[58] **Lin M***, Broadberry RE. Elimination of Rh(D) typing and the antiglobulin test in pretransfusion compatibility tests for Taiwanese. *Vox Sang*,1994; 67: 28-29.

[59] **Lin M***, Chen CC, Hong CC, Lin WS, Cheng YP. Transfusion-associated respiratory distress in Taiwan. *Vox Sang*, 1994; 67: 372-376.

[66] **Lin M***. Broadberry RE. The Lewis phenotype in Orientals (letter). *Vox Sang*, 1995; 68: 68-9.

[69] **Lin M***, Shieh SH, Liang DC, Yang TF, Shibata Y. Neonatal alloimmune thrombocytopenia in Taiwan due to an antibody against a labile component of HPA-3a(Bak[a]). *Vox Sang*, 1995; 69: 336-340.

[71] Wu AM. Duk M, **Lin M**, Broadberry RE. Lisowska E. Identification of variant glycophorins of human red cells by lectinoblotting: application to the Mi.III variant that is relatively frequent in the Taiwanese population. *Transfusion*, 1995; 35: 571-576.

[72] Yu LC, Yang YH, Broadberry RE, Chen YH, **Lin M***. Correlation of a missense mutation in the human secretor alpha (1,2) fucosyltransferase gene with the Lewis(a+b+) phenotype: A potential molecular basis for the weak Secretor allele (Se[w]). *J Bio Chem*, 1995; 312: 329-332.

[73] Broadberry RE, **Lin M***. The distribution of the MiIII (Gp.Mur) phenotype among the population of Taiwan. *Transfusion medicine*, 1996; 6: 145-148.

[74] Broadberry RE, **Lin M***. Comparison of the Lewis phenotypes among the different population groups of Taiwan. *Transfusion Medicine*, 1996; 6: 255-260.

[81] Yu LC, Yang YH, Broadberry RE, Chen YH, **Lin M***. Heterogeneity of the human H blood group alpha (1,2) fucosyltransferase gene among para-Bombay individuals. *Vox Sang*, 1997; 72: 36-40.

[83] **Lin M**, Broadberry RE. Immunohematology in Taiwan. *Transfusion Medicine Review*, 1998; 12: 56-72.

[86] Yu LC, Lee HL, Chu CC, Broadberry RE, **Lin M***. A new identified nonsecretor allele of the human histo-blood group alpha (1,2) fucosyltransferase gene (FUT2). *Vox Sang*, 1999; 76: 115-119.

[89] **Lin M**, Chu CC, Lee HL, Chang SL, Ohashi J, Tokunaga K, Akaza T, Juji T. Heterogeneity of Taiwan's indigenous population: possible relation to prehistoric Mongoloid dispersals. *Tissue Antigens*, 2000; 55: 1-9.

[92] Chu CC, **Lin M***, Nakajima F, Lee HL, Chang SL, Tokunaga K, Juji T. Diversity of HLA among Taiwan's indigenous tribes and the Ivatans in the Philippines. *Tissue Antigens*, 2001; 58: 9-18.

[94] **Lin M**, Chu CC, Chang SL, Lee HL, Loo JH, Akaza T, Juji T, Ohashi J, Tokunaga K. The origin of Minnan and Hakka, the so-called "Taiwanese", inferred by HLA study. *Tissue Antigens*, 2001; 57: 192-199.

[97] Yu LC, Chu CC, Chan YS, Chang CY, Twu YC, Lee HL, **Lin M***. Polymorphism and distribution of the Secretor α (1,2)-fucosyltransferase gene in various Taiwanese populations. *Transfusion*, 2001; 41: 1279-1284.

[98] Yu LC, Twu YC, Chang CY, **Lin M***. Molecular basis of the adult i phenotype and the gene responsible for the expression of the human blood group I antigen. *Blood*, 2001; 98: 3840-3845.

[99] Yu LC, Twu YC, Chang CY, and **Lin M***. Molecular basis of the Kell-null phenotype: a mutation at the splice site of human *KEL* gene abolishes the expression of Kell blood group antigens. *J Bio Chem*, 2001; 276: 10247-10252.

[105] Yu LC, Twu YC, Chou ML, Chang CY, Wu CY, **Lin M***. Molecular genetic analysis for the B^3 allele. *Blood*, 2002; 100: 1490-1492.

[106] **Lin M**, Tseng HK, Trejaut JA, Lee H L, Loo JH, Chu CC, Chen PJ, Su YW, Lim KH, Tsai ZU, Lin RY, Lin RS, Huang CH. Association of HLA class I with severe acute respiratory syndrome coronavirus infection. *BMC Medical Genetics*, 2003; 4: 9.

[107] **Lin M***. Wang CL, Chen FS, Ho LH. Fatal hemolytic transfusion reaction due to a anti-Ku in a K$_{null}$ patient. *Immunohematology*, 2003; 19: 19-21.

[109] Yu LC, Twu YC, Chou ML, Chang CY, Reid ME, Gray AR, Moulds JM, **Lin M***. The molecular genetics of the human I locus and molecular background explaining the partial association of the adult i phenotype with congenital cataracts (Plenary paper). *Blood*, 2003; 101: 2081-2088.

[129] Kataoka S, Kobayashi H, Chiba K, Nakamura M, Shinada, Moritas, **Lin M**, Shibata Y. Neonatal alloimmune thrombocytopenia due to an antibody against a labile component of human platelet antigen-3b (Bak[b]). *Transfu Med*, 2004; 14: 419-423.

[137] Trejaut JA, Kivisild T, Loo JH, Lee CL, He CL, Hsu CJ, Li ZY, **Lin M***. Traces of archaic mitochondrial lineages persist in Austronesian-speaking Formosan populations. *PLoS Biology*, 2005; 3: e247.

[142] **Lin M***. Taiwan experience suggests that RhD typing for blood transfusion is unnecessary in southeast Asian populations. *Transfusion*, 2006; 46: 95-98.

[178] Soares P, Rito T, Trejaut J, Mormina M, Hill C, Tinkler-Hundal E, Braid M, Clarke DJ, Loo JH, Thomson N, Denham T, Donohue M, Macaulay V, **Lin M**, Oppenheimer S, Richards MB. Ancient Voyaging and Polynesian Origins. *Am J Hum Genet*, 2011; 88: 239-247.

[182] Yu LC, **Lin M***. Molecular genetics of the blood group I system and the regulation of I antigen expression during erythropoiesis and granulopoiesis. *Curr Opin Hematol*, 2011; 18: 421-426.

[188] Trejaut JA, Poloni ES, Yen JC, Lai YH, Loo JH, Lee CL, He CL, **Lin M***. Taiwan Y-chromosomal DNA variation and its relationship with Island Southeast Asia. *BMC Genet*, 2014; 15: 77.

[194] Huang JY, Trejaut JA, Lee CL, Wang TY, Loo JH, Chen ZS, Chen LR, Liu KH, Liu YC, Hu CH, **Lin M***. Mitochondrial DNA Sequencing of Middle Neolithic Human Remains of Ling-Ding Site Implication for the Social Structure and the Origin of Northeast Coast Taiwanese. *Journal of Phylogenetics & Evolutionary Biology*, 2018; 6: 6.

[200] **Lin M**. Elimination of pretransfusion RhD typing at Mackay Memorial Hospital, Taiwan-30-year experience (1988-2017). *Vox Sang*, 2021; 116: 234-238.

[202] **Lin M**, Trejaut JA. Diversity and distribution of mitochondrial DNA in non-Austronesian-speaking Taiwanese individuals. *Hum Genome Var*, 2023; 10: 2.

[203] 林媽利. 台灣人的來源— DNA 的探索. *台灣醫界*, 2023. 66: 261-266.

[Please refer to Dr. Marie Lin's conference abstract collection 199]

Lin M, Lee CL, Loo JH, Yen JC, Chu CC, Lee HL, Trejaut JA. More genetic sharing among the populations of Taiwan than expected: a plain tribe (Pinpu) perspective. PNC 2009 Annual Conference, Taipei, Taiwan.

附件
Attachments

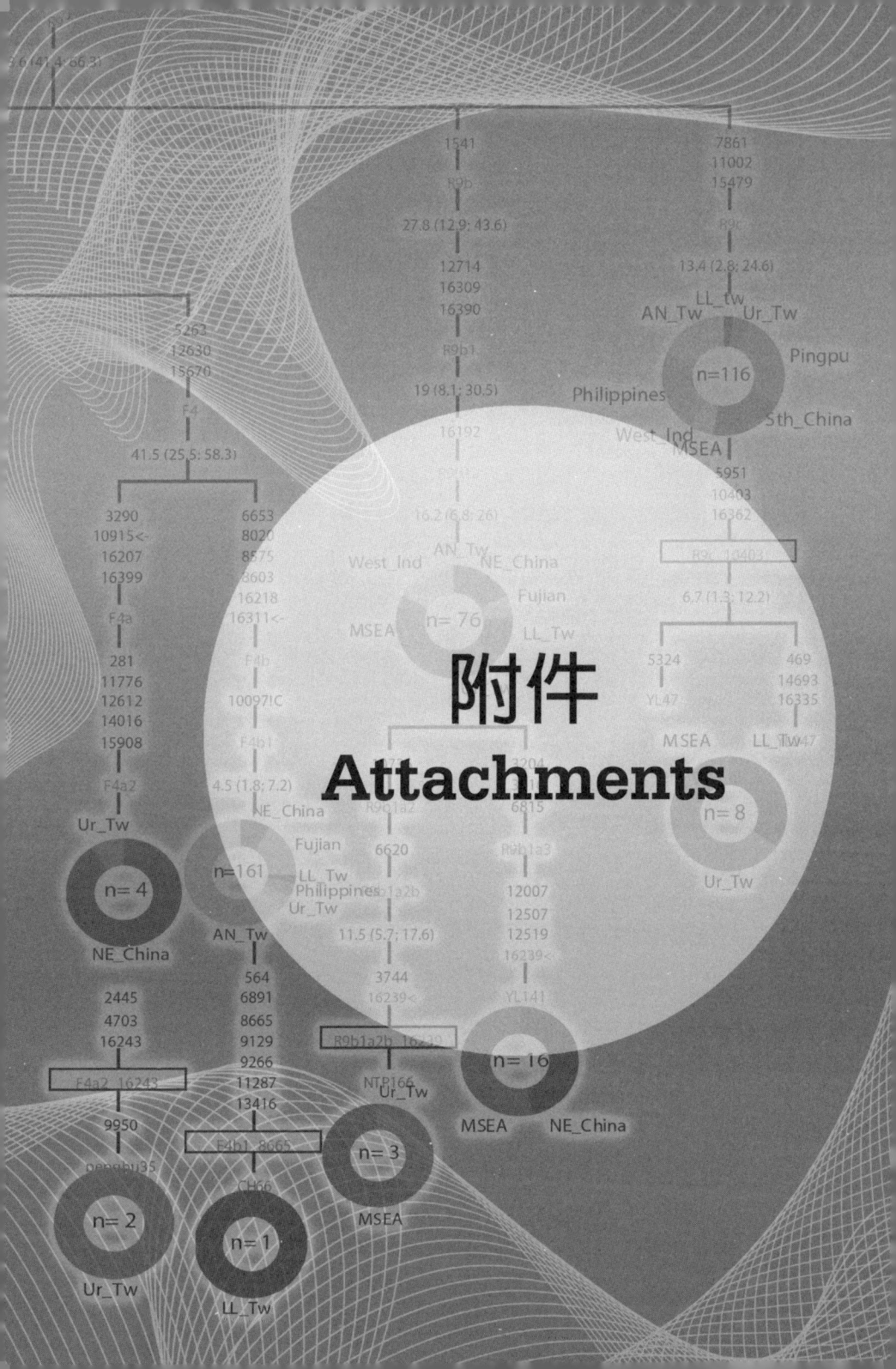

附件 1

Dr. A. Kellner 的信（台灣的國家血液政策，1983）

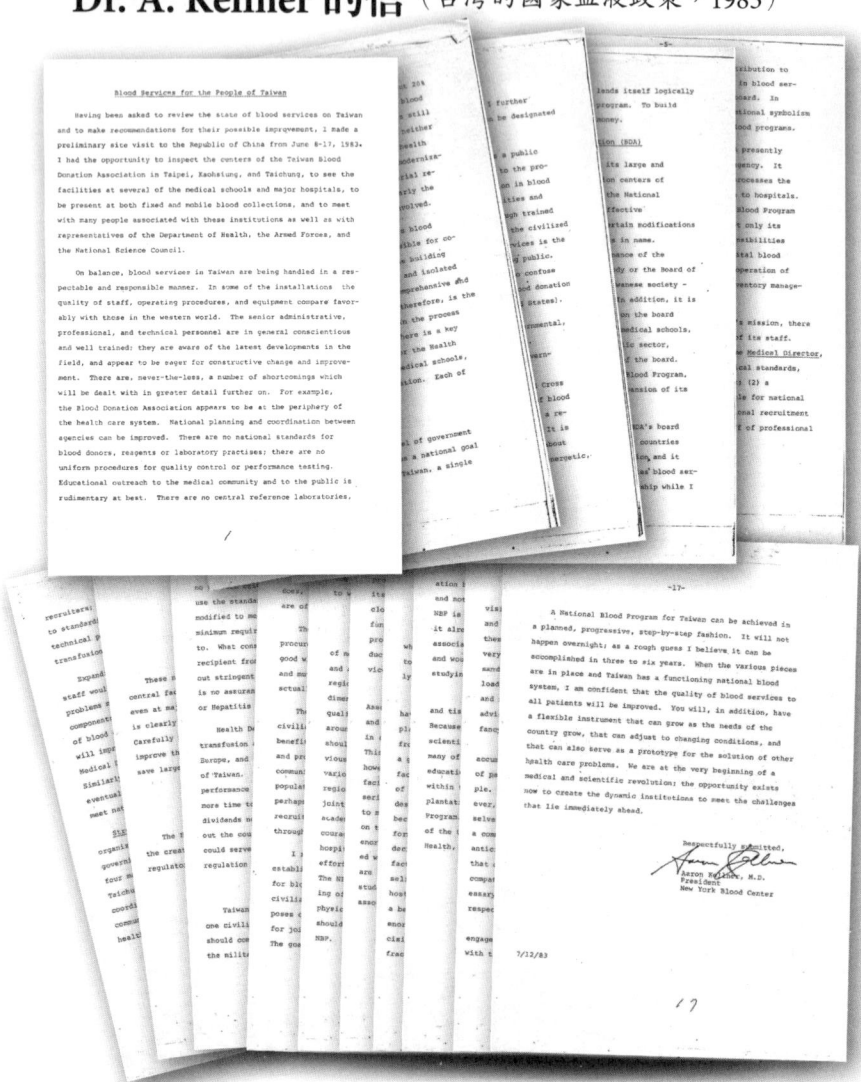

Dr. A. Kellner 的信，原文

【中譯版】

適用於台灣地區人民的血液事業

紐約捐血中心主任
Dr. Aaron Kellner

　　我在1983年6月8日至17日被邀請到中華民國訪問，考察台灣地區的血液事業，並對其可能的改進提供建議。訪問期間，我有機會參觀了中華民國捐血運動協會所屬的台北、高雄及台中捐血中心，並看了幾所醫學院和主要醫院的各項設備，還參觀了團體捐血和巡迴捐血車的血液採集工作，並且會晤了這些機構的許多人員及衛生署、軍方和國科會的代表。

　　台灣的血液事業是以一種審慎而負責的方式來經營，在設備方面，如工作人員的素質、操作的程序以及儀器設備等，皆不亞於西方國家。上級的管理、專家和技術人員都具有敬業精神，且訓練有素，他們都熟知這個事業的最新發展，並企求具有建設性的改進，然而仍然存在一些缺點，留待更進一步的處理。例如：捐血協會似乎與醫療保健系統缺乏聯繫；各單位間全盤性的規劃與合作應可再改進；在捐血人、試藥及檢驗工作方面，沒有國家標準；品質管制和試驗的實施上沒有統一的程序；對於醫療單位和民眾的推廣教育還在初步階段；沒有中央參考實驗室，資料處理的方式既麻煩又落伍；約有20%的血液來自有酬供血者；至於

血液成分的使用,雖然近兩年來有所增加,仍甚低於理想。以上缺點不足爲奇且不很嚴重,在一個快速向現代化擴展的醫療保健系統下是一自然現象,尤其在中華民國擁有可利用的材料資源和優秀人才的條件下,一定能夠克服這些。

　　大致上,台灣血液事業最大的缺點是缺乏一個中央體制來負責協調、計畫、實行等工作,分支機構雖已建立,卻各行其是,沒有結合成一個廣泛且相互交流的系統,因此,我的第一個建議是建立「台灣地區的全國性血液方案」。接著,我想指出在建立全國性血液方案的過程中,決定政策的政府部門、衛生署、軍方、醫院、醫學院及捐血協會所應負的主要任務。

政府的任務

　　我建議政府的適當部門發布一份正式政策性的聲明,做爲一個全國性的目標,就是建立台灣地區的全國性血液方案,爲唯一負責全國血液事業的實體。我更建議可任命現存的捐血協會做爲領導機構,以達成此一目標。血液事業是一種公用事業,一種管制性的壟斷事業,在許多方面與電力、電信服務事業相類似,在血液事業上競爭是一種浪費,會導致儀器設備,尤其是人員上的重複,有經驗人才的不足問題,不僅是在台灣,而且存在於已開發的國家。血液事業最重要的是必須對捐血人做單一而統一的報導,互相競爭的機構所做的競爭性報導,只會混淆民眾且導致已建立的捐血目標的失敗(美國芝加哥就是一個很好的例子)。

　　被任命來發展全國性血液方案的機構,可以是政府、紅十字會或一適當的非營利性私人機構。在台灣,據我的了解,政府正朝著多利用私營機構的力量以達成國民保健的推展,在供血的服

務上，台灣紅十字會似乎只扮演一個次要的角色。捐血協會成立不到十年，已做了一項輝煌的工作，它是一個私營的、非營利性的組織，由一群熱誠、有遠見、有責任感的人士負責經營，現供應全面需血量約 80%，且在繼續成長。因此，它可以很合理的成為全國性血液方案的核心。加強建立現存的力量，可以同時節省時間和金錢。

捐血協會的任務

現存的捐血協會以及分布在台灣主要人口集中地區的四個龐大且繼續擴展的捐血中心，可以做為全國性血液方案的基礎。對捐血協會來說，要發展有成效的全國性血液方案，必須在管理、功能、人員以及名稱方面接受某些改變。

一、捐血協會組織的改變：全國性血液方案的管理，就是決定政策者或理事會應廣泛地包括台灣社會團體──商業界、工業界、勞工界、學生及其他的代表，除此之外，理事會中必須有來自衛生署、軍方、醫學院、主要醫院及醫療團體的高階層代表，公立機構仍應擔任理事會的主體，如果現有的捐血協會要發展成全國性血液方案，它必須同意上述關於理事會的建議。

捐血協會的理事會是否應包括紅十字會的成員，這個問題我無法回答。在許多國家，紅十字會是自願捐血的標誌，同時它在這些國家的血液事業上扮演著支配性角色。我在台灣這段期間，沒有與紅十字會的領導者會面，我不知道他們對血液事業的貢獻及興趣，是否足以加入捐血協會的理事會。大體來說，紅十字會的財源及其國際性的標誌，對發展全國性血液方案而言，是一項很有用的資產。

二、捐血協會的功能及其編制：以目前而言，捐血協會自視其主要功能為一採集血液的機構，它徵募自願的捐血者，採集血液並加以處理，以供各醫院使用。如果捐血協會被任命來實施全國性血液方案，它必須擴展本身的作業範圍，除了目前的作業外，還須負起其他的責任，如醫院血庫技術人員的訓練、執業醫師的教育、中央參考實驗室的操作，尤其是按全國性的比例來計畫及經營存血的調配。為了配合擴展捐血協會的任務範圍，必須進行工作人員的擴充及專業化，關於這一點，至少必須包括：（1）一位專任的醫學主管，受過血庫作業各方面的訓練，能樹立醫學上的權威，提供指導及領導專業性方面的事務。（2）一位負責募集捐血人的主管，負責全國性的計畫、捐血募集工作的協調擴展、公共關係及專業徵募工作人員的訓練。（3）一位負責檢驗和技術性事務的主管，為全國性血液方案中心及各醫院輸血作業從事作業程序標準化，提供品管及訓練技術人員。

擴展捐血協會的功能及人員的專業化，終將解決兩個為台灣居民所熟知的問題，即血液成分的使用不普遍，以及過份依賴有酬供血者。血液成分的使用是教育的一項功能，如果全國性血液方案有一位熱誠的醫學主管能博得執業醫師的尊敬，此情況將自然而快速的改善；同樣地，如果全國性血液方案證明能以一種適時而有效的方式解決全國的血液需求，則對有價供血者的依賴將減少甚至消失。

三、全國性血液方案的架構：全國性血液方案可被視為由現有的捐血協會發展出來的新機構，它在台北有中央管理的主體和行政的機構，且至少在台北、高雄、台南、台中設立四個主要的地區性血液中心，我們可以預見，如果以一種周密計畫和協調的

方式來經營,它將能對醫學界提供一些新的服務,以配合全國性醫療保健系統的需要及成長。

例如:(1)紅血球抗原及 HLA 之諮詢實驗室。(2)中央冷凍血液儲存室及稀有血液之登記。(3)技術人員的訓練及醫師的教育。(4)全國性計畫及預測。(5)存血的運用經營。(6)資料處理。(7)父子關係的鑑定。(8)為較小醫院做機動的血液分離採集術。(9)盡可能的做血漿分成和其他服務。

這些計畫並不需要全部集中在台北,假如大家都認為合適,並已建立適當的協調關係,某些工作可以設置在其他捐血中心,甚至是大醫院。周密計畫和妥善經營可以改善血液事業的品質,且避免重複,以節省大量金錢。

衛生署的任務

衛生署在建立一個全國性的血液事業上具有一個非常重要的任務,下面是其部分的管制工作:

一、建立試藥作業程序和人員素質的標準。

二、建立捐血人標準。

三、給予合格設備之許可證,進行定期檢查和測驗。

四、提供國家標準的品質保證。

以上數點,目前台灣尚未做到,例如:沒有統一的捐血人標準,某些機構使用 AABB(American Association of Blood Banks)的標準加以修改以適合本身的需要,但是缺乏所有的捐血機構都必須遵守的最低標準,且制定什麼樣才是合理的交叉試驗,以避免使受血者產生嚴重反應,各地標準亦不同;缺乏有力的品質管制和定期的測驗,會使例行的作業過程如血型的測定或肝炎檢驗

也失去保證。

在美國和西歐，包括輸血作業各方面的衛生條例已經很完善的建立，且這些條例可以很快的適合台灣的需要，以定期評鑑和測驗來實施這些條例是比較困難，並需要很多時間，但這些努力不僅在改進全國血液事業的品質上可以獲得實質的效益，同時正如班納德博士（Dr. Ivan Bennett）所指出的，還可以做為衛生署管轄下的其他醫療保健範圍的模式。

軍方的任務

台灣目前有兩個主要的捐血機構，一是民間團體，另一是軍方，兩者都是必須的且應相輔相成，平時軍方的血液需求量不多，所以軍方的血源必須且應該支持民間，戰時則兩者角色互易。儘管如此對雙方都有明顯的好處，但是民間和軍方血源的交流卻顯得不協調，在某些地方合作良好且都獲得利益，而在某些地方即使不是敵對，卻也顯得不明確。

關於血液方面，民眾和軍方之間需要一種密切且比較正式的關係，這可使軍方藉著平時和民間的設備與作業之合作，以及彼此之間已經建立的良好聯繫管道而獲得利益；同時對民間有利的是，不只有更穩定的血源，尤其重要的是，可以使在軍中曾經捐過血的人，養成終生繼續捐血的習慣。我建議盡快的成立一個正式的「血液聯絡委員會」，由軍方和民間負責捐血事務的官員組成，這個委員會應定期集會商討捐血、供血配額的計畫和制定，聯合採血計畫及解決問題，其目標應為有效地調整兩個不同體系卻需隨時合作的捐血機構。

醫學院和主要醫院的任務

　　醫學院和主要醫院是國家醫學和科技專家的儲藏庫，因此應該和全國性血液方案及其他地區性血液中心密切而主動的配合，事實上，他們應對全國性血液方案貢獻智慧，因為他們是全國性血液方案人才的來源，也是其與全球尖端科技的連接環，如前文提到的，醫學院和主要醫院應參與全國性血液方案的最高決策委員會，同時也應參加台北和其他地區血液中心之各種專門諮詢委員會。只要有適合的機會，全國性血液方案和鄰近的學術性機構應共同聘用專業性工作人員，同時應鼓勵醫學院人員多利用全國性血液方案的資源從事研究，而那些從事採血的醫院應與全國性血液方案協調來幫助存血的調配。

　　全國性血液方案應與醫學院在訓練年輕醫師和執業醫師的再教育方面密切合作。大體而言，主要的醫學機構和全國性血液方案之間的意見交換，應多加鼓勵，捐血協會現在僅是一個供應血液給醫院病患的周邊機構，如果要轉變成全國性血液方案，必須在醫學方面做更多的努力，成為醫療保健系統不可缺少的一部分，不僅能增加供應臨床所需的血液種類，同時也是臨床專業服務及專業人員的來源。

　　就此而言，正如我曾參觀過的捐血協會、台北、高雄、台中捐血中心及我沒去的台南捐血中心，都是設置於遠離醫院及醫學院的商業大樓，就目前而言，這種安排尚可，但對未來而言，當他們繼續擴展而打算遷移時（勢必會如此），我極力建議，他們應慎重考慮位置緊鄰主要的醫學中心，我所謂的緊鄰，可以說是在醫學中心校區內或隔一條街，血液中心的工作人員可經由這些

機構內有關醫院病患的治療、醫學院的教育、圖書館的利用、研討會、研究生、研究計畫，及其他許多啓發性的活動等，和一個充滿生機的醫學校區帶來的特殊氣氛，而得到相當大的益處。

有待商榷的其他問題

我在台灣期間，參加的許多會議和討論會中，還有許多與血液事業有關的問題，我願意在此提出意見：

一、血漿分成：目前台灣沒有屬於自己的血漿分成設備，必須從日本和美國進口所需的血漿衍生物（凝固因子、蛋白質、免疫球蛋白），我聽說在台灣有一個小組進行審查台灣地區血漿分成設備的成本—效益，特別是在 B 型肝炎疫苗的製造方面。我必須指出，將血漿分成和 B 型肝炎疫苗聯想在一塊兒是不好的，因爲後者是以高度污染的物質爲原料，而前者需要絕對清潔或無菌的環境。這個小組在做決策時，除了成本—效益外，還應考應兩點：(1)自足的問題，這個問題在現在這種充滿敵意的國際現勢，對台灣而言是有些重要性的；(2)是否有機會能在不斷發展的新式生物技術方面居於領導地位，以及這些產品是否能在遠東地區獲得具有潛力而廣大的未來市場。如果決定朝著建立血漿分成廠方面發展，我力勸你們愼重考慮把它列入全國性血液方案的一部分，而不是一種附屬於其他機構的獨立單位。全國性血液方案是血漿的自然來源，是工廠原料的供應處，且對各醫院已有了供應制度，我的同事 Dr. Kenneth Woods 在這方面是大家所公認的專家，他願意與這小組討論研究此事。

二、組織和器官移植：在未來幾年內，器官和組織移植的利用將迅速的發展，因爲血液事業是奠定在與移植術類似的基因和

免疫科學的基礎上，而且因為移植術所需的許多條件，如民眾教育、HLA 型鑑定，以及一個廿四小時的運送系統，已經存在於血液系統裡，因此在全國性血液方案的中央體制下發展移植術是很有意義的。關於這一點，在 1973 年由衛生教育社會福利部長所發表的美國國家血液政策中首先提到。

  國家血液政策：輸血和其他的血液治療法可被視為人體組織移植中最早且不斷高度發展的一面，這個政策專門指導有關血液供應、處理、分配，以及用血方面的問題，其基本原則雖不需要詳細分類，仍可適用於一個即將擴展的系統，以涵蓋所有可移植的人體組織。

  三、自動生化儀器：在我參觀的每一個地區性捐血中心裡，對於自動血液分析儀都相當有興趣，且亟欲獲得這種精密儀器，我建議他們暫緩購買這些自動化儀器，這些儀器很昂貴，且離製造廠很遠，要維護這些儀器的零件可能有困難，各中心的工作量根據成本效益尚可收支平衡，且更新的儀器即將出品，因此各中心在此時人才訓練的投資要比新式的自動化儀器的投資獲益更多。

  四、資料處理：每一個地區性捐血中心都累積了繁多的資料，這些資料都記錄在紙上且以大量的人工處理，他們準備引進電腦來處理資料，然而在採購電腦任憑能說善道的商人擺布之前，我建議他們成立一個委員會來確認他們現在及未來的不同需要，然後選擇一個易操縱的，能隨資料數量、需要、成長而擴展的機型，能使各中心連線作業，並使各中心都能有備用系統。他

們應該迅速發展電腦化作業，但要愼重小心的去做。

　　五、研究：全國性血液方案應該從事本身的研究，並應與醫院和大學做共同的合作實驗研究，現有捐血協會因爲有經濟問題必須優先考慮，所以未能致力於研究工作。總而言之，在從事研究工作的規劃期間，對實驗室、工作人員、經費都應有充分準備，而不宜在事後補救。

　　六、財務狀況：全國性血液方案在財務方面應該能自給自足，其經費來自本身產品及服務所收取的費用，以支付其支出。在全國性血液方案發展的初期，如果政府能支援創立基金，或日後提供建築目的所需的經費，這是很理想的。但大體上而言，全國性血液方案應該在無需政府補助的情況下來經營。

　　關於財務方面，我主張採用開誠布公的原則，一個請求民眾自願捐血的機構，有絕對的義務完全公開如何處理血液及所收取的費用。捐血協會或是全國性血液方案，在政策上應保存其會計帳簿以利主管機關審查，同時至少每年一次對大眾公開詳細的財務狀況，我感覺到這個觀念有些令人難以接受。對大眾坦白，以減少懷疑，以解釋向醫院病患收費的情形，以建立信心和信賴是非常重要的，否則，一個從事捐血的機構是難以成功的。

　　最後我以簡單幾點做個根本的建議：

　　一、由政府的最高階層做個決策以建立一個全國性血液方案。

　　二、任命捐血協會做爲這個方案負責領導的機構。

　　三、開始在捐血協會內做必要的改組，以完成這個擴展的目的。

　　四、開始由捐血協會、衛生署、軍方及其他有關機構從事廣

泛的計畫，以制定目標和實際作業的日程表。

　　台灣地區的全國性血液方案可以一種有計畫的、漸進的方式完成，它不是一夕之間可以做到，粗略的估計，我認為可以在三年至六年間完成，當一切準備都已就緒，台灣有了具有功能的全國性血液制度時，我相信對所有病患供血服務的品質將會改善。此外，你們也將擁有個能隨國家成長需要而發展的有彈性的設施，能適應不斷的改變，且可做為解決其他醫療保健問題的典範。我們正處於醫學和科學革命的開端，應把握現有的機會，建立一強而有力的機構，以迎接即將來臨的挑戰。

1983 年 7 月 12 日

附件 2

前國際輸血學會會長 Contreras 的信，鼓勵別的國家效法台灣血庫的作業

Vox Sanguinis

Editor-in-Chief　C.P. ENGELFRIET, Amsterdam
Section Editors　A.F.H. BRITTEN, Averill Park, N.Y.
　　　　　　　　J.D. CASH, Edinburgh
　　　　　　　　F. DECARY, Montreal
　　　　　　　　W.R. MAYR, Aachen
President,　A. HÄSSIG, Berne
Foundation Vox Sanguinis

International Journal of Transfusion Medicine
Official Journal of the International Society of Blood Transfusion

Dr. M. CONTRERAS
North London
Blood Transfusion Centre,
Colindale Avenue,
London NW9 5BG
Tel: 081 200 7777 Fax: 081 200 3894

M Lin MD FCAP
Transfusion Medicine Laboratory
Mackay Memorial Hospital
92 Sec 2 Chung San North Road
Taipei
Taiwan
Republic of China

MC/ajc/lin

3 March 1994

Dear Marie Lin,

I know, from Paul Engelfriet who is at present staying with me to celebrate Pat Mollison's 80th Birthday, that your **excellent paper on RhD typing in Taiwan has been submitted for publication** in Vox Sanguinis. I welcome this publication. However, now that we have nearly finished editing the Special Issue of Vox Sanguinis, I realise that it would be most useful if we could include a summary of your paper, especially with the practical implications. Jussi Leikola and I would therefore be grateful if you could write a 2 page summary of your paper in double spacing as soon as possible and forward it to me for inclusion in the Special Issue. <u>We think that it is important for other countries to follow your example of breaking away from European and North American traditions/regulations if these are not pertinent or relevant to the population in question.</u>

I hope that you will be able to contribute to the Special Issue.

With warmest regards

Yours sincerely

Marcela Contreras
Review Editor

copy Prof. Leikok

KARGER　Medical and Scientific Publishers
Basel · München · Paris · London · New York
New Delhi · Bangkok · Singapore · Tokyo · Sydney

附件 3

台灣從事常規 Rh 血型篩檢的爭議，
及馬偕醫院血庫的堅持

```
              NATIONAL BLOOD TRANSFUSION SERVICE
                  NORTH LONDON BLOOD TRANSFUSION CENTRE
                                 DEANSBROOK ROAD
                                 EDGWARE, MIDDX
                                        HA8 9BD
Dr. M. CONTRERAS                Telephone: 01-952 5511
Director


MC/mrl                                      24th June, 1985.


Dr. Marie Lin Chu and Mr. R.E. Broadberry,
Mackay Memorial Hospital,
No. 92, North Chung San Road, Sec. 2,
Taipei 104,
TAIWAN.


Dear Dr. Lin Chu and Mr. Broadberry,

Thank you for your interesting letter of 8th June 1985.

We have had a long talk with Professor Mollison about your problem and we
have both come to the conclusion that it is not logical in your population
to type for D when E-typing and c-typing are not done.  The same applies
to anti-Rh(D) immunoglobulin (Rhogam) administration as there is no
anti-Rh(E) or anti-Rh(c) immunoglobulin available.  Your problem (or "non
problem") with D is less than our problem with K and c and yet we do not
type antenatal patients for K and c.  My conscience is quite clear when I
give you this advice that it is ethical to discontinue routine (Rh(D)
typing of recipients and antenatal patients.  I agree with you that you
should selectively test "a proportion" of your donors for Rh(D), Rh(E),
Rh(c), Fya, Jka, Jkb in order to have "antigen negative" blood available
for patients with atypical red cell antibodies in need of transfusion.
We always have "phenotyped" blood on our shelves to supply the needs of
screened blood for prospective recipients with alloantibodies.  However,
if you know of an unsensitized Rh negative antenatal patient, you should
give Rhogam.  Also, caucasians who are pregnant or need blood transfusion
in Taiwan should be Rh(D) typed.

I was glad to hear that Wellcome will help with the shipment of specimens
on ice.

I shall send you the results of the transferase studies in the very near
future.  We shall send the reagents as soon as they are all ready; at
present we are very short of staff in Dr. Lubenko's lab. as one Senior
Scientific Officer is pregnant and a Scientific Officer has just left.

With best wishes,

                                  Yours sincerely,



                                  Dr. Marcela Contreras
                                  Director
```

北倫敦血液中心主任 M. Contreras 的來函，他也贊同台灣不需要做輸血前 Rh 的篩檢

163

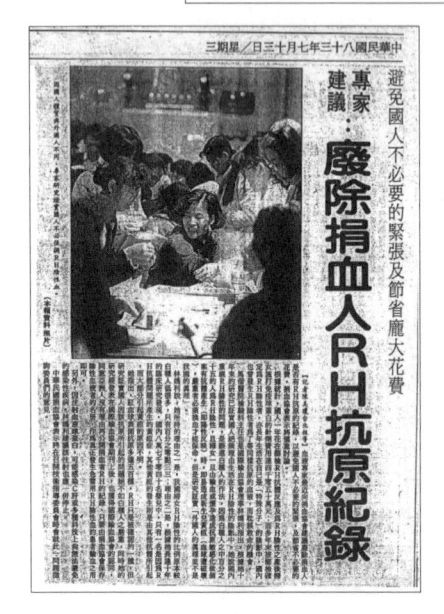

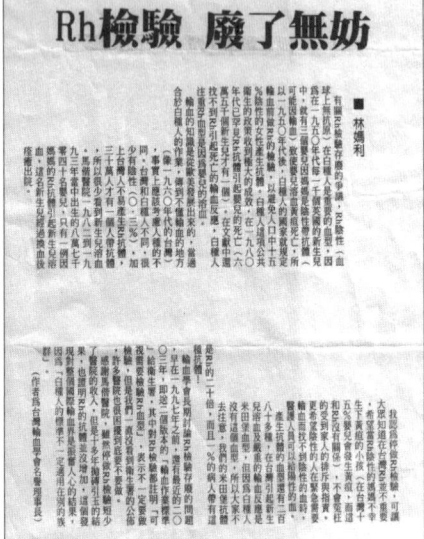

Rh 血型篩檢爭議的相關報導及媒體投書

附件 4

捐血運動 50 週年貢獻獎及得獎感言 [1]

1981 年我結束在美國四年的訓練回到台灣後，被邀到馬偕醫院檢驗科工作，因為當時人事的問題，以致只在血庫工作。發現當時血庫的工作主要是抽血牛的血，這跟我在美國受訓時全部輸血來自自願捐血，在輸血的安全上有很大的落差。另外，當時醫院輸血的作業也太過簡單，以致可能發生危險，讓我不知如何是好。

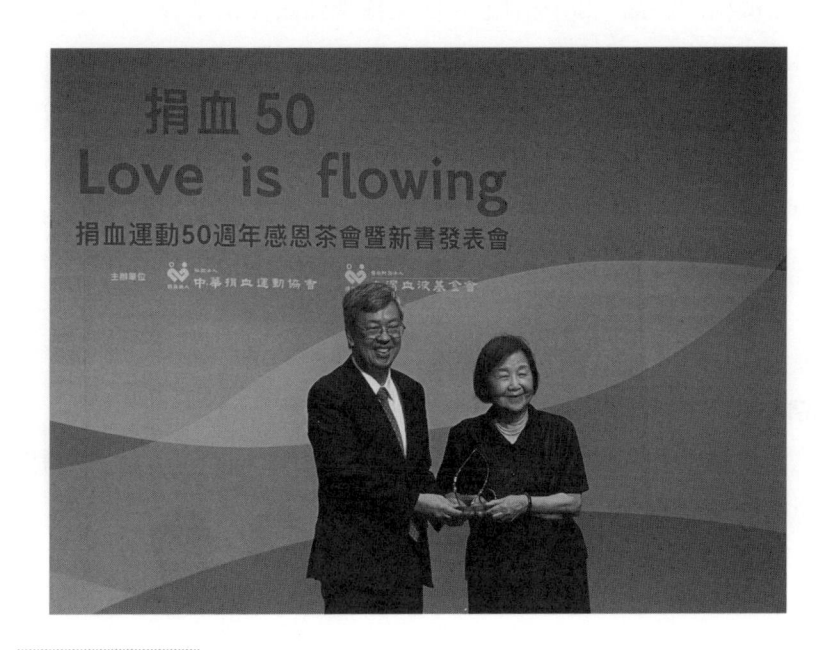

---

[1] 發表於 2024 年 6 月 14 日台灣血液基金會及中華捐血運動協會舉辦感恩茶會暨 50 週年紀念新書發表會。

沒想到，1983年英國的輸血專家同時也是宣教師鮑博瑞先生，在英國家中祈禱時，上帝呼召他到台灣台北馬偕醫院血庫工作，於是最好的同工由天而降，我開始和鮑先生在馬偕醫院進行台灣血型的研究，後因發現許多台灣特有的血型而名噪國際；以及研究尋找最適合台灣的輸血作業而受到國際的肯定。我另一方面同時回應時任衛生署署長許子秋的邀請，參與衛生署的國家血液政策──「用血全部來自捐血，整頓醫院的輸血作業」。我和後來成立的輸血學會會員，包括孫建峰醫師、李正華醫師等，還有衛生署的長官，一起先後進行全台血庫工作人員的在職訓練，也在馬偕醫院血庫成立全台血庫諮詢實驗室，再經過全台醫院及捐血機構的評鑑、隨後制定的作業標準及設置標準等，一步步把捐血及醫院輸血作業導入正軌，這個過程經過了八年。

　　台灣在1992年醫療用血全部來自自願無償捐血，所以台灣在1992年成為沒有血牛的國家。台灣的成就受到國際的肯定，在1996年，著名的輸血月刊把台灣放在全球15個優良輸血的國家之中，與英、美、德、法等國並列。

　　感謝上帝帶領我們完成了這個重要的工作，這個力量是來自每星期一早上和鮑先生一起的禱告，我們把所有的困難排列在上帝的前面，然後重新得力。

　　回顧過去看到上帝的帶領，也感謝使用我們參與了這個重要的工作。

附件 5

2003 年 SARS 期間，我們發現台灣人帶有使 SARS 病人容易轉重症基因的論文，引起國際的重視及評論

自然醫學〔編輯評論〕
(*Nature Medicine*, Vol. 9, no.11, November 2003)

台灣科學家發現基因與 SARS 的關聯性

　　一群台灣的研究者報導說，免疫系統上的某項基因變異，可能導致某一類人較容易染上 SARS。

　　台北馬偕醫院的血液學者林媽利表示，人類白血球抗原 HLA 第一型內的某些基因類型，與嚴重的 SARS 感染有所關聯。

　　林醫師和她的研究團隊抽取了 65 位疑似感染 SARS 的患者的血液檢體（當中的 37 位極可能感染 SARS），將之與 101 位置身於高風險環境、但並未感染 SARS 的醫護人員做比較。他們也以 190 位健康、無關的台灣人的 HLA 資料做為對照組。

　　他們發現，帶有 HLA-B*4601 基因型的人，最可能因染上 SARS 而死亡（參見 *BMC Med. Genet.* 4; 2003）。那 37 位極可能染上 SARS 的患者當中，15 位帶有 HLA-B*4601，而且，將當中 5 位最嚴重的患者與對照組比較時，發現他們帶有 HLA-B*4601 的機率顯著較高。HLA 系統通常是用於研究傳染性疾病的原因或自

體免疫疾病。

大約10%的台灣人身上帶有HLA-B*4601，其他亞洲地區，如中國南方沿海、香港、新加坡及越南部分地區的民眾身上，也可以發現這一基因，而這些地區正是遭SARS嚴重肆虐的地區。相對的，約佔台灣總人口1.5%的原住民，就跟白種人和非洲人一樣，極少帶有HLA-B*4601。

研究人員表示，此一研究結果解釋了SARS的疫情中心為何出現在中國南方。此一發現也與台灣的疫情相符：尚未有原住民染上SARS的案例。這可能也解釋了何以大部分的白種人並未染上SARS，但多倫多是個例外，因為那裡有大量的亞洲移民。

林媽利建議說，為了避免SARS擴散開來，應該要對醫護人員進行篩檢，看看他們身上是否帶有HLA-B*4601。但其他的科學家則對此持疑，認為該項研究的檢體數太小，不足以推論出這項結論。

台灣的國衛院研究員Yuh-Shan Jou表示，「現在談大規模篩檢還言之過早」，「因為林媽利的研究中，並沒有其他遭SARS肆虐地區的數據，所以她的結論還不夠堅強。」

華爾街日報（*The Wall Street Journal*, Wed., Oct. 1, 2003）

研究顯示基因可能揭開 SARS 之謎

　　台灣的科學家表示，他們已找到證據來支持一項令人驚訝、雖是暫時性的假說：SARS 對於帶有某項基因的人們較具致命性，而 10%-15% 的南方漢人的後代帶有這項基因。

　　台北馬偕醫院的研究人員分析了感染 SARS 者及健康者的基因檢體，這些研究對象皆居住在台灣。這項研究的規模過小，還稱不上是決定性的研究，因此這些研究者將他們的發現視為進一步研究的起點，而非重大的科學突破。

　　但如果進一步的研究支持他們的假說，這就可能大大地推進科學家對於 SARS 及其傳播的理解。若出現進一步的研究來確認此項假說，屆時醫護人員可能就要接受基因篩檢，以得知哪些人具有較高的感染風險，所以當往後 SARS 再度席捲而來時，這些醫護人員就得離開 SARS 病房。

　　這篇通過審查、刊登在 *BMC Medical Genetics*（一份線上的生物醫學研究期刊）的論文的作者們表示，他們做這項研究的主要動機，就是希望能設計一套基因篩檢制度，讓醫護人員能免於 SARS 之害。實際上幾乎從未有過這類的基因篩檢制度。一旦要創建此項制度，許多通常只在學院裡討論的倫理問題和法律問題，便會逐一浮上檯面。

　　今（2003）年 5 月，當世界上首次爆發的 SARS 疫情仍肆虐之際，馬偕醫院的研究人員提出了這項研究想法。該院由林媽利醫師領軍的輸血醫學研究室，多年來收集了大量的人類白血球抗

原 HLA 基因的資料，HLA 在人體免疫系統方面扮演了重要的角色。

　　HLA 基因的組合方式因人而異。近年來，許多研究將 HLA 的差異與個人對疾病的不同反應做了聯結。例如，目前已有證據顯示，帶有某些 HLA 基因者較不易染上痲瘋、結核病及人體免疫缺乏症病毒，然而，帶有其他 HLA 基因者則較易受感染。林媽利醫師───一位臨床病理學家───在某次訪問中表示，她想看看能否在 SARS 患者的身上找到相似的機制。

　　SARS 似乎主要在中國南方、台灣、香港、北越和新加坡等地傳播，此一現象令林醫師印象深刻。根據先前的研究，她知道某些特殊的 HLA 基因在這些地區的居民身上相對普遍（這似乎是這些居民具有某些共同遠祖的外在跡象），而這些基因在全球其他地區的居民身上卻很罕見。

　　林醫師及其同事收集了當地 37 位 SARS 患者及三組對照組（未受感染的民眾，共 319 位）的血液，並從血液檢體中抽取 DNA，篩檢是否帶有特殊 HLA 基因。

　　結果令他們大為震驚。該項研究中有六位最嚴重的 SARS 患者，他們在其中五位的身上發現了一種稱作 HLA-B46 的基因。這六位患者都需要使用人工呼吸器，而且最後只有一人倖存。林醫師表示，此一發現「在統計上是顯著的」，因為只有約 10%-15% 的台灣人身上帶有這項基因。她說，因為該研究中的嚴重案例幾乎全帶有 HLA-B46，所以這應該不能用巧合來加以解釋。

　　這一發現也指出了基因與較高的 SARS 感染性之間可能有所關聯。雖然該項研究中的 SARS 患者並沒有全都帶有 HLA-B46，但 12 位 SARS 患者身上帶有 HLA-B46，也就是說，HLA-B46 出

現在SARS患者身上的機率，是出現在未受感染者身上的兩倍。

林醫師表示，「此一基因似乎與SARS的感染率有關，但我們需要多一點的檢體」來確認這項發現。「我真的希望能有人在中國、香港做研究來驗證我的假說，澄清當中的關聯。」林醫師說，HLA-B46出現在中國南方、新加坡、北越及香港民眾身上的比率，大致上與台灣人相似，但這一基因卻極少出現在非洲人及白種人身上。

衛生當局表示，現在要歡呼「SARS基因」的發現還言之過早。世界衛生組織的發言人Dick Thompson不願評論這項研究，他表示，「我們現在剛對SARS有初步的瞭解」，該項研究「可能為我們指出一條有用的研究方向，我們得探索所有的途徑才行」。

塞普勒斯大學（University of Cyprus）的分子生物學家Leondios Kostrikis——他之前曾發表過病患基因與HIV病毒之關聯的研究——表示，台灣的研究看來在科學上是成立的。Kostrikis博士說，「我想它的檢體數足以推論出該項科學假說」，「看看加拿大和其他地區的研究會得出什麼結果，應該是很有趣的。」

當然，即使該項基因真的會影響染上SARS的機率和嚴重性，同樣清楚的是，缺乏該項基因的人還是有染上SARS的可能。最初一批死於SARS的患者中，就有一位義大利人：Carlo Urbani，他是世界衛生組織的醫師。世界上有30個國家爆發了SARS案例。多倫多最早的一批SARS案例中，有一位具有華人血統的婦女，她於2月期間到香港旅遊時，在京華酒店遭到感染。她返回多倫多之後，另一位親人也住院治療，結果，SARS就在各種不同種族的病人、醫護人員和訪客之間快速蔓延開來。

一些科學家已準備要繼續研究這項假說。香港大學的 SARS 專家 K.Y. Yuen 表示,「我們目前還沒有這項資料,但我們會開始進行研究,看看如何確認或推翻這一假說。」

美國有線電視新聞網（CNN, 2003/10/1）

基因突變可能可以解釋 SARS

　　台灣的研究者在本週發表研究報告，認為去（2002）年 SARS 在東南亞肆虐，卻沒在世界上其他地區（多倫多例外）蔓延，這一現象也許可以用基因來解釋。他們發現，某種免疫系統 HLA 的基因變異，會使台灣的 SARS 病患更容易病情加劇。台北的馬偕醫院研究團隊表示，此一基因變異在南方漢人的後裔身上很常見。他們的發現，發表在線上期刊 BMC Medical Genetics，有待其他獨立的研究者來進一步確認。但這個台灣的研究團隊表示，遺傳學可能能夠解釋去（2002）年 SARS 令人迷惑的疫情分布。他們寫道：「自從 SARS 冠狀病毒感染在中國廣東爆發之後，它的傳布方式很令人驚訝，因為它大部分侷限在南亞洲的人口之中（香港、越南、新加坡、台灣）。」

　　美國疾病控制及預防中心（U.S. Centers for Disease Control and Prevention）的感染性疾病負責人 James Hughes 博士說，基因與感染疾病之間的關係，正是他們目前正在研究的一個領域。Hughes 博士在訪問中表示，「帶有某種基因的人，可能較容易引發疾病的併發症。」

　　SARS 最初在 2002 年 11 月於廣東爆發，然後經由受感染的飛機乘客，傳到香港、台灣、越南、北京和新加坡。根據世界衛生組織的最新數據，總共有 8,098 人染上了 SARS，774 人死於 SARS。此一類似流行性感冒的疾病，是由某一種冠狀病毒所引起。冠狀病毒會使家畜生病，有些也會引發人類常見的感冒。

SARS 冠狀病毒具有獨特的基因構造，但中國肉品市場販售的動物身上，找到了幾種相似的冠狀病毒。

林媽利、黃俊雄和其他研究同仁檢視了 37 例疑似 SARS 病患、28 個感冒病患（之後排除掉感染 SARS 的可能性），以及 101 個（可能）接觸過 SARS 冠狀病毒的醫護人員。他們在上述那篇報告中寫道，「他們也用了 190 個無關的健康台灣人來當作對照組。」他們發現，嚴重的 SARS 患者可能帶有 HLA-B4601。他們指出，佔台灣總人口 1.5% 的原住民並沒有出現 SARS 病例，台灣原住民身上並沒有 HLA-B4601。他們補充說，「有趣的是，HLA-B4601 也極少在歐洲人身上看見。」

維吉尼亞大學專長流行性感冒及 SARS 的 Frederick Hayden 博士指出，需要做一個大規模、精心設計的實驗來驗證這項發現。他說，「這的確值得進一步的研究。」在華盛頓舉辦的 SARS 研討會的研究人員表示，他們不確定呼吸性疾病是否會在今年捲土重來，但他們相信應該會，因為其他的冠狀病毒都有季節性的型態。Hughes 在會議上說，「我們可能要再次面對 SARS。」

附件 6

《經濟學人》2005 年評論我們「台灣南島語族（高山原住民）母系血緣粒線體（mtDNA）B4a1a 與波里尼西亞人有直接血緣關係」的發現

經濟學人〔人類學〕（*The Economist*, July 9th 2005）

台灣人與夏威夷人是雙胞胎

波里尼西亞人是變相的台灣人

　　根據毛利人的傳說，波里尼西亞人起源自一處稱作 Hawaiki 的地方。Hawaiki 位在何處，神秘難解。但波里尼西亞人複雜的遷徙歷史——他們可能是歷史上最偉大的航海家——長期吸引著人類學性格的研究者的關注，其中的兩位學者，來自台北馬偕醫院的 Jean Trejaut（尚特鳩）和林媽利，認為他們解開了 Hawaiki 所在之謎：就是台灣。

　　這個答案並不全然出乎意料，因為語言學的證據先前也指出了這個方向。但在這篇剛發表在 *Public Library of Science Biology* 的研究中，Trejaut 博士和林媽利醫師使用現代研究的護身符——遺傳學，讓這個問題塵埃落定。

　　目前台灣有兩千三百萬人口，其中只有 40 萬是島上原住民的後裔（大部分人口是過去 400 年從中國大陸遷徙過來的人的後

裔），這40萬人使用——或者至少在歷史上曾經使用——的語言被歸類為南島語言，南島語言與漢語無關，但波里尼西亞語言也是屬於南島語言。儘管台灣原住民人口稀少，但台灣原住民的語言卻佔了南島語言十大分支中的九支，因此台灣被推測可能就是Hawaiki。

為了檢驗這個推測，Trejaut博士和林媽利醫師決定研究粒線體DNA（mitochondrial DNA）的變異性。粒線體內含DNA，稱為粒線體DNA，存在身體所有的細胞中，尤其最重要的是也在卵細胞中，在受精時，精子的粒線體並不會進入卵細胞，所以所有的人，不管男性或女性的粒線體DNA，都是來自母親，因此母系血緣的研究，可根據人類演化過程中發生的變異容易去追蹤人類遷移的途徑。其他的遺傳基因都在細胞核中，在交配時發生基因重組，以致結果顯得混亂，無法看出遷移的方向。

在一項包含9個台灣原住民族、總共640人的研究中，Trejaut博士和林媽利醫師找到了台灣原住民、波里尼西亞人、美拉尼西亞人（他們也使用南島語言）有三個共同的突變，而且這三個突變未見於其他亞洲人。看來神秘似乎被破解了。但台灣原住民來自何處，則是另一個問題了。

附錄
談悲歡人生

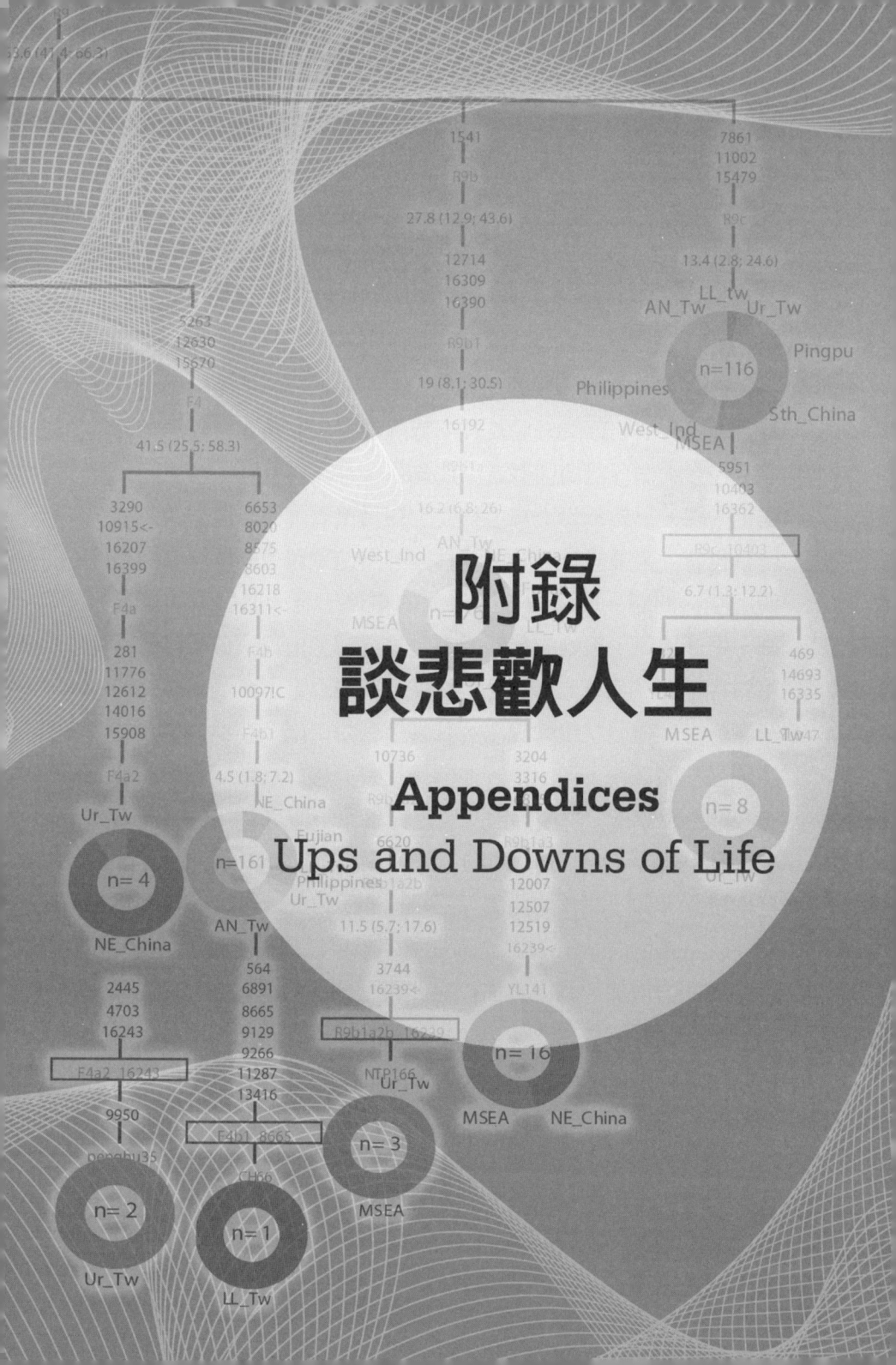

Appendices
Ups and Downs of Life

附錄 1

馬偕醫院的親子鑑定
——台灣親子鑑定檢驗工作的發展史 [1]

1988年，林媽利醫師在馬偕醫院開始了親子鑑定的服務，當時台灣還有法務部調查局及長庚醫院做這項服務。林醫師是因為之前在台大病理科的同事方中民先生，拜託林醫師去台大開親子鑑定的課，另外不少人知道林醫師在馬偕醫院從事血型的研究，所以也有人來拜託林醫師，請林醫師用血型幫他們解決家中有的親子關係問題。影響林醫師最大的事件，是一個智障的年輕媽媽，抱著嬰兒，被她的父親帶來見林醫師，他說這個智障的女兒不只找不到（被否定）嬰兒的父親，還被否定了自己跟嬰兒的母子關係。據這個父親的說法，其實這一對媽媽及嬰兒有真正的母子關係。因為親子鑑定是一件關係社會公義的檢驗工作，需要有人去關心及協助，林醫師因此決定從事親子鑑定。

在1980年代，大家都還不清楚在親子鑑定的檢驗項目中，什麼叫排除非親子關係的能力（power of exclusion, PE），及多項檢驗（Cumulative power of exclusion, CPE）可以讓在非親子關係時使排除的能力增加，且在無法排除非親子關係的時候，這位先生當這個小孩父親的機會有多少（Probability of paternity, PP）。林醫師在1988年之前，一開始除了找資料研究之外，還派陸中衡到

---

[1] 林媽利按：為敘述方便，本篇採第三人稱寫作。

UCLA 的 Dr. Terasaki 的實驗室做短期進修，同時也參考美國血庫協會出版的「親子鑑定」專書。陸中衡設計出一個相當複雜的計算方式。在 1988 年，馬偕醫院開始的親子鑑定已是做多項血型檢驗，隨即加入 HLA 系統及紅血球酵素 PGM1 系統，希望用這三項系統，可以把 99% 以上非親子關係的案例看出來。其實當時這些系統的累積排除的能力（CPE）已到 93.43%，但在最初的幾個案例，就遇到無法排除親子關係的個案，這個案就耗掉林醫師半天到一天的時間計算 PP，經由上述複雜的計算，才把這位先生當真正父親的機會 PP 算出來。因為台灣人血型相似的情形多，所以 PP 常無法很高，但當時有部分個案可來到 98.9%。那時，曾經在台大微生物學科當講師的謝秀花老師跑來幫忙，她看林醫師算得那麼辛苦，就請她先生幫忙設計了一個計算 PP 的電腦程式，所以接下來林醫師就很快得到了許多案例的 PP。後來這個計算 PP 的電腦程式，經過輸血學會舉辦的在職訓練流傳，被廣泛的用在很多台灣醫院的親子鑑定工作上。PP 的計算電腦化以後，在馬偕醫院排隊做親子鑑定的案例，就從要等半年變成一個月。然後經過在輸血學會推動會員做親子鑑定及教授計算的方法，一下子就有好多醫院及生技公司做起親子鑑定了，2000 年代可以說是親子鑑定的全盛時代。2000 年左右，每年全台約有 3,000 件的親子鑑定檢查，大概一半是大陸來台依親的個案。林醫師忙著各處演講親子鑑定，不只在醫院及醫學院，也曾經在台大法律系講課，甚至到法務部調查局，2000 年代林醫師做了好幾年法務部的顧問。

1992 年，馬偕醫院自紐西蘭紅十字會血液中心引進 DNA 的方法，最開始是用耗時的 RFLP-VNTR 法，把 CPE 提高到

99.76%，1998 年被 PCR-VNTR 法取代，最後 1999 年被快速簡易的 PCR-STR 所取代，這時的 CPE 99.9%，PP 至少 99.99% 以上。CPE 99.9% 的意思，是說在非親子關係時，有 99.9% 的機會被看出至少某一項檢驗結果不合而否定親子關係。PP 99.99% 的意思，是說如果是親子關係時，這個父親當真正父親的機會，是隨便一個男人的 10,000 倍。馬偕醫院的親子鑑定，歷年的案例中，約有 1/3 的案例被排除親子關係。因很多醫院做親子鑑定檢查，馬偕醫院在 2000 年以後就不需要排隊，預約就可以做到親子鑑定了。

Paternity Testing in Mackay Memorial Hospital (1999年)
Lin M, Chang SL, Loo JH, Chu CF, Chu CC
Immunohematology Reference Laboratory, Mackay Memorial Hospital, Taipei, Taiwan

Mackay Memorial Hospital (MMH) began paternity testing in 1988. Initally the item tested included RBC'S phenotyping for ABO, Rh, MNSs, P1, Kidd, Duffy and MiIII, and HLA class I phenotyping. Phenotyping for the RBC's enzyme PGM1 was also introduced. However, since the cumulative power of exclusion (CPE) estimated by calculation was only 95% and also because among 40% of cases of non-exclusion the probably of paternity of alleged father was less than 99%, DNA polymorphism testing of RFLP-VNTR (three loci D7S104, D21S112 and D1S47) was introduced in 1992. The observed PE for RFLP-VNTR was found to be 0.98 (estimated PE 0.95), however, higher delta value of 3.09% for D7S104 and 2.51% for both D21S112 and D1S47 with the subsequence of relative lower PI as compared with PCR-STR method was found. The mutation rate for D21S112 locus was 0.483% (2/414), no mutation was found in other 2 loci. Almost all paternity index (PI) value were greater than 99 when RFLP-VNTR was used in conjunction with ABO grouping and HLA class I phenotyping. The observed CPE value (ABO, HLA and DNA) was then 0.9976. Since 1998 RFLP-VNTR DNA polymorphism test was replaced by PCR-VNTR test (three loci D17S5, D1S80 and Apo-B gene), and during 1998 having 76 cases of paternity testing was performed. The observed PE for PCR-VNTR was 0.9474 (estimated PE 0.9736), and the observed CPE value was 0.9975 (estimated CPE 0.9953) when conjunction with ABO grouping and HLA class I phenotyping. In July 1999, PCR-VNTR test was finally replaced by PCR-STR test. Of 535 cases of paternity testing at MMH during the period 1988-1998, 179 cases were excluded as non-father, with an exclusion frequency of 33.5%. For nonexcluded cases, when tested for ABO group, HLA-class I (occationally class II) and RFLP-VNTR or PCR-VNTR, both PE and PI value was acceptable.

親子鑑定 (2000-2001)

馬偕紀念醫 林媽利

親子鑑定是藉著測試遺傳的標誌(記號)，如血型、DNA 等，來看雙親與小孩的關係，一般是測父親(設定父親)與小孩的關係。例如雙親的血型都是 O 型，就不該有 B 型的小孩，所以當母子的關係確定時，設定父親就被排除(否定)。但因 ABO 血型的變異不大，所以在非親子關係時可否定的機會(Power of Exclusion)在台灣只有 19%，所以在尚無 DNA 的時代主要是靠 HLA(組織抗原)排除，其 PE 可達 81%，所以再增加多項其他血型的測試，可將 PE 累積(CPE) 到 96%。另一方面當設定父親無法被否定時，就要計算設定父親當真正父親(生父)的機會有多少，稱 PI 值(Power of Inclusion)，當小孩從設定父親遺傳到在台灣較少見的標誌時，PI 值升高，當多項標誌 PI 的累積結果(CPI)達到 95(即設定父親當小孩父親的機會是隨便一個人該小孩父親機會的 95 倍)時，即使再增加別的標誌，設定父親被否定的機會應減少，這時設定父親當真正父親的機會是 95/95+1=95/96=98.958%。但親子鑑定最主要的精神在於經由變化多端的遺傳標誌而看出非親子的關係，即否定非生父的關係。近年來 DNA 被應用在親子鑑定上，經過幾次方法上的改進，現在已可以在短時間內大量的測試每個人在不同染色體上(至少 13 個染色體上)鹼基(DNA) 短片段的重複次數(STR)，因每個人都有成對的鹼基短片段，一個自父親另一個自母親，所以特定重複的次數也直接得自父母，因每個 STR 基因位上因著不同的人可出現不同次數的重複，所以同時測 13 個不同染色體基因位上 STR 不同重複的次數，而看設定父親的每個 STR 的重複次數是否和小孩的相同，因此 STR 變成強有力鑑定親子關係的方法，CPE 達到 99.9%，CPI 常達百萬，也就是設定父親的機會是隨便一個人的 100 萬倍。
親子鑑定在 20 年前只有在法務部調查局做，每年約 10-30 個案，馬偕醫院

自 77 年開始受理親子鑑定的檢查，當時除法務部調查局外尚有長庚醫院做這項檢查，馬偕醫院自 77 年到 81 年 5 月共做 90 個案的親子鑑定。當時做這項檢查的原因有父親懷疑不是自己的小孩，鑑定私生子的父親，認祖歸宗、報戶口，及懷疑抱錯小孩 (3 個案)，其中以父親懷疑不是自己的小孩為首要原因。

最近台灣每年約有 3000 件的親子鑑定檢查，其中大概有一半是大陸來台依親的個案。統計馬偕醫院最近 100 個案(89 年 6 月到 90 年 8 月)的親子鑑定中首要原因為婚姻中母親的婚姻外小孩(即生母婚外情所生子女)的認定(認祖歸宗)，共 40 個案，如下表：

在馬偕醫院做親子鑑定的原因

89 年 6 月-90 年 8 月 100 個案分析

分類	案數	小計(案數)
生母婚外情所生子女的認定(小孩一歲以內)	16	40
生母婚外情所生子女的認定(小孩一歲以上)	24*	
母親之婚姻情況不明，但否定親子關係	5	5
母親未婚生子，無法否定設定父親(小孩一歲以內)	3	12
母親未婚生子，無法否定設定父親(小孩一歲以上)	6	
母親未婚生子，但否定設定父親(小孩一歲以上)	3	
父親懷疑，但無否定親子關係(小孩一歲以內)	1	12
父親懷疑，但否定親子關係(小孩一歲以上)	11	
大陸來台依親	25	31
領養	1	
更正戶口	5	

*其中 4 例是因法定父親懷疑而做鑑定

附錄 2

「讓二二八受難者遺骸找到回家的路」
工作始末（2011-2019）[1]

　　二二八事件的發生，不僅造成族群撕裂，政治動盪，更造成數以萬計的台灣人無辜犧牲。由於死傷者眾，以及當時實施連坐株連的高壓統治，至今這些人的骸骨，仍然無法回歸家庭，只能散落各處，有的甚至尚未列管。為了安慰遺族、減少社會對立、撫平國家傷痕，尋找二二八受難者的遺骸，並將之歸回家族，是關心台灣的有志之士所共有的心願。馬偕紀念醫院的林媽利醫師，秉持其一生在輸血醫學及親子鑑定、古代DNA研究之專業，透過二二八基金會（附件A）與馬偕紀念醫院的支持，希望能對二二八受難家屬與二二八受難者遺骸進行親子關係配對，藉由此項服務，希望讓二二八受難家屬的心能夠逐漸回復平安，國人的心能夠逐漸放下對立的高牆。

　　這項計畫須完成的工作，將包含（1）從二二八受難者的遺骸中萃取DNA；（2）從二二八受難家屬中採取檢體萃取DNA；（3）從（1）及（2）建立資料庫並相互比較，以期達成骨骸歸回家族之目標。其中，DNA檢測的內容，包括1) 體染色體STR；2) 父系血緣Y-STR；3) 母系血緣粒線體DNA。

　　近年來，馬偕醫院分子人類學實驗室完成了很多台灣人的溯

---

[1] 林媽利按：為敘述方便，本篇採第三人稱寫作。

源檢查以後，讓林醫師想起她父親臨終的遺願：「尋找二二八遇難的朋友林茂生教授的遺骸」，希望尋找二二八受難者的遺骸，並將之歸回家族。林醫師先跟林茂生教授的女兒林詠梅女士聯絡，拿到她的血液檢體，不久也拿到她弟弟的檢體，後來就有從美國回來的幾個受難家屬，陸續來存放血液檢體。林媽利醫師是台灣輸血醫學的先驅，也是台灣第一位發展親子鑑定作業的醫界人士。後來從二十一世紀開始，林醫師再開始一系列的台灣族群血緣的研究，並在2006年開始古代DNA的研究。

實驗室主持人林媽利醫師，於2012年中，即積極規劃二二八受難家屬與二二八受難者遺骸配對計畫。由於二二八受難者遺骸存留之DNA，相較於現生DNA可能太少，相較於古代DNA卻又過多，處理時需規劃另一適當之處所才行，經林醫師積極爭取，馬偕紀念醫院於該年12月底，正式核准近代DNA實驗室之建置，該實驗室比照古代DNA實驗室之規劃，配備正壓調節系統，於2013年完工，相關儀器設備已添購完竣，在淡水馬偕醫院的舊大樓，成立一個專屬做遺骸DNA的實驗室：「近代DNA實驗室」，希望將可能是二二八受難者遺骸（1顆牙或1小塊骨）的DNA萃取、定出序列，再與許多家屬的資料比對，鑑定出遺骸的身份，讓二二八受難者遺骸回家，以安慰死者、家屬及社會。

林醫師積極的和二二八基金會聯繫（附件A），在2014年寫了一個三年經費310,000元的10年計劃（2014-2024年）：「二二八受難家屬與二二八受難者遺骸配對計劃」（附件B），向二二八基金會申請，最後沒有結果。

DNA被應用在個人身份的鑑定上後，俄國尼可拉二世的遺骸被找到（*Nature Genetics* 1994; 6: 130-135），諾曼第許多無名英雄

塚的墓碑上出現名字，本實驗室也已成功把 3,000 多年前遺骸的 DNA 序列定出來。林醫師多次請媒體報導，呼籲受難家屬來馬偕醫院存放血液，也上過民視政論節目呼籲，2015 年也受邀到美國 Orange County 的 FAPA 年會演講呼籲（附件 C），但是效果非常有限。有一年的二二八紀念日，團隊到二二八紀念館去擺攤，結果只有一個人來詢問，但是他後來並沒有來馬偕醫院存放血液。2017 年二二八的 70 週年紀念日，團隊到二二八公園擺攤，共有三個人來抽血。（附件 D）

因為林醫師的父親說過，林茂生教授遺骸可能埋在六張犁山上，所以林醫師在 2016 年 11 月 14 日，和洪維健導演、蔡心女士、馬偕工作人員陸中衡和黃錦源等人上山，除了林醫師在亂葬崗摔了一跤以外，並沒有看出什麼。不久，林醫師家人病重，她需要去照顧，所以沒有多餘的心力再繼續從事二二八的工作。另外，馬偕團隊從 2013 年到 2017 年，只收集到共 11 個家屬的血液檢驗，讓馬偕團隊失去了繼續下去的勇氣。收集到的 11 件家屬的血液檢體，其中 6 件是女兒在尋找父親，3 件是兒子找父親，一件是甥兒找舅舅，另一件是姪兒找叔叔。2019 年，馬偕醫院團隊決定先把 DNA 檢測結果送法醫研究所比對，經林醫師和這 11 位家屬聯繫，只得到其中 5 位寄回同意書，同意馬偕醫院把檢測 DNA 的結果送法務部法醫研究所，檢體檢測的項目含：體染色體 STR、母系血緣 mtDNA、父系血緣 Y-STR 及 Y-SNP。送到法務部法醫研究所，和無名屍的檔案比對，結果沒有找到成功的配對，後來才知道，法醫研究所現有的無名屍只是近 20 年找到的，而二二八事件是早在 70 年前的事，所以找不到配對是可以了解的。（附件 E）

上述工作經驗，讓馬偕團隊深深的感受到二二八的恐怖和陰影，還是深植於台灣島上居民的心中，而且可能的遺骸，即使找到，只有檢察官可以處理，且要經過所有家屬同意、當地縣政府同意，以及二二八基金會同意，才可以去研究比對（附件 A）。這些層層的管制，將阻止研究，呼籲政府相關單位，應該讓後來的研究者較容易取得受難者遺骸的片斷，最好是像越南、韓國及法國，由政府單位做這項工作。衷心期盼以後有人接下去做，讓台灣的社會公義得以伸張，讓二二八的靈魂得到安息，讓二二八受難者家屬的苦難記憶得以平復，讓台灣的社會變得更祥和。

附件 A ｜與二二八基金會會議摘要

林媽利醫師與 228 基金會陳士魁董事長會談希望基金會同意資助本院(林媽利醫師所屬之醫研部輸血醫學組)作 228 受難家屬與 228 受難者遺骸之配對工作

時間：2013 年 12 月 18 日上午 9:00~10:15
地點：台北市徐州路 5 號 16 樓僑務委員會
出席人員：228 基金會董事長陳士魁、228 基金會執行長廖繼斌、本院林媽利醫師、陸中衡助研究員
紀錄：陸中衡助研究員

林媽利醫師：介紹自己的背景：以前的研究項目，包括親子鑑定、父母系血緣檢查、古代 DNA 的研究，因此認為有能力可以為 228 受難家屬與 228 受難者遺骸作配對工作。同時因為朋友及親人的關係，希望這項工作可以安慰現存之 228 受難家屬，及撫平國家社會因為 228 事件所留下的傷痛。林醫師便開始用所帶來的資料向陳董事長說明這項任務該怎樣完成。

林媽利醫師：待解決問題 1，做無名遺骸的 DNA 檢測是否只需要受難者家屬委託即可，還需要檢察官的參與嗎？
陳士魁董事長：因為有牽涉到無名屍的遺骸，檢察官就一定會涉入成立一個無名屍個案，這是無法避免的。
林媽利醫師：228 受難者的遺骸在哪裡？
廖繼斌執行長：目前 228 受難者的遺骸主要存在雲林及嘉義的納骨塔裡面。因為當初那兩個地方有許多 228 受難者死在那邊，遺骸都混在一起，分不出來個人的遺骸。後來政府好不容易將遺骸分成一具一具，便放在當地的納骨塔中，每年由基金會出錢作法事，以紀念他們的犧牲。所以若要打開納骨塔拿出骨骸做檢查，必須 1)所有家屬同意；2)當地縣政府同意；3)228 董事會同意，因此有一定的難度。所以若要做遺骸的 DNA，除非找到目前仍是散在各地尚未列管的 228 受難者遺骸，與受難者家屬做比對才行。

林媽利醫師：待解決問題 2，家屬個人 DNA 資料的保管。
陳士魁董事長：我很贊同 228 受難家屬的 DNA 資料由馬偕醫院保管。

林媽利醫師：待解決問題 3，經費的問題。
陳士魁董事長：由於馬偕醫院已經建立好實驗室，基金會這邊比較沒有立場向內政部申請經費來籌備實驗室，因為不符合採購程序。而且若是由基金會付錢購買儀器或裝修實驗室，這就會變成基金會的財產，將來管理起來會很複雜。最好的方式是由基金會向民間募款來支付這筆費用。陳董事長再與本院楊院長溝通細節。至於骨骸檢體、家屬檢體的檢驗費用，請林醫師實驗室提出專案研究(業務)計畫，我們好向內政部及董事會報請核可。我們希望馬偕做這個動作，因為若是由政府

來做(228基金會為公設財團法人，屬內政部轄管)，家屬會認為政府又在騙人、耍陰謀。家屬信任馬偕、信任林醫師，我們樂觀其成。我認為這是一個很值得作的計畫。

陳士魁董事長：由於228事件對許多家屬而言仍是非常敏感的一件事。所以馬偕若要做此服務，請工作人員對家屬的感受更富同理心。

散會

院長：

副院長：

醫研部主任：

林媽利醫師：

紀錄：

附件 B │「二二八受難家屬與二二八受難者遺骸配對計劃」專題研究計畫申請書

專題研究計畫申請書

一、基本資料：

本計劃名稱	中文	二二八受難家屬與二二八受難者遺骸配對計劃
	英文	
計劃主持人姓名	林媽利	職稱 名譽顧問醫師 身分證編號 XXXXXXXXXX
申請單位	馬偕紀念醫院醫學研究部
執行期限	民國 103 年 8 月 1 日起至民國 113 年 7 月 31 日
計畫類型	A類：□基礎研究 ■應用研究 □技術研究 B類：□前導型 □一般型 □啟發型 □鼓勵型 □輔導型 ■專案型 　　　□ 創作品研發
計畫聯絡人	姓名：陸中衡　　電話：(02)28094661 轉 2384
計畫執行地點	馬偕淡水分院醫研部輸血醫學組

核示	申請人簽章
	日期：
核示結果：□ 通過　□不通過	
金額：　　貳佰零拾陸萬元/每年	

二、申請補助經費：

1. 請將本計劃申請書之研究業務費用填入「其他研究有關費用」欄內。
2. 「小計」欄內請填入上述各項費用之總和，「總計」欄內則為「小計」欄與「研究人力費」之加總。

補助項目	第一年申請補助經費
研究人力費	元
研究設備費	元
其他研究有關費用	耗材費 310,000 元 管理費 10,000 元
小　　計	新台幣參拾貳萬元
中型儀器設備費	0 元
總　　計	新台幣參拾貳萬元

補助項目	第二年申請補助經費
研究人力費	550,000 元
研究設備費	
其他研究有關費用	耗材費 310,000 元 管理費 10,000 元
小　　計	新台幣捌拾柒萬元
中型儀器設備費	0 元
總　　計	新台幣捌拾柒萬元

補助項目	第三年申請補助經費
研究人力費	550,000 元
研究設備費	0 元
其他研究有關費用	耗材費 310,000 元 管理費 10,000 元
小　　計	新台幣捌拾柒萬元
中型儀器設備費	0 元
總　　計	新台幣捌拾柒萬元

三、參與研究人員資料：

姓名	服務機關系所	職稱
Jean A. Trejaut	馬偕紀念醫院醫學研究部	專業副研究員
陸中衡	馬偕紀念醫院醫學研究部	助研究員
王澤毅	馬偕紀念醫院醫學研究部	專業研究員
黃錦源	馬偕紀念醫院醫學研究部	研究助理
陳宗賢	馬偕紀念醫院醫學研究部	助研究員
賴穎慧	馬偕紀念醫院醫學研究部	研究助理
李宛蓉	馬偕紀念醫院醫學研究部	研究助理

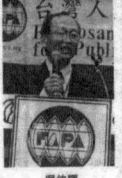

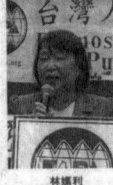

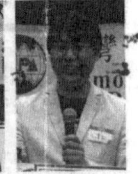

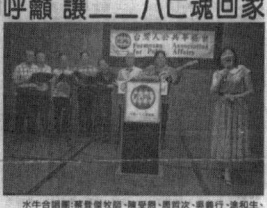

附件 C ｜ 在美國 Orange County 的 FAPA 年會演講的報導

附件 D ｜到二二八公園擺攤宣傳的文件

「讓二二八受難者遺骸回家」草案 12013

前言

「記憶」對每一個人都是重要的：憑著記憶我們憶起過去美好的時光，遙去的人事物又鮮亮的出現在我們腦中，那個人，那件事塑造著我們的生命。可是在我們有限的回憶中，有些回憶甚至會讓我們似見過世界，讓我們疑問為什麼 上帝會允許這件事情發生？

六十九年前的二二八事件以及隨後四五0年代的白色恐怖給台灣人民非常慘酷的回憶：許多逃過險的台灣菁英因為反抗政權統治或發表異議言論而遭到逮捕、殺害；家屬破碎、社會瀰漫恐懼氣氛，台灣人民多數位服於那樣的統治以為自身換來人的生存。那許多二二八受難者家屬而言，他們無法接受自己失去家人的理由，他們甚至無法尋找親人屍體，讓自己記憶中那個家人的身形永遠祕藏妥妥善安置，沒想到只是：一群諫求彩利的買辦。

因此，「讓二二八受難者遺骸回家」對新政府來說「轉型正義」尤其重要：
1. 讓二二八受難者家屬的苦難記憶得以平慰、個人生命可以展現的一頁。
2. 台灣人民可以拒絕過去政權政權的影響，做自己國家的主人。
3. 向國際社會揭發過去政權危害人權的不合法性，並展現新政府的政治能力，帶領台灣走向新的歷史新章。

馬偕醫院林媽利醫師研究團隊從 2011 年開始籌備「讓二二八受難者遺骸回家」相關工作，並於 2013 年 2 月 15 日獲得馬偕醫院的首肯完成為設計計畫所設計的專門實驗室，林媽利醫師以其 30 年的親子鑑定實驗以及分析經驗，再加上 15 年研究台灣族群的血緣（父母系及組織抗原）的專業知識及台灣族群血緣資料庫，近年更延聘基因體研究的博士研究人員，足以擔當「讓二二八受難者遺骸回家」計畫的重責大任。林醫師團隊並由近年的 4500 年前的大坌坑遺址中的遺骸確定出該遺骸的母系血緣。因此由相對近代骨骸中萃取 DNA，並檢測其 DNA 標記，對林醫師團隊來說，並不困難。

作法
1. 研究團隊一：由林媽利醫師帶領的馬偕紀念醫院分子人類學研究團隊
    研究團隊二：由李俊億教授帶領的台大法醫研究所研究團隊
    團隊三：二二八受難家屬代表
2. 由團隊三：二二八受難家屬代表向國家申請尋求可能之二二八受難者遺骸作 DNA 檢驗
3. 由團隊三：二二八受難家屬代表請二二八受難家屬至馬偕醫院留下 DNA 檢體
4. 研究團隊二：受難者遺骸 DNA 檢驗
5. 研究團隊一：做二二八受難家屬 DNA 檢驗
6. 由研究團隊一做受難家屬與遺骸的 DNA 比對
7. 比對結果交由新政府發表

各位二二八受難者家屬平安

時光荏苒，明年我們即將舉行「二二八事件七十周年紀念」。對於許多受難家屬而言，七十年是在忍辱負重的心情下度過。雖然政府首長曾經對事件表達歉意，但是事情的真象到目前為止依然像是曚著厚厚的一層紗。予人過多的操作空間，也因為此，受難者家屬們的心聲，因為莫衷其是的報導，公義未曾回復、平安的心依然未得，緣然新政府有心將公理正義在這個社會恢復，但是家屬們依舊惶惶不安，惟恐七十年前的悲劇再度降臨。

可是七十年對一個人而言是段很長的時間，很多長輩恐怕來日無多。為避免二二八事件的真象無法及時揭露，長輩們盼望逝去，馬偕林媽利醫師建議及諸代們能夠將 DNA 檢體留下來，這樣若將來二二八受難者遺骸可以被檢驗的時候，我們可以將遺骸與家族家訊比起來，從遺骸可以歸靠家族基因，幫助長輩們了卻心中的遺憾。在一生的苦難中安息。我們的報法是：
1. 請二二八受難者家屬留下 DNA 檢體（口腔黏膜刷棒採檢）及與受難者腦資料填寫
2. 二二八受難家屬 DNA 做粒子鑑定套組鑑定、粒線體 DNA、Y 染色體鑑定
3. 將來二二八受難遺骸開放檢驗時，將二二八受難家屬 DNA 檢驗資料予以配對

林媽利醫師團隊將於明年二月二十八日「二二八事件七十周年紀念」大會中擺攤收集各位長輩的 DNA 檢體及填寫委託檢驗的資料。如各位長輩需要提前採檢，也請先與林醫師團隊連絡（連絡電話：02-28094661 轉 2384，email: lockunhun@gmail.com，連絡人：陳中衛、陳宗餐）。以上的檢驗均為免費，所有相關費用馬偕醫院均向二二八基金會申請補助。謝謝您！

馬偕紀念醫院 林媽利醫師 敬上

委託書

本人_____（姓名）為二二八事件受難者_____（姓名）家屬_____（關係）。本人謹委託馬偕紀念醫院醫學研究部輸血醫學組採取本人血液檢體，並由該血液檢體抽取本人的遺傳物質(DNA)，進行粒線體 DNA、Y 染色體 STR (如為女性則無此項檢驗)、及體染色體 STR 的檢查工作，以建立二二八事件受難家屬遺傳標語檔案資料庫。最後再與二二八事件受難者遺骸中所得到的遺傳標語比對，如比對後查出雙方有家族關係，二二八事件受難者遺骸則可以歸回家族來埋，不再流落在外無人照顧。

委託人簽名：_____

西元_____年_____月_____日

附件 E ｜與法務部法醫研究所的聯繫文件

台灣基督長老教會馬偕醫療財團法人馬偕紀念醫院 函

機關地址：104217台北市中山區中山北路2段92號
聯絡人：張富堂28094661
分機3061
Email：bc5046@mmh.org.tw
傳 真：(02)28094679

受文者：財團法人二二八事件紀念基金會

發文日期：中華民國一〇八年三月二十日
發文字號：馬院醫研字第1070005358號
速別：普通件
密等及解密條件或保密期限：
附件：如主旨

主旨：為辦理本院輸血醫學中心主辦之「二二八受難者骨骸回家」活動，檢送有關二二八受難者家屬緘封資料一份，敬請 貴會協助轉發法務部法醫研究所，請 查照。

說明：
一、依 貴會107年10月12日(107)228參字第11070681號函及法務部法醫研究所107年10月08日法醫證字第10700047860號函辦理。
二、依據法務部法醫研究所執行無名比對操作標準，本院其檢送五位二二八受難者家屬所填寫之「法務部法醫研究所親體採樣同意書」及「法務部法醫研究所親緣關係鑑定申請表」，俾利法務部法醫研究所後續進行比對工作。
三、檢送五位二二八受難者家屬之DNA資料經本院輸血醫學中心確認無誤，並依法務部法醫研究所要求增列其中一位家屬粒線體DNA HVII (73-340)序列資料。

正本：財團法人二二八事件紀念基金會
副本：本院醫學研究部

台灣基督長老教會馬偕醫療財團法人馬偕紀念醫院 函

機關地址：104217台北市中山區中山北路2段92號
聯絡人：張富堂28094661
分機3061
Email：bc5046@mmh.org.tw
傳 真：(02)28094679

受文者：財團法人二二八事件紀念基金會

發文日期：中華民國一〇八年七月二十日
發文字號：馬院醫研字第1080008552號
速別：普通件
密等及解密條件或保密期限：普通
附件：如說明二

主旨：敬請 貴金會協助本院輸血醫學中心辦理「二二八受難者骨骸回家」活動計畫，併提請本會中心另一位受難者家屬之遺傳標誌資料及「法務部法醫研究所親體採樣同意書」轉呈至法務部法醫研究所，以為辦理二二八受難者家屬遺傳標誌檔案資料與法務部法醫研究所代為保管存放之無名屍DNA資料進行比對，請 查照。

說明：
一、貴金會辦理本院輸血醫學中心「二二八受難者骨骸回家」活動計畫，已完成五位二二八受難者家屬的遺傳資料與法務部法醫研究所收集之無名屍遺傳資料的比對工作。本院互為處理，相關比對結果，本院已函覆 貴金會及受難者家屬。雖然比對結果並未顯示有配對的結論，但將二二八受難者屬的遺傳資訊保留在資料庫中心確認無誤，期待未來若資料庫中有更多的名基，有基骨骸遺傳資料列入可找到相對的組合，而實慰受難者家屬懷抱的二二八受難者因家的心願。
二、隨函檢送一份二二八受難者家屬遺傳標誌檢測結果暨法務部法醫研究所為保管存放之無名屍DNA資料再比對所填寫的「法務部法醫研究所親體採樣同意書」及「法務部法醫研究所親緣關係鑑定申請表」，以為相關資料比對之用，如蒙惠允，實感德便。
三、本案聯絡人：02-28094661分機轉2383輸血醫學研究組陸中衡小姐。

正本：財團法人二二八事件紀念基金會
副本：本院醫學研究部

受文者：█████████
副本：財團法人二二八事件紀念基金會

主旨：敬覆貴台囑委託本院醫學研究部輸血醫學組比對二二八受難者遺驗結果，請查照。

說明：
一、依據財團法人二二八事件紀念基金會(108)228參字第111080313號函及法務部法醫研究所法醫證字第10800015960號函辦理。
二、台端委託本院醫學研究所輸血醫學組採取DNA檢體，作遺傳標記檢測，而後本院將台端遺傳標記檢測結果送請財團法人二二八事件紀念基金會轉交法務部法醫研究所比對無名屍遺傳資料，以期比對出二二八受難者之遺骸，使二二八受難者遺骸得以回歸家族。
三、由於法務法醫研究所成立時間為1998年，至今不過二十一年，所收集之無名屍遺傳資料皆是在機構成立後才納入管理，因此台端之遺傳標記檢測結果與法醫研究所收集之無名屍遺傳資料比對結果為「未發現具有血緣關聯者」。
四、感謝台端信任本院，使有如此之檢測一比對管道得以構建起來。而望藉二二八受難者檢測一比對管道也將成為安慰受難者家屬歸回安息的重要平台之一。

附錄 | Appendices

附錄 3

從事族群研究的無奈：噶瑪蘭口水事件
——還原歷史真相[1]

　　林媽利醫師在 2005 年到 2008 年參加國科會的大型計劃「南島民族的分類與擴散：人類學、考古學、遺傳學、語言學的整合研究」，林醫師的團隊從事遺傳學的部分。在 2007 年，林醫師的團隊已收集完大部分台灣原住民族群的血液檢體，就差幾個重要的平埔族，如噶瑪蘭的檢體，許多學者認為很可惜。2006 年林醫師另外在進行國人血緣調查的時候，認識了當時已經卸任的游錫堃前院長，他一直主張林醫師應該對噶瑪蘭族的遺傳做調查，並說他在任職時與噶瑪蘭族正名運動的耆老很熟。林醫師便和自己也認識的噶瑪蘭族精神領袖偕萬來長老聯繫，同時聯繫花蓮縣新社村潘金榮頭目、李文勝頭目，期待採檢工作可以順利進行。林醫師團隊研究的目的是「了解噶瑪蘭族的遺傳組成，與鄰近族群的關係，及推論其來源及發展」。以林醫師在各部落採檢的經驗，林醫師通常是以電話說明，然後佐以信件或公文聯繫到可以接觸部落民眾的關鍵人物，如牧師、長老、頭目、村里幹事，然後通過關鍵人物的帶領，再到部落收集檢體。（採檢說明書，見附件 A）

　　2007 年 1 月 12、13 日，林醫師率領兩位專任研究助理何俊

---

[1] 林媽利按：為敘述方便，本篇採第三人稱寫作。

霖、林政賢到花蓮縣豐濱鄉新社村噶瑪蘭部落，抵達後，晚間與潘金榮頭目、李文勝頭目、周智慧鄰長，及原住民代表謝宗修先生聊天，討論第二天如何向族人採檢事宜，他們也討論在林醫師去之前，他們召開部落會議的結果（大部分的人同意林醫師去）。第二天清晨，潘金榮頭目用兩次廣播通知族人前來提供檢體，早晨7點就有族人來，兩位助理依照族人吐口水的時間長短，向他們介紹這次做的研究是什麼，第二天先收集到24個檢體，然後到香蕉絲產業編織工坊去參觀及收集。林醫師在工坊遇到潘朝成，潘朝成質疑林醫師採檢體沒有經過部落會議的同意，潘金榮頭目向潘朝成解釋，確實曾經部落會議的討論及獲得大部分參與會議者的同意參與，林醫師繼而與潘先生解釋約30分鐘。

2月15日，林醫師打電話給噶瑪蘭族精神領袖偕萬來長老時，才知道林醫師回來後兩天，就有三位從台北去的教授（陳叔倬、戴華、邱文聰）去部落調查，月底再去一次與族人開會，在會議時做出結論：族人不應該提供口水給林醫師，族人沒注意到自己的權益，如果讓林醫師發現他們有混血，怕會影響剛剛成功的噶瑪蘭族正名運動（2002年政府公告認定噶瑪蘭族為台灣原住民族之一），偕長老說三位教授的發言，在部落裡引起很大的風波，族人紛紛簽名，要求收回口水。

3月22日，花蓮噶瑪蘭發展協會潘朝成發函馬偕醫院，要求馬偕醫院限期在4月1日拿檢體到噶瑪蘭部落，並在族人面前銷毀口水、DNA檢體。馬偕醫院隨即於4月1日在新社村噶瑪蘭部落面前，銷毀檢體。（向偕長老解釋的信函，見附件B。向國科會解釋的信函，見附件C。花蓮縣噶瑪蘭族發展協會函，見附件D）3月24日，林醫師再打電話給偕長老，偕長老說這個事件演變成這

種結果，不是潘朝成一個人的責任，而是有加入從台北來的三個教授，陳叔倬、戴華、邱文聰共同造成的。

　　林醫師檢討後認為，整個過程如有瑕疵的話，只在於選擇用國科會以前通過的簡易型的舊版本的同意書（舊版採檢同意書，見附件 E），而沒有用新的冗長四頁的同意書（新版採檢同意書，見附件 F），怕引起族人自卑，但舊版也涵蓋簡短的目的、方法、預期試驗效益，參加計劃受試者個人權益受到保護，就是不公開隱私，可隨時退出等。加上當時 2007 年全台的人體試驗委員會管理尚未上軌道，以致林醫師和助理們沒注意到，沒有留下一份拷貝的同意書給族人。（原民會回應，見附件 G。國科會函，見附件 H）

　　「噶瑪蘭口水事件」當下，林醫師選擇保持緘默，主要的原因是當時噶瑪蘭族的總人口數只有 5,000 多人，他們剛好正名成功，林醫師和他們一樣對正名很珍惜，她不想公開取口水時的實況和噶瑪蘭族人對質，讓噶瑪蘭的耆老們尷尬，因此她決定不做任何傷害他們的事情，選擇不為自己辯白，不管排山倒海而來的批判，這件事甚至到現在，還被當成學術倫理的教材在流傳。林醫師相信，這些事的真相，總有一天會攤開在陽光底下。

　　2008 年，林醫師讀到陳叔倬掛名在中國復旦大學人類學院發表的有關「台灣原住民與中國傣族等父系血緣的關係」（*BMC Evolutionary Biology* 2008, 8: 146）的文章，陳叔倬就是前面講的，林醫師在 2007 年 1 月到噶瑪蘭部落採集口水兩天後，隨後去部落調查引起風波的三個教授中的一個。該論文記載，220 名台灣原住民的 DNA 檢體，被送去中國上海的復旦大學分析，這 220 人涵蓋大部分的台灣原住民：阿美族（28 人）、排灣族（22）、

泰雅族（22）、魯凱族（11）、卑南族（11）、鄒族（18）、布農族（17）、賽夏族（11）、巴宰族（21）、西拉雅－馬卡道族（37）、邵族（22）。文章把台灣原住民歸類在中國台灣省，經前原民電視台記者瓦妲先生向慈濟大學人體試驗委員會求證，沒找到同意送檢體到中國的相關資料，在原住民委員會也沒有找到有關同意送檢體到中國的開會紀錄，也就是陳叔倬沒有經過醫學院或原住民委員會的同意，私自把原住民的DNA送到別的國家，而違背了原住民基本法（該法成立於2005年），原住民基本法的第21條第一項是有關學術研究等應取得原住民族的同意等，因此明顯的違背了原住民基本法。同樣這些DNA，也同時被利用在2008年陳叔倬的史丹佛大學的博士論文中。

　　瓦妲先生在原住民電台製作了一個節目「我的血液流向上海」講這件事，在節目中，陳叔倬極力否認他送檢體去中國，而把責任推給慈濟大學許教授（他的老闆），陳說這批DNA是在1996年中研院研討會時，許教授送給中國復旦大學金力教授的DNA。事實上，1996年送檢體當時，林醫師也在場，1996年DNA送到國外尚未被管制，當時，許教授只送給金力教授5個原住民族的檢體：布農族、雅美族、泰雅族、排灣族、阿美族，共58人的DNA（被利用在 Su B, Jin L et al: Polynesian origins insights from the Y chromosome. *PNAS* 2000, 97: 8225-8228），和2008年陳叔倬的11族220人差很多，顯然陳叔倬沒說實話。

　　陳叔倬原先在慈濟醫學院人類學系，在2007年噶瑪蘭口水事件發生的前後時間，他應該是美國史丹佛大學的博士生，但他同時也在中國上海復旦大學考古人類學系的團隊（在當時的網路上可以看到）。1994年陳叔倬進台大醫事技術研究所，因為找不到

老師，由台大微生物學系楊照雄教授拜託林媽利教授收爲學生，在馬偕醫院的血庫研究學習。1996年陳叔倬畢業，拿到碩士學位後，經林醫師幫他在慈濟醫學院人類學系找到工作。

  結論是，整件事看起來，並不像大家在指責的，林醫師有沒有向噶瑪蘭人說清楚研究的種種的「學術倫理」問題，而必須反過來想，是政治問題，因爲製造這個事件的主要原因，最可能是中共怕台灣人知道自己的來源，就是台灣人和平埔族有密切的關係，而不是中國一直在灌輸的「純種北方漢人的後代」，所以林醫師開始做平埔族的研究，就設法阻止，陳叔倬在台灣唱和。有趣的是，陳叔倬的史丹佛大學博士論文是「台灣漢人有多漢？」，說「台灣漢人普遍存在平埔血源的認同想像，台灣國族血統論者甚至主張台灣應藉此獨立」等狹猥的說法（附件I），而顯示了陳叔倬未了解台灣多族群多來源的全貌。藉由這篇文章，希望大家不要再把林醫師說成違反學術倫理，而應該思考陳叔倬是否未完全了解原住民基本法及學術倫理。

附件 A ｜採檢說明書

喀瑪蘭朋友，平安：

我們是由林媽利醫師率領的馬偕紀念醫院醫學研究部輸血醫學研究組的同仁，我們想要請您們慷慨的捐贈您少量的口水或是血液，以供本實驗室做喀瑪蘭族群的研究。

本實驗室是由所收集到的口水或血液中抽取 DNA，然後利用這些 DNA 做父系及/或母系遺傳的標誌鑑定。我們已經做完高山原住民的遺傳標誌鑑定及分析的工作，發現高山原住民在母系及父系遺傳標誌上與台灣漢人有極大的差別，代表他們的起源可能在很久以前即分開了，然後各自發展直到最近才再開始交流。我們用粒線體 DNA 突變的演化趨勢看出台灣原住民可能與波里尼西亞人有血緣的關係，進而推測南島語族在太平洋中各島嶼間的擴散方式。我們將研究成果發表在 2005 年 8 月份的 PLoS Biology 雜誌上，各位如有興趣的話，可以上網查得該篇文獻。

然而，原住民族群僅佔台灣人口約 2%，他們是怎樣與台灣其他 98%的人口互動的？雖然原住民族群一般而言是較孤立於其他的台灣人，但隨著時代的進展，原住民族群中也開始有漢族群的血緣流入，使得我們的研究增加了些困難度。同時我們也需要了解平埔族群在台灣人口中所扮演的角色。雖然平埔族群好像佚失於漢族群之中，但是感謝最近興起的平埔族群復興運動，我們得以收集到西拉雅族及巴宰族的檢體，而對該二族群血緣有了初步的了解。配合有關該二族群的演化歷史(文史工作者提供資料)，我們希望能夠對該二族群的起源及遷徙做深度的探討。喀瑪蘭族在台灣北部平埔族中是很重要的一個族群，數年前本實驗室曾試著採取喀瑪蘭族的血液檢體做族群各項標誌的分析研究，可是並沒有採到很多的檢體(約二十幾個)且多屬於數個家族，致可用的檢體並不多，所以我們對喀瑪蘭族群的研究並不成功。可是我們一直試著聯絡對喀瑪蘭族群熟悉的各界人士，希望能夠將這塊很重要的族群資料補起來。

根據我們在西拉雅及巴宰族群的研究心得，平埔族的遺傳位置似乎是處於高山原住民與漢族之間，而且他們的血緣可以與漢人分享的比例也要比高山原住民高，印證一般民族誌的看法。然而我們認為平埔族的遺傳起源並非來自高山原住民或漢人，而是另有來源，但是仍然必須仰賴個別族群的研究來證實這個假說。由於平埔族群長時間與漢人或其他高山原住民接觸，不論在血緣或生活習慣上皆受到漢人或其他高山原住民極大的影響，因此選擇傳統文化保持良好的社群，應該也是保存平埔族血緣最積極的群體。本實驗室希望能夠取得喀瑪蘭族群沒有血緣關係 50 個檢體。我們期盼在喀瑪蘭復興運動的推展下，各位喀瑪蘭的朋友可以正視自己血緣的問題，找出自己的血緣來源，如此在血緣分析的幫助下，可以對族群的來源有更清楚的了解。

附件 B ｜向偕長老解釋的信函

偕先生，您好：

我是馬偕紀念醫院林媽利醫師的助理陸中衡，很不好意思，上次我們的團隊到噶瑪蘭村落採取口水檢體造成很大的風波，一定對您及族人造成許多的困擾。為了不使您及族人為難，林媽利醫師希望將上次採取的口水檢體，在見證人的見證之下銷毀，以免給人造成印象我們的採檢行動是不符噶瑪蘭朋友意願的印象。可是我們仍然希望願及一些願意及希望我們做噶瑪蘭族血緣調查的朋友的願望，我們則會將他們的口水保留下來，並繼續做後面的分析。因此我們希望您能幫助我們調查在上次收集的個人檢體中，是否仍有人願意將口水給我們做族群血緣的檢查？不論結果如何都請您在所附的表格上打（√），我們會將一份解釋的更詳細的同意書寄上，請那些同意檢查的朋友在同意書上簽名。

造成您的不便，還要請您見諒。我們希望您在一星期內完成本項工作，以便我們籌備後續的銷毀事宜。謝謝您的幫忙，並祝

平安

馬偕紀念醫院 陸中衡 敬上

偕先生，您好：

前一封信曾請您就我們上一次在您的部落中參加我們採檢活動的各位，調查他們是否願意參與我們噶瑪蘭族血緣檢查，否則我們擬將全部所收集的口水檢體銷毀。但是經我們與國家科學委員會的聯繫及我們內部的討論，認為噶瑪蘭族的檢體為國家重要的遺傳資產，不宜由我們單方面決定放棄繼續調查，因此我們衷懇的向您對我上次信件的唐突抱歉，盼望不致造成任何不可彌補的錯誤。

我們希望再次回到您的部落去，親自向您的族人解釋為什麼我們希望做噶瑪蘭族的血緣調查(我們已完成台灣高山原住民，泰雅、賽夏、布農、鄒、魯凱、排灣、太魯閣、阿美、卑南、雅美、邵，平埔族，巴宰、西拉雅、少部分的凱達格蘭，缺乏台灣中的一個重要族群—噶瑪蘭族)，並向族人解釋為什麼我們要用複雜的『受試者同意書』，同意書裡面的內容是什麼，這份受試者同意書可以保護族人什麼樣的權益等等。我們上次去您的部落採集族人的檢體，曾遭受潘朝成理事長質疑我們採檢的正當性，事後並聽說有教授團到您的部落去討論該項採檢事件。當然我們認為我們採檢的行為是正當的，我們也絕對不會做出對貴族人有損傷權益的事情(我們作的是科學研究，目前科學研究的成果尚無法那麼精確的分辨某一個人是否就是噶瑪蘭人，也無法精確的定出噶瑪蘭族特定的遺傳標誌。我們所能做的就是看出噶瑪蘭族與其他族群遺傳距離遠近的程度。族群的認定應是取決於一群人的自由心證，與遺傳的結果沒有太大的關係。)，不過可能在我們進行鼓項活動時一些細節沒有注意，以致造成諸般爭議，因此我們希望能夠再次前往部落向族人解釋，並向他們道歉造成誤解。

我們期盼您能幫忙我們安排一個與族人會面的機會(最好能夠集聚上次如我們收集口水檢體的族人)，我們可以將各項誤會解釋清楚。時間希望定在三月底或四月初，我們並計畫在我們分析完成後，我們得以回到部落向您們報告結果。

非常謝謝您的幫忙，並祝

平安

馬偕紀念醫院 林媽利敬上

198　豐富多彩的台灣

附件 C ｜ 向國科會解釋的信函

紀小姐，您好：

接到您的來函後，我們經過審慎的考慮，認為噶瑪蘭族人的口水/DNA 檢體為國家的資產，似乎不宜由我們單方面決定將採來的檢體銷毀。因此我們決定採用您原先的提議，重新回到噶瑪蘭族部落，向族人清楚解釋我們為什麼要做這一項研究，並向他們解釋我們使用完備的受試者同意書的意義，請他們重新簽署受試者同意書。我們的計畫是：

1. 信件聯絡噶瑪蘭族頭目/長老，解釋我們將要做的事情，請他們幫忙安排會議，我們可派人下去參加會議向族人解釋採檢的目的。時間在 3/11 至 3/17 的禮拜中。
2. 會議時間安排妥當後，派本組人員至花蓮新社參加會議，並請族人重新簽署受試者同意書同時收集檢體並給與同意書副本。時間預定為三月底、四月初。
3. 回台北進行實驗。
4. 待實驗有成果時，回到噶瑪蘭族社區報告結果。

至於以往所進行之研究(本計畫)，由於許多是在目前採用之受試者同意書核定之前執行的，產出許多實驗結果，本組將不重複徵求受試者的同意，簽署新制定的受試者同意書，但會郵寄受試者同意書的副本給每個受試者，以茲參考。

不知您以為何？

　　　　祝

平安

馬偕紀念醫院　林媽利 敬上

附件 D ｜花蓮縣噶瑪蘭族發展協會函

立案字號：花蓮縣政府 92 年 10 月 9 日府社行字第 0920115440 號

檔　號：
保存年限：

花蓮縣噶瑪蘭族發展協會　函

地址：970 花蓮市中美 5 街 73 巷 3 號
電話：0921-037486
聯絡人：偕淑琴

受文者：林媽利女士

發文日期：中華民國 96 年 3 月 27 日
發文字號：(96) 花噶成字第 96014 號
速別：最速件
密等及解密條件：
附件：中英文版切結書

主旨：請　貴院、林媽利女士，切結保證林媽利女士於 96 年 1 月 12、13 日至花蓮縣豐濱鄉新社村，所採集的口水檢體，全數銷毀，亦決無其衍生物質存留，同時保證尚未獲得本會同意之前，決不發表相關研究數據。復請　查照。

說明：
一、中、英文版切結書各乙份，請分別簽章切結。
二、切結書請於 4 月 1 日舉行銷毀檢體時，交給本會。

正本：馬偕紀念醫院、林媽利女士
副本：行政院國家科學委員會、行政院衛生署、行政院原住民族委員會、中央研究院語言學研究所李教授壬癸、花蓮縣衛生局、花蓮縣政府原住民行政局、花蓮縣豐濱鄉衛生所、花蓮縣豐濱鄉新社部落部落會議、花蓮縣原住民健康暨文化研究會、立法委員高金素梅國會辦公室、本會辦公室。

理事長　潘朝成

附件 E ｜舊版採檢同意書

馬偕紀念醫院人體試驗同意書

計畫名稱：噶瑪蘭族的族群研究
計畫編號：

執行單位：馬偕紀念醫院	電話：(02)28094661
主持人：林媽利	轉 2380
聯絡地址：台北縣淡水民生路 45 號	傳真：(02)28094679

自願受試者姓名：	性別： 出生日期：
電話：	病歷號碼：
通訊地址：	

(一)試驗目的：了解噶瑪蘭族的遺傳組成及推論其來源及發展。

(二)試驗方法：我們將對受試者採取約 5cc 的口水，抽取內含的 DNA，再分析。

(三)可能的副作用及危險很少

(四)預期的試驗效益：對於噶瑪蘭族群的遺傳組成及來源發展更加了解。

(五)參加本研究計畫受試者個人權益將受以下保護：
(1)試驗所得資料可能會發表於學術性雜誌，但受試者姓名將不會公布，您的隱私將予以保密。
(2)您在試驗過程中可以隨時撤回同意，退出試驗。如中途退出將不會影響您在馬偕醫院應有的醫療照顧。

自願受試者姓名：＿＿＿＿＿＿　身份字號：＿＿＿＿＿＿
簽名(或法定代理人)：＿＿＿＿＿＿　日期：＿＿＿＿＿＿
見證人簽名：＿＿＿＿＿＿　日期：＿＿＿＿＿＿
研究人員簽名：＿＿＿＿＿＿　日期：＿＿＿＿＿＿

附件 F │ 新版採檢同意書

馬偕紀念醫院醫學研究受試者說明同意書

研究計畫名稱：南島民族的分類與擴散：人類學、考古學、遺傳學、語言學的整合研究－從粒線體DNA、Y染色體及古代DNA的研究看台灣族群的過去與現在

執行單位：馬偕紀念醫院醫學研究部輸血醫學研究組
合作單位：慈濟大學人類學研究所
執行期限：94年8月1日至97年7月31日

主持人：林媽利　　所別：醫學研究部輸血醫學研究組　電話：28094661轉2380
職稱：主治醫師　　組長　　傳真：28094679
協同主持人：陳堯峰、尚特鳩　單位：慈濟大學、輸血醫學組
職稱：助理教授、副研究員　傳真：

1. 研究目的：本研究為跨科學跨領域之整合研究計畫，研究南島民族的分類與擴散。本題目負責遺傳子計畫的部份，由於2005年8月在著名的PLoS Biology上一篇以居住台灣高山原住民血緣體DNA的文章，針對台灣原住民族群的起源與其與其他南島語系族群的關係作了推論。為了了解台灣原住民族群的起源與其與其他南島語系族群的關係有所推論。為了了解台灣原住民族群的起源與其與其他南島語系族群的關係，我們計畫於台灣平埔族及國家遺址的人骨檢體做各種分析作為我們工作的對照，且為了解答以下的問題：1)台灣高山原住民(泛稱原住民族)2)台灣南島民族及其他南島民族群彼此的位置？台灣是否為南島民族的起源？3)台灣平埔族的起源4)台灣原住民族群之間的血緣關係？針對加我們對這些問題的了解，都很重要。研究經費來源：國科會跨領域整合計畫。預定參與試驗人數：1500人。檢測項目包括：粒線體DNA、Y染色體、HLA。

2. 試驗目的及方法：試驗目的：了解台灣族群的起源及與其他族群之關係和屬性；試驗方法：檢測檢體提供者的粒線體DNA、Y染色體及組織抗原粒線體，然後應用結果於族群遺傳方法型理所得到的建議情資訊。檢驗結果是有完全屬於研究性質，檢驗結果是有完全屬於研究性質。

3. 預期試驗效果：了解台灣族群的起源及與其他族群之關係。

4. 受檢者參加本研究所須配合的檢驗或步驟：本研究需由檢驗提供血液(約2cc)或口水(約2cc)，以供實驗操作者分離組織出來的DNA。本研究期間只需要檢體提供者提供一次檢體，但需要檢體提供者蒐集抽出及地及遺傳標記的檢測將，而目前我們的檢測將研究用於粒線體DNA、Y染色體及組織抗原粒線體的檢測，但是我們也希望到將來的DNA檢體能用於將來其他DNA標記(如X染色體及體色體標記)的檢測。

5. 風險：
   (1) 生理風險：本檢驗採用血液檢體或口水檢體作DNA的研究，採取口水檢體並沒有生理方面之風險，可是目前口水分離取出的DNA的數較難達到最佳的標準，因此我們仍希望用血液檢體來分離DNA，抽血難然是很簡單的檢體，但仍然有可能造成檢針位或組織性的不適、疼痛、腫脹、感染等等的的風險等，如有發生您不適的情況下，還是要觀察照顧，請向馬偕紀念醫院負責醫生聯絡。
   (2) 心理風險：本研究之遺傳檢體屬於區別不同族群將持有之遺傳標記，並沒有疾病診斷上之關係，而且研究者將檢測之結果以族群為單位，不會發表個人的資料，個人參與研究可得知自己個人本人的檢測結果，因此不致對個人造成明顯的心理風險。
   (3) 社會風險：本研究若針對台巴自原住族群的檢體供給之，你檢我們的研究員必須在具遵守個人資料保護法上之法律規定，計畫主持人及研究員將很用心來保證您的個人資料檢測結果內中。有關如何檢體試驗者本人取得資料及需要資訊的標明，請參本第16條。

6. 測試結果：本研究的目的在找出族群特殊的檢體，與疾病研究沒有關係，因此檢驗結果不會告知受試者。

7. 補償：如依本研究所訂試驗計畫所引發之身體、心理上之不良反應、副作用或傷害，本院將免費提供受試者專業醫療照顧及醫療諮詢。

8. 受益：受試者將不因參與試驗而獲得任何利益或獎勵。

9. 檢體的多用途性及儲存：檢體將儲存於馬偕紀念醫院醫學研究部輸血醫學研究組，只用於檢體，研究員及本研究部輸血醫學研究組群負責保管。但您亦若同意將檢體人類族群相關族群體其他族群有關的研究，檢體將抽取DNA儲存於馬偕紀念醫院醫學研究部輸血醫學研究組負責保存，保存期限20年。

10. 使用檢體及檢體相關資訊之同意：本研究將於計畫主持人及其所屬實驗室及協同主持人及所屬實驗室的實驗室所有人員執行所有實驗及分析步驟，不會將檢體及檢測結果讓其他檢驗使用。

11. 參與試驗之個人報酬：無

12. 受檢者自費之費用：無

13. 研究結束後檢驗處理方式：
    研究結束後之檢體，原則本執行單位為馬偕紀念醫院醫學研究部輸血醫學研究組負責銷毀。但若您同意，可另選擇下列方式處理：

---

1. 以去名化（不記名）方式提供其他研究之對照組使用。
   若您同意此選項，請在此簽名：＿＿＿＿＿
2. 願意繼續提供馬偕紀念醫院內其他族群方面研究。
   （所有相關研究計畫，必須通過馬偕紀念醫院研究倫理委員會審查通過，並且得時轉再次您的同意簽名）
   若您同意此選項，請在此簽名：＿＿＿＿＿

14. 捐贈檢體的使用權及智慧財產權：您同意參與本計畫，馬偕紀念醫院及其合作單位仍保留到您的授權來儲存及使用所提供的檢體進行研究，此研究成果若直接或間接衍生出具有商業價值的產物，智慧財產權屬於馬偕紀念醫院及馬偕紀念醫院合作單位，而不屬於受試者。

15. 排除條件：本計畫將收集台灣各地區鄰近國家非本人的人民及台灣地區平埔族群，若在收集以後，研究者發現您是不符合研究的場所，您會被認的檢體，並刪除您的資料。

16. 參加本醫學研究計畫之個人權益將受以下保護：
    （一）本計畫將依機續隨機的方式在試驗治療的中應用之權益上。
    （二）隱密權：研究過程中其研究員將設法保密，除非標明將無法解開您檢驗資訊，並且在未能同意的情況下，為您他人醫院不會透漏任何使您們們被辨識的訊息等。研究所收集的同個結果，實驗數據會分別供機密非特個體保存：除非出由您的書面授權或法律程序所要，否則我們不會將您取得您的個人資訊，也會經由電話與網路語傳行公布。此研究結果會以綜合結論的方式公布，但不包括可辨識個人資料(可辨識個人資料: 如姓名、照片…等)，將予以絕對保密。
    （三）終止參與權：在計畫進行時中，您有權退出本研究計畫。這個步驟只收請有正式表格便您使用。只要您告知研究員。研究員身以電確認您的意願後即刪除相關資料，請您先期所提供的檢體以即刪除您的資料。
    （四）如依本研究所訂試驗計畫所引發之身體、心理上之不良反應、副作用或傷害，本院將免費提供受試者專業醫療照顧及醫療諮詢。

17. 其他檢體採集及使用有關之重要事項：若需先檢體遺失或受損，受試者被研究單位要求提供第二份檢體或使用如超過原先所訂定之範圍，則會重新向受檢者取得同意。

18. 同意書中所述馬偕紀念醫院「合作單位」為慈濟大學。

試驗計畫主持人簽名：＿＿＿＿＿　　日期：＿＿＿＿＿

同意書

本人在詳細閱讀此馬偕紀念醫院南島民族的分類與擴散：人類學、考古學、遺傳學、語言學的整合研究－從粒線體DNA、Y染色體及古代DNA的研究看台灣族群的過去與現在的計畫之同意書後，確實瞭解以上所有內容，本人願意參加此研究計畫。
本人有任何疑問隨時可和馬偕紀念醫院醫學研究部輸血醫學研究組計畫主持人，林媽利醫師 02-28094661轉2380聯絡。本人並且保留於計畫進行期間內，本人有權終止參與此研究計畫。本人可以保留一份此同意書的複印本。

姓名(簽名)：＿＿＿＿＿　　簽署日期：＿＿＿＿＿
未成年受試者之法定代理人簽名：＿＿＿＿＿　關係：＿＿＿＿＿　簽署日期：＿＿＿＿＿
研究護士(助理)簽名：＿＿＿＿＿　簽署日期：＿＿＿＿＿
受試者家屬簽名：＿＿＿＿＿　簽署日期：＿＿＿＿＿　關係：＿＿＿＿＿
處見證人簽名：＿＿＿＿＿　簽署日期：＿＿＿＿＿

受試者為成年者不識字，請研究助理先見證人人親筆寫明對個案解釋後再請簽字，受試者蓋手印於簽名欄。

附件 G ｜原民會的回應

原民會回應：

一、　本會認為該協會此一主張，符合聯合國人權委員會於 2006 年通過之「聯合國原住民族權宣言」（UNITED NATIONS DECLARATION ON THE RIGHTS OF INDIGENOUS PEOPLES）第 31 條規定「原住民族有權維持、控制、保護並發展其...基因資源」之精神，該條規定基因屬於原住民族之集體權。馬偕醫院採納噶瑪蘭族人之建議，銷毀所採集之唾液檢體，有助於原住民族權之保障，並可惕勵在原住民族地區進行相關研究之研究人員。

二、　自 95 年度部落會議即為本會重要推動工作之一，凡部落事務應透過部落會議機取得共識，而此共識應為各機關單位所尊重。對於本案噶瑪蘭族透過部落會議機制，展現民族集體意志，作為提出主張之基礎，本會表示支持與尊重。對馬偕醫院能尊重部落決議，在族人面前銷毀唾液檢體，使本事件和諧落幕，亦深感欣慰。

三、　為避免類似情形再度發生，宜建立統一規範，或請相關學術研究之主管機關責請各學術團體於進行研究時，應先提出明白易懂之計畫，事先提請部落會議討論。

附件 H ｜ 國科會函

檔　號：
保存年限：

行政院國家科學委員會　函

地址：台北市和平東路 2 段 106 號
聯絡電話：(02)2737-7568
聯絡人：魏淑美
傳真電話：(02)2737-7924
電子信箱：mswei@nsc.gov.tw

受文者：

發文日期：中華民國 96 年 8 月 21 日
發文字號：臺會綜二字第 0960043279 之 1 號
速別：最速件
密等及解密條件或保密期限：密（公佈後解密）
附件：

主旨：有關　台端至花蓮縣豐濱鄉新社村噶瑪蘭部落，在未讓被採集人充分知悉研究相關資訊，又未留下同意書讓被採集人存查之情況下，採集 29 件口水檢體乙案，復如說明，請　查照。

說明：案經本會召開專案學術倫理審議委員會議審議結果，請　台端就以下事項予以改進：

一、受試者告知同意書之內容，應依行政院衛生署 95 年 8 月 18 日衛署醫字第 0950206912 號函公布之「研究用人體檢體採集與使用注意事項」第五條之規定辦理。告知之方式與內容，尤須斟酌原住民族在文化及社會上之特殊處境，以落實告知同意的精神。

二、未來如從事與原住民族有關之研究，應切實依據原住民族基本法第 21 條規定辦理。

正本：林媽利醫師
副本：本會人文處、生物處、綜合處

行政院國家科學委員會

附件 I ｜ 2008 年陳叔倬的史丹佛大學的博士論文摘要

臺灣漢人有多漢？平埔血源流入臺灣漢人的比例及其對臺灣國族認同的影響

陳叔倬 史丹佛大學人類科學系博士

摘要

受到俗諺「有唐山公無唐山媽」的影響，台灣漢人普遍存在平埔血源的認同想像。加上一些錯誤的遺傳數據誇大了台灣漢人帶有原住民血源的比例，台灣國族血統論者甚至主張台灣應該藉此獨立。事實上平埔血源從未被正式研究，藉由日治時期戶籍資料的輔助，平埔後裔的遺傳特性首次被揭露，指出平埔後裔仍保有完整的原住民族遺傳特性，但台灣漢人帶有平埔血源者幾希，間接實證清末移民潮稀釋了平埔血源的假說。此外藉由一個同宗家戶認同自漢轉番的參與觀察，以及平埔/漢人雜居村落認同集體轉變的量化分析，進一步驗證認同不根植於血源。

【英文版】

Postscript to the "Kavalan Saliva Incident"— Restoring Historical Truth[1]

Text and images by Dr. Marie Lin

Mackay Memorial Hospital, Department of Transfusion Medicine and Molecular Anthropology Research

From 2005 to 2008, Dr. Lin participated in a large-scale research project funded by the National Science Council (NSC) titled *Classification and Dispersal of Austronesian Peoples: An Integrated Study of Anthropology, Archaeology, Genetics, and Linguistics*. Dr. Lin's team was responsible for the genetics aspects of the study.

By 2007, the team had already collected blood samples from most of Taiwan's Indigenous ethnic groups, except for a few crucial Plains Indigenous groups (Pinpu), including the Kavalan. Many scholars considered this a significant omission. During a separate genetic lineage investigation in 2006, Dr. Lin met former Premier Yu Shyi-kun, who had already left office at that time. He strongly advocated for Dr. Lin to conduct a genetic study on the Kavalan people, mentioning that he had developed close ties with the elders leading the Kavalan ethnic identity movement during his tenure.

---

1 Translated by Dr. T. Burnouf.

Dr. Lin then reached out to the Kavalan spiritual leader, Elder Chieh Wan-lai, whom she had known previously. She also contacted community leaders in Xinshe Village, Hualien County, including Chief Pan Jin-rong and Chief Li Wen-sheng, hoping for a smooth sample collection process. The research objective was to "understand the genetic composition of the Kavalan people, their relationship with neighboring ethnic groups, and to infer their origins and development."

Based on past experience collecting samples in various Indigenous communities, Dr. Lin typically first explained the study over the phone, followed by sending official letters or documents to key local figures, such as pastors, elders, chiefs, and village representatives, who could facilitate community engagement. Once a local leader provided support, the research team would visit the village to collect samples.

The Sample Collection Process

On January 12-13, 2007, Dr. Lin, along with two full-time research assistants, Ho Chun-lin and Lin Cheng-hsien, traveled to the Kavalan settlement in Xinshe Village, Fengbin Township, Hualien County. Upon arrival, they met with Chief Pan Jin-rong, Chief Li Wen-sheng, neighborhood representative Chou Chih-hui, and Indigenous community representative Hsieh Tsung-hsiu to discuss the sample collection process for the next day. The local leaders also informed Dr. Lin of the outcome of a prior community meeting, where the majority had agreed to participate in the study.

The following morning, Chief Pan Jin-rong made two public announcements, inviting community members to provide samples. By 7 a.m., villagers began arriving. As the research assistants collected saliva samples, they explained the study's purpose based on the time each participant took to provide a sample. That day, they collected 24 samples. Later, the team visited a banana fiber weaving workshop to observe local industry and collect additional samples.

While at the workshop, Dr. Lin encountered Pan Chao-cheng, who questioned the legitimacy of the sample collection process, claiming it had not been approved by a community meeting. Chief Pan Jin-rong explained that a community meeting had indeed been held and that a majority of participants had consented. Dr. Lin further clarified the research purpose to Pan Chao-cheng in a 30-minute discussion.

Backlash and Community Retraction

On February 15, Dr. Lin called Elder Chieh Wan-lai and learned that, two days after the sample collection, three professors from Taipei—Chen Shu-chuo, Tai Hua, and Chiu Wen-tsung—visited the Kavalan community to investigate the research. At the end of February, they held another meeting with the villagers. During this meeting, they argued that the community should not have provided saliva samples, claiming that villagers were unaware of their rights. They also expressed concerns that if the research revealed genetic admixture, it could undermine the recently successful Kavalan ethnic recognition movement.

Elder Chieh reported that these professors' statements caused significant turmoil in the community, leading villagers to sign petitions demanding the return of their saliva samples.

On March 24, Dr. Lin called Elder Chieh again. He informed her that the incident had escalated beyond Pan Chao-cheng's individual concerns, as the three Taipei professors had also become involved. On March 22, the Kavalan Development Association of Hualien, led by Pan Chao-cheng, sent an official letter to Mackay Memorial Hospital, demanding that all collected samples be returned and destroyed in front of the community by April 1.

In compliance with this request, Mackay Memorial Hospital publicly destroyed the saliva and DNA samples in Xinshe Village on April 1.

Reflection and Ethical Considerations

Upon reflection, Dr. Lin concluded that the only procedural flaw was the use of a simplified consent form previously approved by the National Science Council, rather than the newer, more detailed four-page version. She had opted for the shorter form to avoid making participants feel overwhelmed. However, the version used still included essential details, such as the study's purpose, methods, anticipated benefits, participant rights (including privacy protection and the option to withdraw at any time).

At that time, in 2007, Taiwan's Institutional Review Board (IRB) regulations were still in their infancy. Consequently, neither Dr. Lin nor her research assistants realized they had failed to leave a copy of the consent form with the participants.

During the *Kavalan Saliva Incident*, Dr. Lin chose to remain silent. She understood that the Kavalan community, with only around 5,000 members, had just achieved official recognition. She cherished this milestone as much as they did and did not wish to embarrass the elders by publicly disputing the facts. To avoid harming them, she refrained from defending herself, despite the overwhelming criticism. Even today, the incident continues to be cited as a case study in research ethics. However, Dr. Lin believes that the truth will eventually come to light.

DNA Sent to China—A Larger Ethical Issue

In 2008, Dr. Lin came across a paper co-authored by Chen Shu-chuo, published under Fudan University's Anthropology Department in China. The article, titled *Taiwan Indigenous Peoples and Patrilineal Relationships with the Dai Ethnic Group in China* (*BMC Evolutionary Biology*, 2008, 8: 146), reported the analysis of DNA samples from 220 Taiwanese Indigenous individuals at Fudan University in Shanghai. The samples covered various Indigenous groups, including:

- Amis (28)
- Paiwan (22)
- Atayal (22)

- Rukai (11)
- Puyuma (11)
- Tsou (18)
- Bunun (17)
- Saisiyat (11)
- Pazeh (21)
- Siraya-Makatau (37)
- Thao (22)

The paper classified Taiwan's Indigenous peoples under "China Taiwan Province." Investigations by a former Indigenous television reporter, Watan, found no evidence that neither Tzu Chi University's IRB nor the Indigenous Affairs Council had records of any such approval. This meant Chen had violated Taiwan's *Indigenous Peoples Basic Law* (enacted in 2005), which ban on sending DNA of Indigenous peoples abroad for genetic research. Additionally, the same DNA samples were later used in Chen's doctoral dissertation at Stanford University.

In response, Watan produced a radio program titled *My Blood Flowed to Shanghai,* exposing the case. On the program, Chen denied sending the samples to China and attempted to shift responsibility to Professor Hsu from Tzu Chi University. He claimed that the DNA had been transferred in 1996 during an Academia Sinica seminar when there was no regulation for transferring DNA across the border. However, Dr. Lin, who was present in 1996, confirmed that only 58

DNA samples from five ethnic groups (Bunun, Yami, Atayal, Paiwan, and Amis) were sent to China, making Chen's claim inconsistent.

Conclusion

The *Kavalan Saliva Incident* was not merely an academic ethics issue but a politically motivated one. The Chinese government likely sought to suppress research that could prove Taiwan's Indigenous people (Pinpu) were genetically closely related to Taiwanese with the consequency of the Taiwanese distinct from Han Chinese. Chen Shu-chuo's Stanford dissertation, *How Han are the Taiwanese Han?*, suggested that Taiwan's population generally having imagination of having Indigenous ancestry, a finding that could politically fuel Taiwan's independence movement. Dr. Lin hopes this article will end the unjust accusations against her and redirect attention to the real ethical breaches in Indigenous DNA research.

||【法文版】||

Post-scriptum à l'« Incident de la salive Kavalan »—Rétablir la vérité historique[1]

Texte et images par Dr. Marie Lin

Mackay Memorial Hospital, Department of Transfusion Medicine and

Molecular Anthropology Research

De 2005 à 2008, le Dr Lin a participé à un projet de recherche de grande envergure financé par le Conseil national des sciences (NSC), intitulé *Classification et dispersion des peuples austronésiens: une étude intégrée en anthropologie, archéologie, génétique et linguistique*. L'équipe du Dr Lin était responsable des aspects génétiques de l'étude.

En 2007, l'équipe avait déjà collecté des échantillons sanguins de la plupart des groupes ethniques autochtones de Taïwan, à l'exception de quelques groupes autochtones des plaines (Pinpu), y compris les Kavalan. De nombreux chercheurs considéraient cela comme une omission importante. Lors d'une enquête séparée sur les lignées génétiques en 2006, le Dr Lin a rencontré l'ancien Premier ministre Yu Shyi-kun, qui n'était plus en fonction à ce moment-là. Il a fortement plaidé pour que le Dr Lin mène une étude génétique sur le peuple Kavalan, mentionnant qu'il avait tissé des liens étroits avec les anciens

---

1 Translated by Dr. T. Burnouf.

menant le mouvement d'identité ethnique Kavalan durant son mandat.

Le Dr Lin a ensuite contacté le leader spirituel des Kavalan, l'Aîné Chieh Wan-lai, qu'elle connaissait déjà. Elle a également pris contact avec les chefs de communauté du village de Xinshe, dans le comté de Hualien, notamment le chef Pan Jin-rong et le chef Li Wen-sheng, dans l'espoir que le processus de collecte d'échantillons se déroule sans encombre. L'objectif de la recherche était de « comprendre la composition génétique du peuple Kavalan, sa relation avec les groupes ethniques voisins, ainsi que d'inférer ses origines et son développement ».

Sur la base de son expérience passée dans la collecte d'échantillons dans diverses communautés autochtones, le Dr Lin expliquait généralement d'abord l'étude par téléphone, avant d'envoyer des lettres officielles ou des documents aux figures locales clés, telles que des pasteurs, des anciens, des chefs et des représentants de village, qui pouvaient faciliter l'engagement de la communauté. Une fois le soutien d'un leader local obtenu, l'équipe de recherche se rendait dans le village pour collecter les échantillons.

Le processus de collect d'échantillons

Les 12 et 13 janvier 2007, le Dr Lin, accompagnée de deux assistants de recherche à temps plein, Ho Chun-lin et Lin Cheng-hsien, s'est rendue dans l'établissement Kavalan du village de Xinshe, dans le canton of Fengbin, comté de Hualien. À leur arrivée, ils ont rencontré le chef Pan Jin-rong, le chef Li Wen-sheng, le représentant du quartier

Chou Chih-hui et le représentant de la communauté autochtone Hsieh Tsung-hsiu pour discuter du processus de collecte d'échantillons prévu pour le lendemain. Les chefs locaux ont également informé le Dr Lin du résultat d'une réunion communautaire antérieure, où la majorité avait accepté de participer à l'étude.

Le lendemain matin, le chef Pan Jin-rong a fait deux annonces publiques, invitant les membres de la communauté à fournir des échantillons. À 7 heures du matin, les villageois ont commencé à arriver. Pendant que les assistants de recherche recueillaient les échantillons de salive, ils expliquaient l'objectif de l'étude en fonction du temps que chaque participant mettait à fournir un échantillon. Ce jour-là, ils ont collecté 24 échantillons. Plus tard, l'équipe a visité un atelier de tissage de fibres de banane pour observer l'industrie locale et collecter des échantillons supplémentaires.

À l'atelier, le Dr Lin a rencontré Pan Chao-cheng, qui a remis en question la légitimité du processus de collecte d'échantillons, affirmant qu'il n'avait pas été approuvé par une réunion communautaire. Le chef Pan Jin-rong a expliqué qu'une réunion communautaire avait bien eu lieu et que la majorité des participants avait donné son consentement. Le Dr Lin a ensuite clarifié l'objectif de la recherche auprès de Pan Chao-cheng lors d'une discussion de 30 minutes.

Réactions et rétractation de la communauté

Le 15 février, le Dr Lin a appelé l'aîné Chieh Wan-lai et a appris que, deux jours après la collecte des échantillons, trois professeurs de

Taipei — Chen Shu-chuo, Tai Hua et Chiu Wen-tsung — avaient visité la communauté Kavalan pour enquêter sur la recherche. Fin février, ils ont organisé une autre réunion avec les villageois. Lors de cette réunion, ils ont affirmé que la communauté n'aurait pas dû fournir d'échantillons de salive, soutenant que les villageois n'étaient pas conscients de leurs droits. Ils ont également exprimé des inquiétudes sur le fait que si la recherche révélait un mélange génétique, cela pourrait nuire au mouvement de reconnaissance ethnique Kavalan, qui venait tout juste de réussir.

L'Aîné Chieh a rapporté que les déclarations de ces professeurs avaient provoqué une grande agitation dans la communauté, amenant les villageois à signer des pétitions exigeant la restitution de leurs échantillons de salive.

Le 24 mars, le Dr Lin a de nouveau appelé l'Aîné Chieh. Il l'a informée que l'incident avait pris une ampleur dépassant les préoccupations individuelles de Pan Chao-cheng, car les trois professeurs de Taipei s'étaient également impliqués. Le 22 mars, l'Association de développement Kavalan de Hualien, dirigée par Pan Chao-cheng, a envoyé une lettre officielle à l'hôpital Mackay Memorial, exigeant que tous les échantillons collectés soient restitués et détruits devant la communauté avant le 1er avril.

En réponse à cette demande, l'hôpital Mackay Memorial a publiquement détruit les échantillons de salive et d'ADN dans le village de Xinshe le 1er avril.

Réflexions et considérations éthiques

Avec le recul, le Dr Lin a conclu que la seule faille procédurale résidait dans l'utilisation d'un formulaire de consentement simplifié, précédemment approuvé par le Conseil National des Sciences, au lieu de la version plus détaillée de quatre pages récemment introduite. Elle avait choisi le formulaire plus court pour éviter de dérouter les participants. Cependant, cette version incluait toujours les détails essentiels, tels que l'objectif de l'étude, les méthodes, les bénéfices anticipés, les droits des participants (y compris la protection de la vie privée et la possibilité de se retirer à tout moment).

En 2007, les réglementations des comités d'éthique (IRB) à Taïwan en étaient encore à leurs débuts. Par conséquent, ni le Dr Lin ni ses assistants de recherche n'avaient réalisé qu'ils n'avaient pas laissé une copie du formulaire de consentement aux participants.

Lors de l'*Incident de la salive Kavalan*, le Dr Lin a choisi de rester silencieuse. Elle comprenait que la communauté Kavalan, qui comptait seulement environ 5000 membres, venait d'obtenir une reconnaissance officielle. Elle chérissait cette réussite autant qu'eux et ne souhaitait pas embarrasser les anciens en contestant publiquement les faits. Afin d'éviter de leur causer du tort, elle s'est abstenue de se défendre, malgré les critiques virulentes. Encore aujourd'hui, cet incident continue d'être cité comme une étude de cas en éthique de la recherche. Toutefois, le Dr Lin croit que la vérité finira par éclater au grand jour.

L'ADN envoyé en Chine—Un problème éthique d'une plus grande envergure

En 2008, le Dr Lin est tombée sur un article co-écrit par Chen Shu-chuo, publié sous l'égide du département d'anthropologie de l'Université Fudan en Chine. L'article, intitulé *Taiwan Indigenous Peoples and Patrilineal Relationships with the Dai Ethnic Group in China* (*BMC Evolutionary Biology*, 2008, 8: 146), rapportait l'analyse d'échantillons d'ADN de 220 individus autochtones taïwanais à l'Université Fudan, à Shanghai. Ces échantillons couvraient plusieurs groupes autochtones, notamment :

- Amis (28)
- Paiwan (22)
- Atayal (22)
- Rukai (11)
- Puyuma (11)
- Tsou (18)
- Bunun (17)
- Saisiyat (11)
- Pazeh (21)
- Siraya-Makatau (37)
- Thao (22)

L'article classait les peuples autochtones de Taïwan sous la catégorie "Province de Taïwan, Chine". Une enquête menée par un ancien journaliste de télévision autochtone, Watan, a révélé qu'aucun document officiel ne prouvait que l'Université Tzu Chi ou le Conseil des Affaires autochtones avait approuvé l'envoi de ces échantillons. Cela signifiait que Chen avait enfreint la *Loi fondamentale sur les peuples autochtones de* Taïwan (promulguée en 2005), qui interdit l'envoi d'ADN des peuples autochtones à l'étranger pour des recherches génétiques. De plus, ces mêmes échantillons d'ADN ont ensuite été utilisés dans la thèse de doctorat de Chen à l'Université Stanford.

En réponse à cette révélation, Watan a produit une émission radio intitulée *Mon sang a coulé jusqu'à Shanghai*, exposant l'affaire. Lors de l'émission, Chen a nié avoir envoyé les échantillons en Chine et a tenté de rejeter la responsabilité sur le professeur Hsu de l'Université Tzu Chi. Il a affirmé que ces échantillons d'ADN avaient été transférés en 1996 lors d'un séminaire de l'Academia Sinica, à une époque où aucune réglementation ne régissait le transfert transfrontalier d'ADN. Cependant, le Dr Lin, qui était présente en 1996, a confirmé que seuls 58 échantillons d'ADN provenant de cinq groupes ethniques (Bunun, Yami, Atayal, Paiwan et Amis) avaient été envoyés en Chine, ce qui rendait les affirmations de Chen incohérentes.

Conclusion

L'*Incident de la salive Kavalan* n'était pas seulement une question d'éthique académique, mais aussi une affaire politiquement motivée. Le gouvernement chinois aurait cherché à empêcher des recherches pouvant prouver que les peuples autochtones de Taïwan (Pinpu) avaient des liens génétiques étroits avec les Taïwanais, ce qui pourrait remettre en question la narration selon laquelle les Taïwanais descendent uniquement des Han. Le Dr Lin espère que cela mettra fin aux accusations injustes portées contre elle et recentrera l'attention sur les véritables violations éthiques dans la recherche sur l'ADN autochtone.

附錄 4

台灣人可能沒有古老的 M174 父系血緣 [1]

　　最近盛傳台灣主要的父系血緣是 M174（D-M174），約五萬年前發生，所以台灣人是屬於比中國人更古老的族群，讓大家很高興。事實上 M174 父系血緣主要分布在藏族（43%）、日本人（28%）、羌族（16%）和回族（11%）。

　　在馬偕醫院七千多人血緣的檢測中，做父系血緣的研究（Y-SNP, Y-STR），包含 1,608 名台灣人（閩、客、平埔及高山原住民）、12 名日本人以及泰國人、越南人、中國人、菲律賓人及印尼人（886 人），共 2,506 人。我們在這 2,506 人中，共發現 11 人是 M174 父系血緣，這 11 人分別為 6 名日本人、3 名泰國人、一名越南人及一名台灣客家人。

　　因我們對這個新竹的客家人並沒有詢問其父母親的資料，所以我們並不清楚他有沒有日本人的祖先？因此很難說台灣有或沒有 M174 血緣，如果有的話，也是很少。

　　台灣主要的父系血緣是屬於 M175（O-M175），時間比較淺，形成在約三萬五千年前，台灣人大部分是屬於 M175 演化下的 O1-M119、O2-P31、O3-M122 血緣，因為父系血緣在台灣及亞洲大陸（包括中國）都很相似，而且父系血緣的研究時間相當短，許多問題尚待研究。

1　本文原刊於 2024/07/30《自由時報》「自由廣場」。

母系血緣 三千年前就在台灣

　　但請大家不要氣餒,我們研究室做古代遺骸的 DNA 研究,經母系血緣證明,台灣人的祖先早在 3,000 年前新石器時代晚期就已定居台灣,比我們一般的認知「四百年前唐山公的移民」,更早更早。

附錄 5

馬祖居民的粒線體 DNA 遺傳多樣性及其歷史淵源 [1]

馬祖人群與周邊東亞人群的關係，是一個多層次且豐富的故事。通過對粒線體 DNA（mtDNA）部分及完整序列的分析，我們得以揭示，馬祖人群並未展現與東亞、東南亞或東北亞某一特定人群的專屬母系親緣關係。相反地，其基因結構展現出高度遺傳多樣性，並包含來自不同亞洲地區的多樣且獨特的單倍群。這些遺傳特徵反映出，馬祖人群的形成，是一個持續重新定居的歷程。

這種重新定居的過程，可追溯至末次冰河時期結束時。隨著海平面上升，馬祖群島從中國東南沿海陸地分離出來。自此，馬祖逐漸成為一個人口流動的樞紐，吸引來自不同地區的移民。這一過程持續至上個世紀，使得遺傳漂變未對馬祖人群形成顯著影響，也未賦予其特定的遺傳特徵。

古代與現代遺傳連結

馬祖群島（包括亮島）的首次人類定居，可能發生在全新世早期，距今約 8,000 年。亮島考古遺骸的粒線體 DNA 分析顯示，

---

1 本篇由陳宗賢執筆。

當時人群的單倍群為R9/pre-F與E1a。然而，在現代馬祖人群中，這些前新石器時代特徵的單倍群（如亮島人中的 pre-E1a 或 R9/pre-F）並未被觀察到，表明馬祖現今的遺傳構成，主要是新石器時代及之後移民所形成的。

新石器時代以來，馬祖人群的基因構成，深受中國沿海和內陸地區人群的影響。此外，東北亞的基因流入（如 D 或 G 單倍群）和島嶼東南亞的基因流入（如 F1 或 M7 單倍群），進一步支持了馬祖做為多元文化與基因交流交匯點的地位。

馬祖與其他人群的母系遺傳分布

林媽利醫師的研究，通過多維尺度分析（FST）檢測馬祖與其他亞洲人群之間的母系遺傳分布。從50位馬祖居民的樣本中，觀察到38種獨特的粒線體 DNA 單倍型，其中29種單倍群僅出現一次。在較低的分類層次上，8個單倍群（D4、D5、F1、F2、G 和 M7）的頻率超過5%，佔總多樣性的64%。其中，D4、D5、F2 和 G 的亞型在現代東北亞人群中較為常見，而 F1（如 F1a1'、F1a1a、F1a1c、F1a4a 和 F1c1a1）和 M7（如 M7c1'、M7c1b2b 和 M7c1c2）的亞型則多見於東南亞地區。

馬祖人群高單倍群多樣性及大量獨特單倍型表明，其基因結構中存在相對高比例的核苷酸變異，顯示這是一個自新石器時代以來，經歷多次基因流動的種族異質性人群。

馬祖與台灣原住民的關聯性

馬祖人與台灣原住民的母系血緣關聯性，並不特別顯著。在研究中，僅有單倍群 B4c1b2a 和 F1a4a 表現出與東亞島嶼類似的

分布模式,這些單倍群在台灣漢族中頻率較低,但在台灣原住民與菲律賓中更為常見。其他如 F1c1a1 和 N9a1'3,在台灣閩南人與平埔族中稍微常見,但整體而言,馬祖單倍群在台灣的分布並不突出。

遺傳特徵與人口動態分析

錯配分布分析(見彩圖 13 Ⓑ)顯示,在 5 至 25 個鹼基對差異間呈現平坦且寬的單峰曲線,其平均差異為 14.5 鹼基對。這些結果拒絕了突發人口擴張的假設,表明馬祖單倍群的歧異,來自多個亞洲起源群體的基因混合,而非單一人口擴張事件。

結論

綜上所述,馬祖人群的遺傳特徵,展現出一個由多次移民與基因流動共同塑造的動態歷史。馬祖人群並未與某一特定人群形成專屬關係,而是受多元地區基因影響,反映出自新石器時代以來,東亞遺傳多樣性的縮影。做為中國東南沿海的一個島嶼樞紐,馬祖在新石器時代及其後期的人口遷徙中,吸納了來自東北亞、東南亞及東亞其他地區的基因,成為多元文化與基因交流的交匯點。

附錄 6

1990 年代與國際輸血專家學者的討論往返書信，可以看到台灣在 10 年當中，輸血醫學趕上歐美國家的軌跡

MRC
Medical Research Council

MRC Blood Group Unit
Wolfson House
University College London
4 Stephenson Way
London NW1 2HE

telephone 01-388 7752

reference

26th January 1990

Dr Marie Lin-Chu
Mackay Memorial Hospital
No.92 North Chng San Road
Sec 2
Taipi
Taiwan

Dear Marie,

                    Chou Su Sz Bwo

Thank you very much indeed for sending blood from this mother whose baby had HDN. This is a very hasty note to say that we had problems with her s group: her cells gave weak positive reaction although they were S-, her U antigen appeared normal. Carole tested Chou's cells with antibodies to Miltenberger antigens: all were negative except one multispecific reagent (Pe). Carole has not been able to identify the culprit antibody and has very few cells left. Please could we have another sample?

We know that we should be looking at her antibody and Carole will be sending you a report in due course. We always MNSs phenotype cells of markers of Miltenberger antibodies and had not expected to meet a problem.

With best wishes

Yours sincerely

Patricia

Patricia Tippett

MRC
Medical Research Council

Dr. P. Tippett
MRC Blood Group Unit
Wolfson House
University College London
4 Stephenson Way
London NW1 2HE

telephone 071-388 7752
fax   071-388 2374

reference

29 May 1990

Mr. R. Broadberry
30 Bourne Avenue
Shirley
Southampton SO1 5NU

Dear Richard,

<u>Cho Su Sz Bwo</u>

A brief report of Carole's recent work with this antibody. She has done some of the adsorption/elution tests that she promised.

She used MiI, MiII, MiVI and MiIX cells. MiIX are the new class which only express Mur of the known antigens, unfortunately these cells were group A. Absorption with MiI cells removed the antibody against MiI cells but did not appear to affect the activity with MiII and MiVI cells. The eluate from MiI cells used for the absorption only reacted with MiI cells. Conclusion anti-Vw is present (no sign of anti-Mi^a).

Absorption with MiII cells, removed antibody against MiII cells but left activity against MiI (presumably anti-Vw) and MiVI cells; the eluate from MiII cells reacted with MiII and MiVI cells but not MiI or MiIX cells. Absorption with MiVI cells removed activity against its own cells, weakened the antibody against MiII cells and left anti-Vw; the eluate from MiVI cells reacted with MiII and MiVI cells but not MiI or MiIX cells (that same specificity as eluate from MiII). Absorption with group A MiIX cells removed antibody against MiIX cells; eluate contained anti-A and antibody against MiVI cells but not MiI or MiII cells.

Conclusion: this serum contains anti-Vw plus probably anti-Hut (Giles definition) and possibly anti-Mur (because of reaction with MiIX), anti-Mut (this has same specificity as Hut of Cleghorn, Race and Sanger p112, 6th edition) and tentatively anti-Hil.

Carole now has less than $^1/_4$ml left. Please could she have some more of this interesting serum, she would like to 'solve' its specificities. Anti-Vw, which cannot have caused the HDN, is the only specificity of which she is certain.

Have a good trip home.

Yours sincerely

Patricia

Patricia Tippett

↑ Patricia Tippett 做上述抗體的詳細評估及分析。(1990-05-29)

← 與英國的醫學研究委員會 MRC（Medical Research Council）血型專家 Patricia Tippett 討論米田堡血型母親 Chou Su Sz Bwo 的抗體引起新生兒溶血症的血型問題。(1990-01-26)

附錄 | Appendices   227

Form: AL-06

馬偕紀念醫院
MACKAY MEMORIAL HOSPITAL
No. 92, NORTH CHUNG SAN ROAD, Sec. 2
TAIPEI 104, TAIWAN

Cable Address:
"MACKAY TAIPEI"

T E L: 5433535
Fax 886 .2 5433638

Aug 3, 1990

Dr. Patricia Tippett
MRC Blood Group Unit

Dear Patricia,

    Thank you so much for the results of the Lewis samples. I am especially pleased that you were able to confirm the Le(a+b+) samples. However, I was woundering that if you still have any saliva left, could you possibly test the Le(a+b+) salivas with Ortho anti-Le^b which is anti-Le^{bL}. You will discover that the amount of Le^b in these cases is about the same as for Le(a-b+) salivas which is quite different from Caucasian Le(a+b-) where there is no Le^b. This together with our paraBombay findings has led us to wonder whether the Lewis of RBC (plasma) and saliva are inherited differently.

    Interesting that you have found one of your own Le(a-b-) to inhibit anti-Le^a. This phenomenon was reported by Dr. Gunson in Vox Sang 22, 344, 1972. Salmon et al from these observations (CRC Handbook Series in Clinical Laboratory Science Section D: Blood Banking Volume 1 page 311) hypothesized that the le gene may not be completely inert but an inefficient Le gene. In fact we have found some Le(a-b-) saliva to neutralize neat anti-Le^a and anti-Le^b and if the anti-Le^a and anti-Le^b is diluted almost all our Le(a-b-) salivas can be shown to have at least some Le^a and Le^b.

    Now comes an even more strange phenomenon. We were given some different caucasian Lewis phenotypes from USA and England and discovered some anomalies:

```
RBC                   Saliva
O  Le(a+b-)           Lea Leb (neutralized neat Ortho anti-Leb); also a small amount of H.
O  Le(a+b-)           Lea (Leb) (   "     1:8   "    "    )
O  Le(a+b-)           Lea no Leb
A1 Le(a+b-)           Lea (Leb) (   "     1:8   "    "    )
A1 Le(a+b-)           Lea (Leb) (   "     1:4   "    "    )
A2 Le(a+b-)           Lea (Leb) (   "     1:8   "    "    )
O  Le(a-b-) sec       H Lea (Leb) (  "    1:16  "    "    )
C  Le(a-b-) sec       H Lea (Leb) (  "    1:16  "    "    )
A1 Le(a-b-) sec       AH Lea Leb  (  "    neat   "    "   )
A1 Le(a-b-) sec       A H(Lea)no Leb
A1 Le(a-b-) non sec   Lea only
O  Le(a-b-) non sec   —
```

↑→ 與 Patricia Tippett 討論我們篩檢台灣沒有但在白種人出現的 Le(a+b-) 血型的結果，與亞洲特有的 Le(a+b+) 血型比較，提及意外的發現。（1990-08-03）

Form: AL-06

Cable Address:
"MACKAY TAIPEI"

馬偕紀念醫院
MACKAY MEMORIAL HOSPITAL
No. 92, NORTH CHUNG SAN ROAD, Sec. 2
TAIPEI 104, TAIWAN

TEL: 5433535
Fax 886 2 5433638

As you will notice the above findings of various amounts of Le^b in the saliva of Le(a+b-) Caucasians is different to previous reports. Perhaps this is because of the anti-Le^b used and also because small amounts are not detected if the anti-Le^b were not diluted. Therefore, I am wondering whether or not you might like to do some testing of your own Caucasian Le(a+b-) salivas using doubling dilutions of Ortho anti-Le^b to see whether or not our results are correct. If our findings are correct then I'm not sure how to explain them. Do you have any suggestions?

Sorry to hear about the Mi III donor's sample being **hemolysed**. I am going to try and get a whole unit today from this donor to sent to you as you previously requested Richard for a whole unit of Mi III. So if everything goes smoothly you should get it within a couple of weeks.

I haven't forgotten about sending some other Mi III samples to you, it's just that the Lewis research has kept us busy.

I would be grateful if you could send any results or answers to our questions as soon as possible without meaning to give you any pressure.

Thanking you so much for your kind help,

yours sincerely,

Marie Lin-Chu MD FCAP

MRC
Medical Research Council

'anti - Mi a'
→ anti - 'Mi a'

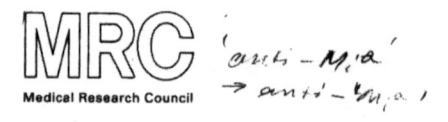

MRC Blood Group Unit
Wolfson House
University College London
4 Stephenson Way
London NW1 2HE

telephone 071-388 7752
fax   071-388 2374

reference

24 October 1990

Dr. Marie Lin-Chu
Mackay Memorial Hospital
No. 92 North Chung San Road
Sec. 2. Taipei
Taiwan

Dear Marie,

                      Miltenberger paper

Thank you very much for sending a copy of your manuscript about the clinical significance of anti-Mi^a. Carole and I would certainly like to join you as co-authors but there is a great problem. We no longer believe that Mi^a exists as a specific antigen! We think that 'anti-Mi^a' is always a mixture of antibodies; varying mixtures of anti-V^w, anti-Hut, anti-Mur and so on. Therefore, it would not be honest to be co-authors on a paper about anti-Mi^a. There are two possibilities. 1) Carole and I will not be authors and you can go ahead with it as it is. I do not know if our disbelief about Mi^a is shared by everyone although I know that many agree. 2) Carole and I are co-authors and we put in more detail about the specificities demonstrated by absorption/elution tests. The text could be reworded so that anti-Mi^a was not the antibody blamed. Carole is away to-day so I cannot summarise the work she has already done. I think it would be sufficient to give details of the two sera which gave clinical problems and say that the other sera were found by screening with Mi.III cells, but not call the antibody anti-Mi^a. I imagine that we have not tested all the antibodies and do not think it necessary to do so.

I am not sure if the tests that you have done are sufficient to claim that all antibodies are clinically significant. A referee might require more sophisticated tests, such as macrophage assays or IgG subclassing.

I realise that this is not a very helpful letter. I have only had time to read the manuscript quickly but thought that I should write to you in case we have time to discuss it in Los Angeles. Let me know if you would like to do it as anti-Mi^a or have some input by Carole and I. In any case I shall not have time to do anything to it until I return from the ISBT meeting, I am still preparing my lectures!

Hope to see you in Los Angeles,

With best wishes,

Patricia

Dr. Patricia Tippett

與Patricia Tippett討論米田堡血型抗體的命名及我們將發表該抗體的臨床意義。(1990-10-24)

INTERNATIONAL SOCIETY OF BLOOD TRANSFUSION
SOCIÉTÉ INTERNATIONALE DE TRANSFUSION SANGUINE

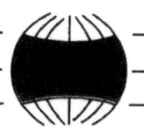

HHG/LB

18th September 1992

BY FAX

Dr. M. Lin,
President,
The R.O.C. Society of Blood Transfusion,
Mackay Memorial Hospital,
No. 92, North Chung San Road, Sec. 2,
Taipei,
TAIWAN , 10449 R.O.C.

Dear Marie,

    I am pleased to inform you that you have been elected as an ISBT Councillor.

    Your term of office will commence after the ISBT General Assembly on Monday 12th October 1992 when the results of the election will be announced.

    I look forward to your attendance at the Council meeting on Tuesday 13th October if you are attending the Congress in Sao Paulo. An agenda for this meeting will follow.

    With kind regards.

Yours sincerely,

H.H. GUNSON,
President and
acting Secretary-General

Central Office: National Directorate of NBTS, NWRHA, Gateway House, Piccadilly South, Manchester. M60 7LP.
Tel: 061-236 2263 Fax: 061-236 0519　　England

國際輸血學會 ISBT（International Society of Blood Transfusion）主席 Harold Gunson 通知我選上 ISBT（1992-1994）的理事。（1992-09-18）

```
                    The Canadian Red Cross Society
                    La Société canadienne de la Croix-Rouge
                    1800 Alta Vista Drive
                    Ottawa, Ontario, Canada K1G 4J5
                    Telephone: (613) 739-3000
                    Cable: CANCROSS Ottawa
                    Telex: 05-33784
                    FAX: (613) 731-1411
                    National Office/Siège social


                                                      May 12, 1993

Dr. Marie Lin
Transfusion Medicine Laboratory
National Health Research Institute
Mackay Memorial Hospital
92, Sec.2, Chung San North Road
Taipei
Taiwan, R. O. C.


Dear Marie:

        In response to your letter of May 5, 1993, I have two separate donors
who may be of interest to you. One group A donor with anti-Sc1 and -K, and
another donor, group O, with anti-Sc1. How many mL of antisera do you think
you need or how many phenotypings do you plan to do?

        I do not have anti-Sc2.

        I'll be attending the European Congress of the ISBT in June. Perhaps
I'll see you there.

              Kind regards.


                                              Sincerely yours,


                                              Amy Chung, PhD
```

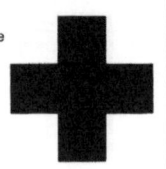

與加拿大紅十字會 Ottawa 血液中心技術主任 Amy Chung 通信，訊問能否給我們 anti-Sc1 & anti-Sc2 抗體。（1993-05-12）

OSAKA RED CROSS BLOOD CENTER

4-43, MORINOMIYA, 2-CHOME,
JOTO-KU, OSAKA, 536
JAPAN.
Fax: 06-968-4900
Tel: 06-962-7001

May 28, 1993

Dr. Marie Lin
Transfusion Medicine Laboratory of
National Health Research Institute
Mackay Memorial Hospital
92, Sec. 2, Chung San North Road
Taipei, Taiwan, R.O.C.

Dear Dr. Lin,

   I'm sending anti-Di^a and anti-Di^b to you by your request. We have not enough anti-Di^b because it is very rare in Japan.

   Anti-Di^a: group A, 3ml×4tubes
   anti-Di^b: group B, 1ml×3tubes

I attended the meeting of Japanese Society of Transfusion Medicine held in Tokyo this week. The meeting was a great success (over 1,600 people attended).

   With best wishes,

                     Yours sincerely,

                     Y. Okubo
                     Yasuto Okubo

日本紅十字會大阪府血液中心副主任大久保康人是幫助我們最多的國際知名血型專家，在 1993 年我們遇到世界罕見的 anti-Di^b 引起的新生兒溶血症，我們為確認我們的發現，請他送給我們 anti-Di^b、anti-Di^a 的抗血清。（1993-05-28）

NBTS
NATAL BLOOD TRANSFUSION SERVICE
(incorporated association not for gain)
Registration no. 05/19482/08
Incorporating THE NATAL INSTITUTE OF IMMUNOLOGY and THE NATAL FRACTIONATION CENTRE

3 June, 1993

Dr Marie Lin
Mackay Memorial Hospital
92 Chung San North Road
Taipei, Taiwan, O.O.C.

Dear Dr Lin

Thank you very much for the sample of Jk(a-b-) cells and anti-Jk3 plasma you sent recently. The sample arrived here in fair condition and is a useful addition to our reference collection.

Yours sincerely,

Elizabeth Smart (Mrs)
Section Supervisor, Serology

1990 年代從事血型研究者，都經過 Gamma 公司主辦的全球稀有血型血球及血清交換組織 SCARF（約有 30 個著名的實驗室參加）做交換，台灣因在短期內發表許多新的血型，所以馬偕醫院血庫常常被要求做血清血球的交換，這封信是南非 Natal Blood Transfusion Service 寄來的感謝函。（1993-06-03）

HOKKAIDO RED CROSS BLOOD CENTER

November 8, 1993

Dr. Marie Lin
President
The R.O.C. Society of Blood Transfusion
Director
Transfusion Medicine Laboratory of
National Health Research Institute
Mackay Memorial Hospital
92, Sec.2, Chang San North Road
Taipei, Taiwan, R.O.C.

Dear Dr. Lin,

    Thank you very much for your letter of October 28th regarding your invitation to Dr. Takahashi to the Annual Meeting of the R.O.C. Society of Blood Transfusion which will be held on November 12th, 1993 in Taipei. I am pleased to send Dr. Takahashi to the meeting.

    I appreciate you that you kindly recommended me as the ISBT Counciller. I am also running for the ISBT Regional Counciller. I always appreciate your kindness.

    With very best wishes.

Sincerely yours,

Sadayoshi Sekiguchi, M.D.
Director
Hokkaido Red Cross Blood Center

ADDRESS : YAMANOTE 2-2, NISHI-KU
SAPPORO 063, JAPAN
TEL : 011-613-6121
FAX : 011-613-4131

與日本北海道紅十字會血液中心主任關口教授連繫，有關邀請高橋醫師來台，在台灣輸血學會演講事宜。（1993-11-08）

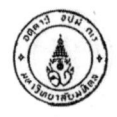

ภาควิชาเวชศาสตร์การธนาคารเลือด คณะแพทยศาสตร์ศิริราชพยาบาล มหาวิทยาลัยมหิดล
Department of Transfusion Medicine, Faculty of Medicine Siriraj Hospital, Mahidol University
2 ถนนพรานนก ต. ศิริราช อ. บางกอกน้อย กทม. 10700 Fax no. 4128419
Bangkok 10700 Tel. 4110273, 4112424, 4110241-9 ext. 2156, 2157, 2159, 5086
THAILAND

December 1, 1993

Marie Lin M.D., FCAP
President
The ROC Society of Blood Transfusion
Director of Transfusion Medicine Laboratory
National Health Research Institutes ROC
Mackay Memorial Hospital
92, Sec 2,
Chung San N Road
Taipei Taiwan ROC.

Dear Marie,

    It was really very nice to see you and renew our friendship. I think about the trip to Taipei and Hualien often and have many wonderful memories of all the things I saw, the people I met and the many unique experiences we shared.

    Enclosed herewith please find anti Mur, anti Anek and MI, III and VI positive cells. Which I promise to send you.

    With best personal regards.

Yours sincerely,

Dasnayanee

Dasnayanee Chandanayingyong, M.D.
(Professor and Chairperson)

Encl:
DC/hj

我們在 1983 年發現米田堡血型，接下來有許多國際知名的血型專家參與協助和研究，其中有泰國 Siriraj 醫院 Chandanayingyong 教授贈送我們 anti-Mur、anti-Anek、MI、MIII、MVI 的細胞。（1993-12-01）

CENTRAL BLOOD CENTRE
JAPANESE RED CROSS SOCIETY

Dr Marie Lin   14th February 1994
Director of Transfusion Medicine Laboratory
National Health Research Institutes R.O.C.
Mackay Memorial Hospital
92,Sec.Chung San N.RD.
Taipei
R.O.C.

Dear Dr Lin,

I am happy to share our reagents for red cell antigens with you. I hope these reagents are usuful for your work.

anti-Mur	KAMIYA	A	albumin at RT(should be use undiluted serum)
-Hil	KOBAYASHI	AB	antiglobulin (titer 256)
-Anek	IBE	O	antiglobulin (titer 256)
murine monoclonal			
$-Le^a$(504A)			enzyme at RT
$-Le^b$(609F-4F5)			enzyme at RT
-Ge(glycophorin C)(908-42)			saline at RT
-DAF(CD55)(907-3G2)			saline,enzyme,antiglobulin
-CD59(9102-38)			saline, antiglobulin
human monoclonal			
-D(D6)	IgM		saline
-E(E9)	IgG		enzyme

I am sorry that MiX red cells are not good condition, I am going to send another MiX cells to you later.
I am looking forward to seeing you again.

Sincerely yours,

Makoto Uchikawa
Makoto Uchikawa, PhD.

日本紅十字會血液中心（在東京）的內川誠教授，也是國際知名血型專家，贈送我們許多我們需要的血型抗體。（1994-02-14）

DEPARTMENT OF TRANSFUSION MEDICINE & IMMUNOHEMATOLOGY
FACULTY OF MEDICINE THE UNIVERSITY OF TOKYO

HONGO 7-3-1, BUNKYO-KU
TOKYO 113, JAPAN
PHONE:(81)-3-3815-5411 EX.5160
FAX: (81)-3-3816-2516

Dr.Marie Lin

Director

Transfusion Medicine Laboratory of

National Health Research Institute

Mackay Memorial Hospital

92, Sec. 2,,Chung San North Road

Taipei, Taiwan, R.O.C.

19, May,1994.

Dear Dr.Lin

Thank you very much for your fax letter of 17, May,1994.

I think that your work is very important in platelet serology.

I willingly accept your proposal.

I will receive your samples(PRP) on May 30th., 1994.

And I will do platelet-phenotyping these samples as soon as I can.

I am looking forward to seeing you at the meeting.

Sincerely yours,

Yoichi Shibata M.D.

Dept.of Transfusion Medicine and

Immunohematology

Faculty of Medicine, Tokyo University

日本東京大學輸血醫學部主任柴田洋一教授協助我們做血小板的研究。（1994-05-19）

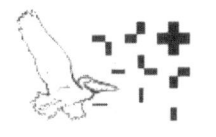

CLB

amsterdam 18-07-1994

central
laboratory
of the
netherlands red cross
blood transfusion
service

Dr M.Lin, MD FCAP,
Tr.Med.Lab.of Nat. Health Research Inst.,
Mackay Memorial Hospital
92, Sec. 2, Chung San North Road,
Taipei, Taiwan, R.O.C.

plesmanlaan 125
1066 CX amsterdam
PO box 9190
1006 AD amsterdam
telephone 20 - 5129222
telefax 20 - 512 3332

department bloodgroupserology
reference anti-Jr(a)
your reference

direct telephone number 205123373
telefax number 205123474

Dear Marie,

It was good to see you at the ISBT congress.
As promised I am sending you 10 vials of anti-Jr(a) serum.
This serum is suited for the bloodgroups O and A and the antibodies react in the IAGT with added bovine albumin and in the PEG IAGT.

Do let me know if the package arrived safely.
With best wishes,
yours sincerely,

Marijke Overbeeke

荷蘭紅十字會血液中心實驗室（CLB）血型部主任 Marijke Overbeeke 送給我們 anti-Jr(a) 血清，去分析診斷一個困難的輸血個案。我在 1992 年 7 月為了解決當時有時遇到的輸血引起的呼吸窘困症，整個月都待在 CLB 的白血球研究室，荷蘭人都很親切，讓人有賓至如歸的感覺，我到現在還記得他們給人感受的溫暖，我還記得我常常告訴他們說「荷蘭是我的第二個故鄉」。（1994-07-18）

TRANSFUSION
The Journal of the American Association of Blood Banks

July 25, 1994

Marie Lin, M.D.
National Health Research Institute
Transfusion Medicine Laboratory
Mackay Memorial Hospital
92, Chung San North Road, Sec 2
TAIPEI, TAIWAN, R.O.C.

Dear Marie,

Thank you for sending me your response to Dr. Feng's letter about the possible HDN case caused by anti-Mi^a. I believe that your comments are pertinent and correct and provide a suitable answer to Dr. Feng's letter. I will make a few changes at the editing stage as per your request. It seems to me that perhaps a suitable solution to the problem would be to replace one of the screening cells in a current three cell set, with one carrying the same (Rh, Kidd, etc) antigens, that was from an Mi.III donor. It would seem that with your high incidence of such donors, finding a suitable replacement would be possible. This would ensure that anti-Mi^a was found in antibody-screening tests on potential transfusion recipients, the alternative would seem to be a full IAT crossmatch for all patients, clearly more wasteful than specialized screening. By running screening tests at 37C, clinically insignificant examples of anti-Mi^a would not be a problem (we deliberately miss many examples of cold-reactive anti-P$_1$ in our patients). There seems to me to be no doubt that some examples of anti-Mi^a can cause in vivo red cell destruction and hence transfusion reactions and HDN. I will consult with the Editor to see if perhaps an editorial comment covering these points should be added after the two letters.

Based on our current production schedule, Dr. Feng's letter and your reply should appear in the January 1995 issue of the journal. However, space availability occasionally results in letters appearing one issue earlier or one issue later than originally planned.

↑→ 當我們在 1994 年發表 anti-Mi^a [53] 的臨床意義後，香港衛生部病理研究所的 Chi. S. Feng 即去信 *TRANSFUSION*，認為再增加抗體篩檢細胞的抗原項目太麻煩，於是我們和香港的 Dr. Feng 在 *TRANSFUSION* 打筆戰 [57]。（1994-07-25）

Thank you for your interest in TRANSFUSION and your prompt reply to Dr. Feng's letter. It was good to see you in Amsterdam.

All best wishes,

Peter

Peter D. Issitt, Ph.D.
Associate Editor for Correspondence

PDI/meo

HONG KONG RED CROSS
BLOOD TRANSFUSION SERVICE

No. 15 King's Park Rise
Yaumatei
Kowloon
Hong Kong

Telephone : 710 1333
Telegram : BLOODTRANS
Telex : 60160 BRCHK HX
FAX : 780 1862

24th August 1994

Dr. Marie Lin, MD FCAP,
Mackay Memorial Hospital,
92, Sec. 2, Chung San North Road,
Taipei, Taiwan,
Republic of China.

Dear Dr. Lin,

Anti-Mi^a which have caused HDN or HTR

Thank you very much for your FAX dated 24.8.94.

We also expected to obtain a positive result on your serum which caused TR, but contrary to expection we obtained negative results by performing the test twice; hence I attempted to ascribe the cause of the TR to the ability of the serum to activate complement. The following are the specificities of our Miltenberger antibodies (anti-Mi's), together with our other Lab. findings:

Case No.	Specificity	MMA % Reactivity	Serological findings RT	SIAT	SIAT titre
Donors					
6	Anti-Mur+Hut	10	V	V	4
12	-do-	4	-	V	8
27	-do-	12	V	V	16
Patient					
Our HTR case	Anti-Mur+MUT (mainly anti-Mur)	16	+	+++	16

Key: V=visual agglutination. SIAT: saline antiglobulin test
RT= room temperature phase. Ref.range of MMA: 1-3%

We do not know whether the addition of sodium azide would affect the MMA, but if the preservative has not yet been added, I would suggest that this be not done. 2-3 ml. of a sample would be adequate, though we would prefer larger volumes. We would like to perform the MMA test even if sodium azide has been added. We would like to have samples which have caused HDN or HTR, with which to standardize our MMA. On the other hand, samples which merely contain anti-Mi^a, but which lack such clinical data are of little value, as we also have quite a number of these samples.

Dr. Leong and Dr. Lin would like thank you for your kind assistance and would like to join me in extending to you our best wishes and kindest regards.

Yours sincerely,

K. H. Mak,
Chief Technologist.

P.S. We found that treatment of sample by heat, 56°C for 60 min. so as to convert plasma to serum, would render a positive MMA to become negative, presumably due to denaturation of the immunoglobulin

香港紅十字會輸血服務處的來函，在 1980 年代香港已是捐血的國家（沒有血液買賣），所以受到國際重視，K. H. Mak 也是著名的輸血專家。（1994-08-24）

The University of Texas Medical Branch at Galveston

DIVISION OF
HEMATOLOGY/ONCOLOGY

4.164 John Sealy
301 University Boulevard
Galveston, Texas 77555-0565
(409) 772-1164
FAX (409) 772-3533

Jack B. Alperin, M.D.
Acting Chief

Sanjay Awasthi, M.D.
J. David Bessman, M.D.
Frank H. Gardner, M.D.
Donna J. Griebel, M.D.
James T. Lin, M.D.
Suzanne McClure, M.D.

January 3, 1995

Marie Lin, M.D.
Mackay Memorial Hospital
92, Sec. 2, Chung San North Road
Taipei, Taiwan, R.O.C

Dear Marie:

    Thank you for your Season's Greetings letter. It was good to hear from you. It is good to know that you continue to be a regular contributor to Vox Sang and Transfusion. I have read some of your recently published papers. Sorry to learn that you acquired hepatitis C, but I am glad to know that interferon has been an effective therapy. I am also sorry to learn that your father had passed away. The painting "Hawaiian Sea" exhibits serenity and grace. You continue to impress me with your intelligence and sense of beauty.

    Lynn and I have been very busy this past year. Both in our professional activities and in our travels. Among other things, I made a two week visit to Antarctica for a vacation that was greatly needed and truly relaxing.

    Let us know when you will next come to the United States. Lynn and I would very much like to visit with you. Best wishes for the New Year.

Sincerely yours,

Jack

Jack B. Alperin, M.D.
Professor, Department of
Internal Medicine
Acting Chief, Division of
Hematology-Oncology

JBA/cah

1978-1981 年我在美國德州墨西哥灣（現改為美國灣）中的一個小島 Galveston 上的德州大學醫學分院的病理部（The University of Texas Medical Branch）接受住院醫師的訓練，當時我已經是台大病理研究所的副教授，所以有些時候不太習慣，這位 Jack B. Alperin 教授很佩服我有始有終的把他每週一個案例的試題做完，後來我們變成好朋友，所以有時他和夫人邀請我和我兩個兒子一起去享用愉快的晚餐，我們一直保持聯繫約 30 多年，直到兩年前為止。
（1995-01-03）

Vox Sanguinis

Copy to be sent to author(s)

(Note to referees: Please do not put your name or signature on this form. If necessary attach additional sheets. Please return the original and two copies to the editor.)

Reference No.   94/157

Title manuscript: NEONATAL ALLOIMMUNE THROMBOCYTOPENIA IN TAIWAN DUE TO AN ANTIBODY AGAINST A LABILE COMPONENT(S) OF HPA-3a (BAK[a])

Author(s): Marie Lin, Shiow-Hua Shieh, Der-Cherng Liang, Ting-Fan Yang, Yoichi Shibata

Referee's comments: #1

This paper is of interest to laboratories investigating possible cases of neonatal alloimmune thrombocytopenia.

General comments:

Antigenicity of HPA-3a is strongly influenced by glycosylation HPA-3a antibodies from different individuals vary in their reactions with asialo-GPIIb (Take et al, BJH 1990;76,395; Goldberger et al, Blood 1991;78,681). The paper would be considerably more interesting if the changes which affect reactivity of fixed or stored platelets with the reported antibody could be determined. For example, is there loss of sialic acid residues with storage, and does treatment of fresh platelets with neuraminidase lead to loss of reactivity?

Recommendations for minor revision:

The main point of the paper is the importance of using "fresh" platelets for detecting this particular antibody. Therefore, more details should be given in the material and methods section regarding the timing of specimen donation, platelet preparation, and performance of the test. Details of platelet fixation in the SPRCA should also be mentioned in the methods section.

The MAIPA and immunoblot assays done should be mentioned briefly in the methods. Were these tests done with fresh platelets? Did the known anti-HPA-3a serum (Fujiwara) react in these tests?

KARGER Medical and Scientific Publishers
Basel · Freiburg · Paris · London · New York
New Delhi · Bangkok · Singapore · Tokyo · Sydney

433/03

努力七年證明「只和新鮮血小板」反應的抗體，解決國際長久以來無法證明存在的血小板抗體的論文 [69]「Neonatal alloimmune thrombocytopenia in

Vox Sanguinis

Copy to be sent to author(s)

(Note to referees: Please do not put your name or signature on this form. If necessary attach additional sheets. Please return the original and two copies to the editor.)

Reference No. 94/157

Title manuscript: NEONATAL ALLOIMMUNE THROMBOCYTOPENIA IN TAIWAN DUE TO AN ANTIBODY AGAINST A LABILE COMPINENT(S) OF HPA-3a (BAK[a])

Author(s): Marie Lin, Shiow-Hua Shieh, Der-Cherng Liang, Ting-Fan Yang, Yoichi Shibata

Referee's comments: #2

I found this report interesting. The detection of platelet-specific antibodies is still hampered by the lack of one definitive test that can be both sensitive and specific.

This report helps to emphasize the need to interpret with caution any negative result based on one assay alone.

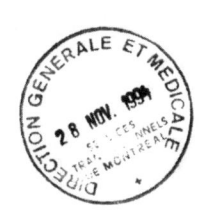

KARGER Medical and Scientific Publishers
Basel · München · Paris · London · New York
New Delhi · Bangkok · Singapore · Tokyo · Sydney

433/03

Taiwan due to an antibody against a labile component of HPA-3a(Bak[a])」，國際輸血學會月刊 *Vox Sanguinis* 編輯部的評論。（1994-11-28）

> Secretariat
> The 8th Asia-Pacific Regional Congress of ISBT
> Chinese Society of Blood Transfusion
> No.37 Beisanhuan Zhonglu
> Beijing, 100088
> People's Republic of China
> Tel: (010) 62382363
> Fax: (010) 62382363
>
> October 28, 1996
>
> Dr. Marie Lin
> Dept. of Laboratory Med.
> Mackay Memorial Hospital
> 92 Sec.2. Chuong Shan North Road
> Taipei
>
> Dear Dr. Lin,
>
> The 8th Asia-Pacific Regional Congress of the International Society of Blood Transfusion will be held in Beijing, China on October 30 to November 2, 1997. The Congress takes great pleasure in inviting you to be vice chairman of educational committee.
>
> Please confirm your participation at your earliest convenience.
>
> With kind regards,
>
> Yours sincerely
>
> Kai-rui Hu
> Secretary-General

1990年左右，我參與國際輸血學會幫助中國輸血發展的團隊，前往中國三次。中國輸血學會決定1997年主辦亞太地區國際輸血學會，當時天津血液中心的HU Kai-rui 擔任大會秘書長，他代表大會邀請我擔任將召開的國際輸血學會教育委員會的副主席，但因發生中共飛彈試射（1996），讓我驚醒過來，就以工作忙碌為由婉拒。（1996-10-28）

附錄 7

演講記錄（2006-2016）

陸2015每年平均有一場輸血相關的演講

2010 以前

2006 (14)

檔名	備註	日期	類型	大小
Taiwan population genetics(TUSO 2006).ppt	成大臺灣生物海外研習營	2006/2/7 下午 03...	Microsoft Office...	14,424 KB
粒線體DNA及Y染色體的研究(NSC, 1-2006).ppt	國科會	2006/2/21 下午 0...	Microsoft Office...	14,413 KB
台灣原住民基因的研究(慈濟醫學院)060303.ppt		2006/3/2 下午 03...	Microsoft Office...	11,041 KB
台灣原住民基因的研究(Rotary meeting)060307.ppt	扶輪社	2006/3/7 下午 03...	Microsoft Office...	11,066 KB
台灣族群的遷移 200612.ppt	台灣科學國際會議(中央圖書館)	2006/5/16 上午 1...	Microsoft Office...	21,849 KB
台灣族群遺傳基因的過去與現在-1.ppt	各中學化學會	2006/5/19 下午 0...	Microsoft Office...	18,492 KB
Taiwan population genetics, past and present 5-30-06 and med assoc 6-30-06.ppt		2006/5/30 下午 0...	Microsoft Office...	31,267 KB
Taiwan population genetics, past and present(醫學會).ppt		2006/7/7 上午 11...	Microsoft Office...	30,612 KB
Taiwan population genetics - 2006 KMUAA.ppt	高醫校友會	2006/8/17 下午 0...	Microsoft Office...	26,287 KB
Taiwan population genetics - 2006 TUSO.ppt		2006/8/29 下午 0...	Microsoft Office...	41,835 KB
多樣性台灣.ppt	國科會	2006/9/27 下午 0...	Microsoft Office...	7,438 KB
Perspectives of mtDNA, Y and aDNA.ppt	?中研院史語所	2006/10/12 下午...	Microsoft Office...	1,479 KB
Taiwan population genetics (culture dept)- 9-30-2006.ppt	民俗賞文化部	2006/11/28 上午...	Microsoft Office...	45,404 KB
中山醫會 11-29-2006.ppt		2006/11/29 下午...	Microsoft Office...	19,652 KB

2007 (10)

檔名	備註	日期	類型	大小
population genetic (Taichung) 12-15-2006.ppt	台中輸血會	2006/12/15 下午...	Microsoft Office...	37,151 KB
population genetic, Yang-Ming U 3-16-2007.ppt	陽明醫學院	2007/3/19 上午 1...	Microsoft Office...	30,433 KB
Taiwan population genetics, health and diseases, TUSO 3-24-2007.ppt		2007/3/24 下午 0...	Microsoft Office...	19,478 KB
台灣族群的遺傳基因台灣導讀 03-21-2007.ppt		2007/4/3 下午 03...	Microsoft Office...	15,840 KB
population genetic (Kyoto) 04-14-2007.ppt	京都國際妊娠分娩協會	2007/4/14 下午 0...	Microsoft Office...	31,406 KB
公視.ppt	節目	2007/7/10 下午 0...	Microsoft Office...	3,339 KB
Perspectives of mtDNA, Y and aDNA-Academia Sinica 7-2007.ppt	中研院	2007/8/17 上午 1...	Microsoft Office...	4,216 KB
Genetic structure of Taiwanese-Taita Pathol Institute.ppt	台大病理研究所	2007/11/9 上午 0...	Microsoft Office...	12,456 KB
永恆的西拉雅族.ppt	台南縣文化局	2007/12/3 下午 0...	Microsoft Office...	10,320 KB
Non Abor Taiwanese-MMH_2 007.ppt	馬偕醫院(即原住民台灣人)	2007/12/25 下午...	Microsoft Office...	6,311 KB

2008 (10)

檔名	備註	日期	類型	大小
NATaiwanese-MMH_2 (modified).ppt		2008/1/4 下午 01...	Microsoft Office...	6,814 KB
Classification and dispersion of Austronesian-Academia Sinica 2-2008 (2).ppt	中央研究院	2008/2/14 下午 0...	Microsoft Office...	15,374 KB
97-02-15 Lin (Taitong MMH metabolic syndrome).ppt	台東基督教民健康研討會	2008/3/7 下午 03...	Microsoft Office...	1,260 KB
Non Abor Taiwanese-TSBT 2008 (2).ppt		2008/6/12 下午 0...	Microsoft Office...	21,145 KB
Taiwan Abo genetic 1-26-08 (Puyuma meeting) (2).ppt		2008/6/12 下午 0...	Microsoft Office...	34,707 KB
Non Abor Taiwanese-MMH_2 007 (2).ppt	馬偕醫院國際生殖研討會	2008/6/12 下午 0...	Microsoft Office...	6,365 KB
The genetic profiles of Taiwanese -KMU 2008.ppt		2008/8/25 下午 0...	Microsoft Office...	35,441 KB
The genetic profiles of Taiwanese -Taipei, September 2008(Taiwan Union).ppt	外省國民黨榮團(娃娃事件)	2008/9/1 下午 03...	Microsoft Office...	34,515 KB
The genetic profiles of Taiwanese -Taipei, November 2008(Pu-zi).ppt	北投教育文化協會	2008/11/18 下午...	Microsoft Office...	31,940 KB
The genetic profiles of Taiwanese -Taichung, December 18, 2008 (Pu-Kong-ln).ppt	埔光英語營	2008/12/18 下午...	Microsoft Office...	28,255 KB

2009 (5)

檔名	備註	日期	類型	大小
Classification and dispersion of Austronesian-Academia Sinica 1-2009 (plain tribes)_980113.ppt		2009/1/16 下午 0...	Microsoft Office...	1,630 KB
Silaya meeting 2009 05 30.ppt		2009/5/27 下午 0...	Microsoft Office...	578 KB
Taiwan population genetic (National Library) Aug 15, 2009.ppt	國家圖書館平埔研究 台大生物多樣性研究室 國語中央圖書	2009/8/15 下午 0...	Microsoft Office...	30,263 KB
More genetic sharing among the populations of Taiwan sept 14.ppt	這是太平洋血緣學會	2009/9/14 下午 0...	Microsoft Office...	4,796 KB
Taiwan population genetic-Chinan University October 29, 2009.ppt	長榮大學	2009/10/28 下午...	Microsoft Office...	26,419 KB

2010 (10)

檔名	備註	日期	類型	大小
Taiwan population genetic-Tokyo 11-20- 2009 (2).ppt	東京熊本大學	2010/1/19 下午 0...	Microsoft Office...	25,827 KB
human migration and Taiwan populations 2010.ppt	同郷會	2010/1/19 下午 0...	Microsoft Office...	22,833 KB
Taiwan population genetic-Forensic Medicine, NTU, June 2, 2010.ppt	台大法醫學研究所	2010/6/2 下午 12...	Microsoft Office...	27,282 KB
Human Migration, Forensic Medicine NTUH 2010.ppt		2010/6/11 下午 0...	Microsoft Office...	12,864 KB
白藜因專人類的遷移 Sin-Yian-Kuan 20090721.ppt	新眼光電視錄影	2010/6/14 下午 0...	Microsoft Office...	4,307 KB
National Yang_Ming_University_Mt_Workshop_091028.pptx		2010/8/25 下午 0...	Microsoft Office...	12,891 KB
Human Migration, Dept of Surgery, KMU 2010-July (2).ppt		2010/8/30 上午 1...	Microsoft Office...	12,617 KB
我們留著不同的血液 -2010 Austin.ppt	台灣同郷會德州 Austin 年會	2010/9/1 下午 0...	Microsoft Office...	29,216 KB
我們留著不同的血液, Shih-Lin Church-2010-10-7.ppt	士林教會文化	2010/10/5 下午 0...	Microsoft Office...	21,049 KB
我們留著不同的血液, Abor TV, 2010-10-14 (1) .ppt		2010/12/20 下午...	Microsoft Office...	13,251 KB

010 我們流著不同的血液出版

2011

檔名	日期	類型	大小
The genetic profiles of Taiwanese -Taipei, September 2008(Taiwan Union).ppt	2011/1/21 下午 1...	Microsoft Office...	31,730 KB
我們留著不同的血液, Teichung Medical Association 2011-04-24ppt.ppt	2011/4/12 上午 1...	Microsoft Office...	18,767 KB
我們留著不同的血液 -1, Teichung Medical Association 2011-04-24ppt.ppt	2011/5/20 下午 0...	Microsoft Office...	20,217 KB
Mackay Medical College international mtDNA meeting.ppt	2011/6/13 上午 1...	Microsoft Office...	288 KB
我們留著不同的血液 -1, Kaohsiung Medical Univ. 6-1-2011.ppt	2011/7/15 上午 1...	Microsoft Office...	18,884 KB
Kaohsiung Chang Keng Hosp mtDNA international meeting -1 08062011.ppt	2011/9/13 上午 0...	Microsoft Office...	17,229 KB
KMUAA 08-20-2011 Chicago.ppt	高醫校友會	2011/10/17 下午...	Microsoft Office...	29,374 KB

2012

File	Date	Type	Size
我們留著不同的血液-2010-12 Susanhan museum.ppt	2012/2/10 下午 0...	Microsoft Office...	29,958 KB
Taipei Art University 2012-03-19 (2) _馬水龍.ppt	2012/3/27 上午 1...	Microsoft Office...	30,932 KB
Western Rotary Club Regional Meeting 2012-04-25.ppt	2012/4/24 下午 0...	Microsoft Office...	25,060 KB
Tainan Art Association 12-15-2011 ppt.pptm	2012/4/26 下午 0...	Microsoft Office...	20,863 KB
KMU pharcogenetic 2012-04-06.ppt	2012/4/26 下午 0...	Microsoft Office...	29,701 KB
Formosan Med. Assoc. for presentation 2011-11-13.ppt	2012/4/26 下午 0...	Microsoft Office...	22,170 KB
Taiwan perspective Shilin Church 2011-11-17 .ppt	2012/4/26 下午 0...	Microsoft Office...	2,557 KB
KMU General Education 2012-06-13ppt.ppt	2012/6/7 上午 11...	Microsoft Office...	31,839 KB
VGH, NTUH joint meeting 2012-07-07.ppt	2012/7/7 上午 06...	Microsoft Office...	23,590 KB
Shin-Chu Comunication University 2012-05-17.ppt	2012/8/3 上午 10...	Microsoft Office...	31,850 KB
Hualien Sun Shine Asso 2012-8-25 (2).ppt	2012/8/25 上午 0...	Microsoft Office...	28,942 KB
Mackay Memorial Hospital 2012-9-1 (2).ppt	2012/8/31 下午 0...	Microsoft Office...	33,761 KB

2013

File	Date	Type	Size
Tao Yuan Steel Association-1 2013-1-17 (2).ppt	2013/1/16 下午 0...	Microsoft Office...	30,597 KB
Cheng-Wei Publisher 2013-1-26.ppt	2013/1/26 上午 1...	Microsoft Office...	31,048 KB
Taiwanesse, Ping-tong An-Tai Hospital 2013-3-7 (2).ppt	2013/3/5 下午 05...	Microsoft Office...	33,577 KB
讓二二八受難者追戲回家 (2).ppt	2013/3/12 下午 0...	Microsoft Office...	16 KB
Tai-ta alumni association 2013-3-23 (2).ppt	2013/3/23 上午 1...	Microsoft Office...	25,864 KB
Chi-Long Chang Keng Hospital 2013-07-12 (2).ppt	2013/7/15 下午 0...	Microsoft Office...	25,745 KB
NATWA 2013-04-20 (2).ppt	2013/7/15 下午 0...	Microsoft Office...	28,761 KB
TWA TV 2013-07-2 (2).ppt	2013/8/2 下午 02...	Microsoft Office...	7,760 KB
識校的原住民博物館 (2).ppt	2013/8/2 下午 02...	Microsoft Office...	3,150 KB
尋找228事件遇南的追戲 (2).ppt	2013/11/26 下午...	Microsoft Office...	155 KB
MMH Christian Medical Association 2013-11-27.ppt	2013/11/27 下午...	Microsoft Office...	23,663 KB
Public hearing- Taiwan plain tribe heritage 2013-08-28 (2).pptx	2013/11/29 下午...	Microsoft Office...	11,349 KB
Kaohsiung Medical Univ. 2013-12-18.ppt	2013/12/10 下午...	Microsoft Office...	31,018 KB

2014

File	Date	Type	Size
Kan-San Library 2014-2-8.ppt	2014/2/7 下午 03...	Microsoft Office...	39,259 KB
2014-3-26 Kaohsung Medical University.pptm	2014/3/21 上午 1...	Microsoft Office...	42,674 KB
TV Ming-Shu interview 2014-4-7 人類遷移 (2).ppt	2014/4/7 下午 02...	Microsoft Office...	4,057 KB
2014-04-18 Kaohsung Shieu-Kang Hospital.pptm	2014/4/17 下午 0...	Microsoft Office...	43,149 KB
2014-05-21 Mackay Memorial Hospital.pptm	2014/6/24 下午 1...	Microsoft Office...	27,525 KB
2014-07-3 Dr. Saji's HLA Lab The origin of Taiwan population.pptm	2014/7/1 下午 05...	Microsoft Office...	30,551 KB
new power point for lectures-Pu Chi H (2).ppt	2014/7/28 下午 0...	Microsoft Office...	70,823 KB
Hua-Lien Tong-Hua Univ 2014-11-3 .ppt	2014/11/3 上午 0...	Microsoft Office...	25,028 KB
Kaohsiung Medical Univ. 2014-12-10.ppt	2014/11/11 上午...	Microsoft Office...	21,591 KB

2015

名稱	修改日期	類型	大小
Kaohsiung Medical Univ. 2014-12-10 classmate reunion.ppt	2015/7/21 下午 0...	Microsoft Office...	21,582 KB
讓228事件遇害的遠戚回家-2015-10-3_1 LA.pptx	2015/10/3 下午 1...	Microsoft Office...	463 KB
Japanese Red Cross Annual Meeting 2015-10-6.ppt	2015/10/12 下午...	Microsoft Office...	555 KB
2015-11-2 Nei Fu Rotary Club meeting.pptx	2015/10/26 下午...	Microsoft Office...	69,583 KB
溯源台灣_20151104_內湖.pptx	2015/11/3 下午 0...	Microsoft Office...	14,362 KB
Chong-San Church 2015-11-18.ppt	2015/11/17 下午...	Microsoft Office...	22,304 KB
VA General Hospital 2015-12-16.pptx	2015/12/15 下午...	Microsoft Office...	30,685 KB
Taichuan Tatong Rotary 2015-12-31.pptx	2015/12/29 上午...	Microsoft Office...	22,022 KB

2016

名稱	修改日期	類型	大小
讓228事件遇害的遠戚回家-2015-10-3 LA.pptx	2016/2/22 下午 1...	Microsoft Office...	876 KB
DNA分析 二二八 _Japanese version.ppt	2016/2/26 下午 0...	Microsoft Office...	16,690 KB

林媽利教授簡介

出生年月日：1938.05.30　出生地：台灣宜蘭
現職：馬偕紀念醫院輸血醫學暨分子人類學名譽顧問醫師
E mail: marielin0530@gmail.com

學經簡歷

高雄醫學院醫學系學士	1957-1964
國立台灣大學醫學院病理研究所碩士	1964-1967
台灣大學醫學院病理系助理、講師、副教授	1965-1980
美國德州德州大學醫學院 Galveston 分校病理科住院醫師	1972-1973;1978-1981
美國病理學會研究員（Fellow, FCAP）	1981-
台灣及美國病理專科醫師	1981-
台灣文化學院榮譽博士	2001
國立台灣大學法醫研究所兼任教授	2004-
台灣馬偕紀念醫院檢驗科主任	1981-1998
台灣馬偕紀念醫院醫學研究部輸血暨分子人類學研究組組長	1988-2013
台灣馬偕紀念醫院醫學研究部輸血暨分子人類學研究組榮譽顧問醫師	2013-

榮譽獎項

教育部四維獎章	1975
台灣輸血學會理事長及秘書長	1987-1996
王明寧研究貢獻獎	1992
國際輸血學會理事（學會地址在倫敦）	1992-1996

衛生署國家血液政策衛生獎章	1994
國際輸血學會西太平洋地區分支第十屆大會主席	1999
主辦瑞士日內瓦大學「東亞及台灣島上人類的遷徙」國際研討會	2003
國家衛生研究院研究獎章	2009
高雄醫學院2010年榮譽校友獎	2010
台灣醫學會杜聰明博士紀念獎	2011
巫永福文化評論獎	2011
2011年國際輸血學會獎	2011
立法院厚生基金會醫療奉獻獎	2017
北美洲台灣人教授協會廖述宗教授紀念獎	2017
北美洲台灣人醫師協會林一雄醫師紀念獎	2022
中華捐血運動協會「捐血運動50週年感謝獎」	2024

About Professor Dr. Marie Lin

Date of birth: May 30, 1938
Place of birth: Yilan, Taiwan
Current position: Honorary consultant in Transfusion medicine and Molecular anthropology at Mackay Memorial Hospital

Curriculum Vitae

Kaohsiung Medical College   1957-1964
Graduate School of Pathology, School of Medicine, NTU, M.S. 1964-1967
Assistant (1965-1969), Lecturer (1969-1976), Associate professor (1976-1980) in Department of Pathology, NTUH   1965-1980
Residency in Pathology, UT Med. Branch, Galveston, Texas
  1972-1973; 1978-1981
Board of Clinical and Anatomical Pathology, US and Taiwan   1981-
Fellow of American College of Pathology (FCAP)   1981-
Honorary Doctorate of Taiwan Culture Collage   2001
Visiting Professor, Institute of Forensic Medicine, National Taiwan University   2004-
Director of Lab. Medicine, Mackay Memorial Hospital (MMH), Taiwan
  1981-1998
Director of Transf. Med. and Molecular Anthropology Lab., MMH
  1988-2013
Honorary consultant in Transf. Med. and Molecular Anthropology at MMH
  2013-

Awards and Honors

Su-Wei Awards, Minister of Education	1975
President and Secretary General of the Taiwan Society of Blood Transfusion	1987-1996
Wang Ming-Ning Research and Contribution Award	1992
Counselor of the International Society of Blood Transfusion (ISBT)	1992-1996
Wei-Shen Award for contribution to National Blood Program, Ministry of Health	1994
President of 10th Regional Congress of ISBT, Western Pacific Region, Taipei	1999
Research award, National Health Research Institute, Taiwan	2009
Outstanding Alumni Award, Kaohsiung Medical University	2010
Honorary President of 22th ISBT, Western Pacific Region, Taipei	2011
Dr. Tu Chong-Ming Memorial Award for Basic Med. Science from FMA	2011
ISBT (International Society of Blood Transfusion) Award	2011
Wu Yong Fu Literature Commentary Award	2011
Medical Dedication Award from The Welfare Foundation, Legislative Yuan	2017
Contribution Award from NATPA「廖述宗教授紀念獎」	2017
Lin I-Yang Memorial Award from North American Taiwanese Medical Association	2022
Contribution Award from 50 years Anniversary of Taiwan Blood Donation Association	2024

林媽利教授（Marie Lin, Lin M）學術著作

一、專書

1. 林媽利　《輸血醫學》中文版　台北：健康文化，第 1 版 1990 年；第 2 版 1997 年；第 3 版 2005 年；第 4 版 2018 年（總校閱）；第 5 版 2021 年（總校閱）；第 6 版 2023 年（總校閱）。

2. A. Sanchez-Mazas, R. Blench, M. D. Ross, I. Petros and M. Lin. *Past Human Migrations in East Asia, matching Archaeology, Linguistics and Genetics*. Routledge Curzon, 2008.

3. 林媽利　2010　《我們流著不同的血液》　台北：前衛出版社。

4. 林媽利　2018　《圖解台灣血緣─從基因研究解答台灣族群起源》　台北：前衛出版社。

5. Marie Lin "Chapter Seven: Retracing the Han among the Taiwanese" in Shyu-Tu Lee and Jack F. Williams eds. *Taiwan's Struggle*. Rowman & Littlefield, 2014.

二、期刊論文集（＊責任作者）

1. Hung CR, **Lin M**, Hsu KY, Chen CM. Left atrial myxoma. *J Surg Soc ROC*, 1968; 1: 1-12.

2. **Lin M***. Pathological study in reticulum cell sarcoma. *Transaction of the Pathological Society of ROC*, 1969; 45-64. (Master thesis)

3. Chen WJ, Chen KM, **Lin M***. Colon perforation in amebiasis. *Arch Surg*, 1971; 103: 676-680.

4. **Lin M***. Lympholoma with "starry sky" pattern in children in Taiwan. *Transaction of the Pathological Society of ROC*, 1971. (遺失)

5. **Lin M***, Lin WSJ, Yoshida T, Chu SH, Lin TY. Demonstration of alpha-fetoglobulin in hepatoma tissue by fluorescent antibody technique. *Cancer*, 1974; 34: 268-273.

6. **Lin M***, Hsu HC. Two cases of pneumocystis pneumonia with electron microscopic study. *J Formosan Med Assoc*, 1975; 74: 48-53.
7. Yang CS, **Lin M**, Hsu MM. Malignant histiocytosis with aural manifestations--report of a case. *J Surg Soc ROC*, 1976; 11: 25-30.
8. **Lin-Chu M***, Yao TY, Pai IF. Malignant histiocytosis with special reference to involvement of the liver and spleen. *J Formosan Med Assoc*, 1977; 7: 402-408.
9. Chen WY, Chuang CY, Chen DS, Wang TH, Yen TS, Hsieh BS, **Lin-Chu M***. HBsAg, HBsAb, immunoglobulins and C3 in primary nephritic syndrome. *J Formosan Med Assoc*, 1978; 7: 378-385.
10. **Lin-Chu M***, Marshall RB. Ultrastructural localization of immune complex in kidney diseases by immunoenzyme technique. *J Formosan Med Assoc*, 1978; 77: 497-507.
11. Hung WT, Chen WJ, **Lin-Chu M***. A study on the diagnosis of Hirschsprung's disease. Primary report of anorectal manometric study and acetylcholinesterase stain for Hirschsprung's disease. *Acta Paed Sinica*, 1979; 20: 93-98.
12. **Lin-Chu M***, Chang TW, Chuong CM, Lin WSJ. Immunoelectron microscopic study on alphafetoprotein synthesis. *J Formosan Med Assoc,* 1982; 81: 127-134.
13. **Lin-Chu M***, Lin WSJ, Lin TY. Ultrastructural of primary carcinoma of the liver. *J Formosan Med Assoc*, 1982; 81: 1514-1523.
14. Luo WF, Jee SH, **Lin-Chu M***. Angioimmunoblastic lymphadenopathy. *Dermatol Sinica*, 1983; 1: 51-56.
15. **Lin M***. Blood bank procedure. *J Med Technology ROC*, 1983; 2: 73-75.
16. Chen HS, Yeh JC, Yang CS, Lin JF, **Lin M***. Acute interstitial nephritis associated with renal failure induced by rifampin--a case report. *Taiwan J Formosan Med Assoc*, 1984; 83: 1053-1057.
17. **Lin-Chu M***. Experience with the manual Polybrene method in Taiwan (letter). *Transfusion*, 1984; 24: 543.
18. **Lin-Chu M***. The Rhesus blood group in Taiwan. *J Formosan Med Assoc*, 1984; 83: 796-799.
19. **Lin-Chu M***, Broadberry RE, Chang FJ. Serological investigation on autoimmune hemolytic anemia. *J Formosan Med Assoc*, 1984; 83: 942-946.

20. Hwang FY, **Lin-Chu M**, Broadberry RE, Chen KY, Yuang WL. A study of ABO incompatibility in Chinese neonates. *Acta Paed Sinica*, 1985; 26: 430-435.

21. Liang DC, Huang FY, **Lin-Chu M***. Macrophage reaction in fulminant hepatic failure. *J Formosan Med Assoc*, 1985; 84: 823-827.

22. **Lin-Chu M***, Broadberry RE, Yen LS. An appraisal of Rh(D) typing in Chinese. *J Formosan Med Assoc*, 1986; 85: 196-198.

23. **Lin-Chu M**, Broadberry RE, Chang FJ, Yang TF, Huang FY. Blood group antibodies and ABO hemolytic disease of the newborn. *J Formosan Med Assoc*, 1986; 85: 799-806.

24. Chang MC, Shih CC, **Lin-Chu M**, Huang WC. Acquired immunodeficiency syndrome related comples. *J Formosan Med Assoc*, 1986; 85: 890-897.

25. Hwang FY, Yang WL, Lee HC, **Lin-Chu M**, Broadberry RE. T antigen and anaerobic infections. *Acta Paed Sinica*, 1986; 27: 52-56.

26. Liang DC, **Lin-Chu M**, Shih CC. Reactive histiocytosis in acute lymphoblastic leukemia and non-Hodgkin's lymphoma. *Cancer*, 1986; 58: 1289-1294.

27. **Lin-Chu M***, Broadberry RE, Chiou FW. The B_3 phenotype in Chinese. *Transfusion*, 1986; 26: 428-430.

28. **Lin-Chu M**, Broadberry RE, Tsai SJ. Incidence of ABO subgroups in Chinese in Taiwan. *Transfusion*, 1987; 27: 114-115.

29. **Lin-Chu M***, Broadberry RE, Chyou SC, Hung HY, Shen EY, Hsu CH, Ho HY. Hemolytic disease of newborn due to maternal irregular antibodies in Taiwan. *J Formosan Med Assoc*, 1987; 86: 645-648.

30. **Lin-Chu M***, The para-Bombay phenotype in Chinese persons. *Transfusion*, 1987; 27: 388-390.

31. **Lin-Chu M***, Broadberry RE. Heterogeneity of the ABO subgroups among Chinese in Taiwan. *Revue Francaise de Transfusion et Immunohematologie*, 1987; 30: 563- 568.

32. Shyur SD, Shih CC, Hung HY, **Lin-Chu M**, Liang DC, Lan CC. Nonhydropic cases in homozygous alpha-thalassemia: report of 3 cases. *J Formosan Med Assoc,* 1987; 86: 438-441.

33. **Lin-Chu M***. Inspection and continuing education on blood banking in Taiwan. *Excerpta Medica*, *Current Clinical Practice Series*, 1988; 47: 249-253.

34. Lee CS, Tsan KW, **Lin-Chu M**, Shih CC, Yang JP. Thrombotic thrombocytopenic purpura--report of a case. *Chin Med J (Taipei)*, 1988; 41: 81-84.

35. **Lin-Chu M***, Broadberry RE, Chang FJ. The distribution of blood group antigens and alloantibodies among Chinese in Taiwan. *Transfusion*, 1988; 28: 350-352.

36. Linag DC, Ms SW, **Lin-Chu M**, Lan CC. Granulocyte/macrophage colony-forming units from cord blood of premature and fullterm neonates: its role in ontogeny of human hemopoiesis. *Pediatric Research*, 1988; 24: 701-702.

37. **Lin-Chu M***, Lin SJ, Chang SL, Tsai LSJ, Yang TF. HLA antigens among Chinese in Taiwan: association of Cw1 and Cw3 on the same haplotype. *Human Heredity*, 1989; 39: 89-93.

38. **Lin-Chu M***, Broadberry RE. 血型. *J Formosan Med Assoc*, 1989; 88: 385-390.

39. **Lin-Chu M***, Lee EC, Ho MY. Malignant mesothelioma in infancy: a case report. *Arch Pathol Lab Med*, 1989; 113: 409-411.

40. **Lin-Chu M***, Broadberry RE. Blood transfusion in the para-Bombay phenotype. *Brit J Hemat*, 1990; 75: 568-572.

41. **Lin-Chu M**, Tsai SJL, Watanabe J, Nishioka. The prevalence of anti-HCV among Chinee voluntary blood donors in Taiwan. *Transfusion*, 1990; 30: 471-473.

42. **Lin-Chu M***, Yen CT. The prevalence of hepatitis B surface antigen among Chinese voluntary blood donors in Taiwan. *Excerpta Medica, Current Clinical Practice Series*, 1990; 57: 183-185.

43. Liu YJ, Lee BF, Lin YZ, Chen W, Wu KW, **Lin-Chu M**. Hemolytic disease of the newborn caused by maternal irregular antibody anti-E: report of a case. *Acta Pediatric Sinica,* 1990; 31: 332-335.

44. Brodberry RE, **Lin-Chu M***. The Lewis blood group system among Chinese in Taiwan. *Human Heredity*, 1991; 41: 290-294.

45. Chien SF, **Lin-Chu M**. The conversion of group B RBC to group O by α-galactosidase. *Carbohydrate Research*, 1991; 217: 191-200.

46. Hayward MA, **Lin-Chu M***. Phosphoglucomutase-1 (PGM1) W23 and W26 variants detected in the Taiwanese Chinese population. *Human Heredity*, 1991; 41: 411-412.

47. **Lin-Chu M**, Broadberry RE, Tanaka M, Okubo Y. The i phenotype and congenital cataracts among Chinese in Taiwan. *Transfusion*, 1991; 31: 676-677.

48. **Lin-Chu M***, Loo JH, Hayward MA. Phosphoglucomutase-1 polymorphism among Chinese in Taiwan. *Human Heredity*, 1991; 41: 22-25.
49. Lee PH, Lai HS, **Lin-Chu M**, Chen YC, Hu RH, Lee CS, Chen KM, Chu TH. Acquired hemolytic anemia after ABO-unmatched liver transplantation. *Transplantation Proceedings*, 1992; 24: 1477-1478.
50. Chen CC, Chang FJ, Ting F, **Lin M***. Hemolytic disease of the newborn due to maternal anti-Di^b in a Chinese infant. *Chin Med J (Taipei)*, 1993; 52: 262-264.
51. **Lin M***, Shieh SH, Yang TF. Frequency of platelet-specific antigens among Chinese in Taiwan. *Transfusion*, 1993; 33: 155-157.
52. **Lin M***. The development of transfusion medicine in Taiwan. *Transfusion Today*, 1993; 17: 7-8. (遺失)
53. Broadberry RE, **Lin M***. The incidence and significance of anti-"Mi^a" in Taiwan. *Transfusion*, 1994; 34: 349-352.
54. **Lin M**. The national blood program of Taiwan, ROC (letter). *Vox Sang*, 1994; 66: 299.
55. **Lin M***, Broadberry RE. The modification of standard Western pretransfusion testing procedures for Taiwan. *Vox Sang*, 1994; 67: 199- 202.
56. **Lin M***, Broadberry RE. An intravascular hemolytic transfusion reaction due to anti-"Mi^a" in Taiwan. *Vox Sang*, 1994; 67: 320.
57. **Lin M***, Broadberry RE. The clinical significance of anti-'Mi^a' (letter). *Transfusion*, 1994; 34: 1013-1014.
58. **Lin M***, Broadberry RE. Elimination of Rh(D) typing and the antiglobulin test in pretransfusion compatibility tests for Taiwanese. *Vox Sang*, 1994; 67: 28-29.
59. **Lin M***, Chen CC, Hong CC, Lin WS, Cheng YP. Transfusion-associated respiratory distress in Taiwan. *Vox Sang*, 1994; 67: 372-376.
60. **Lin M***, Chen CC, Wang CL, Li HL. The frequencies of neutrophil specific antigens among Chinese in Taiwan. *Vox Sang,* 1994; 66: 247.
61. **Lin M***, Shieh SH. Postnatal development of red cell Lea and Leb antigens in Chinese infants. *Vox Sang*, 1994; 66: 137-140.
62. **Lin M***. The national blood program of Taiwan, ROC. *Japanese Journal Transfusion Medicine,* 1994; 40: 766-768.
63. McOmish F, Yap PL, Dow BC, Follett EAC, Seed C, Kelleer Aj, Cobain TJ, Krusius T, Kolho E, Naukkarinen R, Lin C, Lai C, Medgyesi GA, Hej-

jas M, Kiyokawa H, Fukada K, Cuypers T, Saeed AA, Alrasheed AM, **Lin M**, and Simmonds P. Geographical distribution of hepatitis C virus genotypes in blood donors: an international collaborative survey. *J Clin Microbiol*, 1994; 32: 884-892.

64. 林媽利. 台灣產前檢查及輸血前配合試驗中Rh血型的篩檢是必要的嗎? *當代醫學*, 1995; 22: 815-818.

65. Chen SH, Liang DC, **Lin M***. Treatment of platelet alloimmunization with intravenous immunoglobulin in a child with aplastic anemia. *Am J Hematol*, 1995; 49: 165-166.

66. **Lin M***, Broadberry RE. The Lewis phenotype in Orientals (letter). *Vox Sang*, 1995; 68: 68-9.

67. **Lin M***, Broadberry RE. ABO hemolytic disease of the newborn is more severe in Taiwan than in white populations (letter). *Vox Sang*, 1995; 68: 136.

68. **Lin M***, Shieh SH, Huang FY. The Lea antigen and neonatal hyperbilirubinemia in Taiwan. *Vox Sang*, 1995; 69: 131-134.

69. **Lin M***, Shieh SH, Liang DC, Yang TF, Shibata Y. Neonatal alloimmune thrombocytopenia in Taiwan due to an antibody against a labile component of HPA-3a(Bak^a). *Vox Sang*, 1995; 69: 336-340.

70. **Lin M***, Broadberry RE. Simplification of compatibility testing procedures for Taiwan. *Transfusion Today*, 1995; 24: 8. (遺失)

71. Wu AM, Duk M, **Lin M**, Broadberry RE, Lisowska E. Identification of variant glycophorins of human red cells by lectinoblotting: application to the Mi.III variant that is relatively frequent in the Taiwanese population. *Transfusion*, 1995; 35: 571-576.

72. Yu LC, Yang YH, Broadberry RE, Chen YH, **Lin M***. Correlation of a missense mutation in the human secretor alpha (1,2) fucosyltransferase gene with the Lewis(a+b+) phenotype: A potential molecular basis for the weak Secretor allele (Se^w). *J Bio Chem*, 1995; 312: 329-332.

73. Broadberry RE, **Lin M***. The distribution of the MiIII (Gp.Mur) phenotype among the population of Taiwan. *Transfusion medicine*, 1996; 6: 145-148.

74. Broadberry RE, **Lin M***. Comparison of the Lewis phenotypes among the different population groups of Taiwan. *Transfusion Medicine*, 1996; 6: 255-260.

75. Liu YJ, Chen W, Wu KW, Broaberry RE, **Lin M***. The development of ABO isohemagglutinins in Taiwanese. *Human Heredity*, 1996; 46: 181-184.
76. Wei CH, **Lin M**, Hsieh RK, Tseng CH, Liu JH, Fan S, Chiou TJ, Chen PM. Selective IgA deficiency and anaphylactoid transfusion reaction: a case report. *Chin Med J (Taipei)*, 1996; 57: 165-8.
77. Yu LC, Broadberry RE, Yang YH, Chen YH, **Lin M***. Heterogeneity of the human Secretor α(1,2) fucosyltransferase gene among Le(a+b-) non-secretors. *Biochem Biophys Res Commun*, 1996; 222: 390-394.
78. **Lin M***. Blood groups and transfusion medicine in Taiwan. *J Formos Med Assoc*, 1997; 96: 933-942.
79. **Lin M**, Broadberry RE. Immunohematology in Taiwan. *Transfusion Today*, 1997; 32: 3-6.
80. Yu LC, Hsiao YL, Yang YH, **Lin M**, Chen YH. The genomic structure of a mouse seminal vesicle autoantigen. *Biochem Biophys Res Commun*, 1997; 231: 106-110.
81. Yu LC, Yang YH, Broadberry RE, Chen YH, **Lin M***. Heterogeneity of the human H blood group alpha (1,2) fucosyltransferase gene among para-Bombay individuals. *Vox Sang*, 1997; 72: 36-40.
82. Broadberry RE, Chang FC, **Lin M***. The distribution of the red cell St[a] (Stones) antigen among the population of Taiwan. *Transfusion Medicine*, 1998; 8: 57-58.
83. **Lin M**, Broadberry RE. Immunohematology in Taiwan. *Transfusion Medicine Review*, 1998; 12: 56-72.
84. Rana BK, Hewett-Emmett D, Jim L, Chang BH-J, Sambuughin N, **Lin M**, Watkins S, Bamshad M, Jorde LB, Ramsay M, Jenkins T, Li W-H. High polymorphism at the human melanocortin 1 receptor locus. *Genetics*, 1999; 151: 1547-1557.
85. Yu LC, Lee HL, Chan YS, **Lin M***. The molecular basis for the B(A) allele: an amino acid alteration in the human histoblood group B alpha-(1,3) galactosyltransferase increases its intrinsic alpha-(1,3)-N-acetylgalactos-aminyltransferase activity. *Biochem Biophys Res Commun*, 1999; 262: 487-493.
86. Yu LC, Lee HL, Chu CC, Broadberry RE, **Lin M***. A new identified nonsecretor allele of the human histo-blood group alpha (1,2) fucosyltransferase gene (FUT2). *Vox Sang*, 1999; 76: 115-119.

87. Chen SH, Liang DC, Liu HC, **Lin M***. Treatment of neutropenia with intravenous immunoglobulin in autoimmune neutropenia of childhood. *Int J Pediatr Hematol/Oncol,* 2000; 6: 347-353.

88. **Lin M**, Engelfriet CP, Reesink HW. The detection of alloantibodies against red cells in patients with warm-type autoimmune haemolytic anaemia. In International Forum, *Vox Sang*, 2000; 78: 200-207.

89. **Lin M**, Chu CC, Lee HL, Chang SL, Ohashi J, Tokunaga K, Akaza T, Juji T. Heterogeneity of Taiwan's indigenous population: possible relation to prehistoric Mongoloid dispersals. *Tissue Antigens*, 2000; 55: 1-9.

90. Yu LC, Chang CY, Twu YC, **Lin M***. Human histo-blood group ABO glycosyltransferase genes: Different enhancer structures with different transcriptional activities. *Biochem Biophys Res Commun*, 2000; 273: 459-466.

91. Chu CC, Lee HL, Chu TW, **Lin M***. The use of genotyping to predict the phenotypes of the human platelet antigen systems 1-5 and neutrrphil antigens in Taiwan. *Transfusion*, 2001; 41: 1553-1558.

92. Chu CC, **Lin M***, Nakajima F, Lee HL, Chang SL, Tokunaga K, Juji T. Diversity of HLA among Taiwan's indigenous tribes and the Ivatans in the Philippines. *Tissue Antigens*, 2001; 58: 9-18.

93. Daniels GL, Anstee DJ, Catron JP. Dahr W, Fletcher A, Garratty G, Henry S, Jorgensen J, Judd WJ, Kornstad L, Levene C, **Lin M**, Lomas-Francis C, Lubenko A, Moulds JJ, Moulds JM, Moulds M, Overbeeke MER, Rouger P, Scott M, Sistonen P, Smart E, Tani Y, Wendel S, Zelinski T. International Society of Blood Transfusion working party on terminology for red cell surface antigens. *Vox Sang*, 2001; 80: 193-196.

94. **Lin M**, Chu CC, Chang SL, Lee HL, Loo JH, Akaza T, Juji T, Ohashi J, Tokunaga K. The origin of Minnan and Hakka, the so-called "Taiwanese", inferred by HLA study. *Tissue Antigens*, 2001; 57: 192-199.

95. **Lin M**, Loo JH, Chu CC. Paternity testing in Taiwan. *Transfusion Today*, 2001; 48: 7-9.

96. **Lin M***. Transfusion-related acute lung injury (TRALI). In International Forum, *Vox Sang*, 2001; 81: 269-283.

97. Yu LC, Chu CC, Chan YS, Chang CY, Twu YC, Lee HL, **Lin M***. Polymorphism and distribution of the Secretor α (1,2)-fucosyltransferase gene in various Taiwanese populations. *Transfusion*, 2001; 41: 1279-1284.

98. Yu LC, Twu YC, Chang CY, **Lin M***. Molecular basis of the adult i phenotype and the gene responsible for the expression of the human blood group I antigen. *Blood*, 2001; 98: 3840-3845.

99. Yu LC, Twu YC, Chang CY, and **Lin M***. Molecular basis of the Kell-null phenotype: a mutation at the splice site of human *KEL* gene abolishes the expression of Kell blood group antigens. *J Bio Chem*, 2001; 276: 10247-10252.

100. **Lin M**. The origin of Taiwan indigenous peoples--DNA study. *Language and Linguistics*, 2001; 2: 241-246.

101. Lee JC, **Lin M**, Tsai LC et al. Population study of polymorphic microsatellite DNA in Taiwan. *Forensic Sci J (Taipei)*, 2002; 1: 31-37.

102. Schanfield MS, Okuda K, **Lin M**, Shyu R, Gershowitz H. Immunoglobulin allotypes among Taiwan aborigines: evidence of malarial selection could affect studies of population affinity. *Human Biology*, 2002; 74: 363-379.

103. Tsai LC, Yuen TY, Hsieh HM, **Lin M**, Tzeng CH, Huang NE, Linacre A, Lee JCI. Haplotype frequencies of nine Y-chromosome STR loci in the Taiwanese Han population. *Int J Legal Med*, 2002; 116: 179-183.

104. Wu KH, Chang JK, **Lin M**, Shih MC, Lin HC, Lee CC, Peng CT, Tsai CH. Hydrops foetalis caused by anti-Mur in first pregnancy--a case report. *Transfusion Medicine*, 2002; 12: 325-327.

105. Yu LC, Twu YC, Chou ML, Chang CY, Wu CY, **Lin M***. Molecular genetic analysis for the B^3 allele. *Blood*, 2002; 100: 1490-1492.

106. **Lin M**, Tseng HK, Trejaut JA, Lee H L, Loo JH, Chu CC, Chen PJ, Su YW, Lim KH, Tsai ZU, Lin RY, Lin RS, Huang CH. Association of HLA class I with severe acute respiratory syndrome coronavirus infection. *BMC Medical Genetics*, 2003; 4: 9.

107. **Lin M***, Wang CL, Chen FS, Ho LH. Fatal hemolytic transfusion reaction due to a anti-Ku in a K$_{null}$ patient. *Immunohematology*, 2003; 19: 19-21.

108. Sun CF, Yu LC, Chen DP, Chou ML, Twu YC, Wang WT, **Lin M***. Molecular genetic analysis for the A^{el} and A^3 alleles. *Transfusion*, 2003; 43: 1138-1144.

109. Yu LC, Twu YC, Chou ML, Chang CY, Reid ME, Gray AR, Moulds JM, **Lin M***. The molecular genetics of the human *I* locus and molecular background explaining the partial association of the adult i phenotype with congenital cataracts (Plenary paper). *Blood*, 2003; 101: 2081-2088.

110. Chang FJ, Chan YS, Wang CL, Chiou PY, HO KN, **Lin M***. Frequency of alloantibodies in patients in Mackay Memorial Hospital. *Formosan J Med*, 2004; 8: 755-759.

111. Chen ZX, Tsan SG, Dang CW, Chu CC, **Lin M**, and Lee YJ. Identification of two new HLA-DRB1 alleles: HLA-DRB1*1350 and DRB1*140502. *Tissue Antigens*, 2004; 64: 300-303.

112. Chu CC, Lee HL, Hsieh NK, Trejaut J, **Lin M***. Two novel HLA-DRB1 alleles identified by sequence based typing: HLA-DRB1*1443 and DRB1*1351. *Tissue Antigens,* 2004; 64: 308-310.

113. Chu CC, Lee HL, **Lin M***. Identification of a new HLA-DRB1 allele, HLA-DRB1* 0436. *Tissue Antigens,* 2004; 63: 279-281.

114. Chu CC, Lee HL, Trejaut J, Chang HL and **Lin M***. HLA-A, -B, -Cw and -DRB1 Allele Frequencies in an Ami population from Taiwan. *Human Immunology*, 2004; 65: 1102-1107.

115. Chu CC, Lee HL, Trejaut J, Chang HL and **Lin M***. HLA-A, -B, -Cw and -DRB1 Allele Frequencies in an Atayal population from Taiwan. *Human Immunology*, 2004; 65: 1107-1112.

116. Chu CC, Lee HL, Trejaut J, Chang HL and **Lin M***. HLA-A, -B, -Cw and -DRB1 Allele Frequencies in a Bunun population from Taiwan. *Human Immunology*, 2004; 65: 1112-1117.

117. Chu CC, Lee HL, Trejaut J, Chang HL and **Lin M***. HLA-A, -B, -Cw and -DRB1 Allele Frequencies in a Hakka population from Taiwan. *Human Immunology*, 2004; 65: 1118-1123.

118. Chu CC, Lee HL, Trejaut J, Chang HL and **Lin M***. HLA-A, -B, -Cw and -DRB1 Allele Frequencies in a Minnan population from Taiwan. *Human Immunology,* 2004; 65: 1123-1128.

119. Chu CC, Lee HL, Trejaut J, Chang HL and **Lin M***. HLA-A, -B, -Cw and -DRB1 Allele Frequencies in a Paiwan population from Taiwan. *Human Immunology*, 2004; 65: 1129-1134.

120. Chu CC, Lee HL, Trejaut J, Chang HL and **Lin M***. HLA-A, -B, -Cw and -DRB1 Allele Frequencies in a Pazeh population from Taiwan. *Human Immunology*, 2004; 65: 1134-1139.

121. Chu CC, Lee HL, Trejaut J, Chang HL and **Lin M***. HLA-A, -B, -Cw and -DRB1 Allele Frequencies in a Puyuma population from Taiwan. *Human Immunology*, 2004; 65: 1139-1145.

122. Chu CC, Lee HL, Trejaut J, Chang HL and **Lin M***. HLA-A, -B, -Cw and -DRB1 Allele Frequencies in a Rukai population from Taiwan. *Human Immunology*, 2004; 65: 1145-1150.

123. Chu CC, Lee HL, Trejaut J, Chang HL and **Lin M***. HLA-A, -B, -Cw and -DRB1 allele Frequencies in a Saisiat population from Taiwan. *Human Immunology* 2004; 65: 1150-1155.

124. Chu CC, Lee HL, Trejaut J, Chang HL and **Lin M***. HLA-A, -B, -Cw and -DRB1 Allele Frequencies in a Siraya population from Taiwan. *Human Immunology*, 2004; 65: 1155-1161.

125. Chu CC, Lee HL, Trejaut J, Chang HL and **Lin M***. HLA-A, -B, -Cw and -DRB1 Allele Frequencies in a Tao population from Taiwan. *Human Immunology*, 2004; 65: 1161-1166.

126. Chu CC, Lee HL, Trejaut J, Chang HL and **Lin M***. HLA-A, -B, -Cw and -DRB1 Allele Frequencies in a Taroko population from Taiwan. *Human Immunology*, 2004; 65: 1166-1171.

127. Chu CC, Lee HL, Trejaut J, Chang HL and **Lin M***. HLA-A, -B, -Cw and -DRB1 Allele Frequencies in a Thao population from Taiwan. *Human Immunology*, 2004; 65: 1171-1176.

128. Chu CC, Lee HL, Trejaut J, Chang HL and **Lin M***. HLA-A, -B, -Cw and -DRB1 Allele Frequencies in a Tsou population from Taiwan. *Human Immunology*, 2004; 65: 1176-1181.

129. Kataoka S, Kobayashi H, Chiba K, Nakamura M, Shinada, Moritas, **Lin M**, Shibata Y. Neonatal alloimmune thrombocytopenia due to an antibody against a labile component of human platelet antigen-3b (Bak[b]). *Transfu Med*, 2004; 14: 419-423.

130. **Lin M***. Compatibility testing without a centrifuge: the slide Polybrene method. *Transfusion*, 2004; 44: 410-413.

131. Liu CJ, Shih YN, Chu CC, **Lin M***. Identification of two novel HLA-DRB1 alleles. DRB1* 0903 and DRB* 1145. *Tissue Antigens*, 2004; 64: 99-101.

132. Trejaut JA, Tsai ZU, Lee HL, Chen ZX, **Lin M***. Cytokine gene polymorphisms in Taiwan. *Tissue Antigens*, 2004; 64: 492-499.

133. Chu CC, Lee HL, Chen ZX, **Lin M***. Anewly identified HLA-C allele: CW*1210, and confirmation of HLA-CW*080102. *Tissue Antigens*, 2005; 66: 61-63.

134. Hung SI, Chung WH, Liou LB, Chu CC, **Lin M**, Huang HP, Lin YL, Lan JL, Yang LC, Hong HS, Chen MJ, Lai PC, Wu MZ, Chu CY, Wang KH, Chen CH, Fann CSJ, Wu JY, Chen YT. HLA-B*5801 allele as a genetic marker for severe cutaneous adverse reaction by allopurinol. *PNAS*, 2005; 102: 4134-4139.

135. **Lin M**, Hou MJ, Twu YC, Yu LC. A novel A allele with 664G>A mutation identified in a family with the A$_m$ phenotype. *Transfusion*, 2005; 45: 63-69

136. **Lin M**, Pan SH, Wu IC, Chang SL, Hong CC, Lee MC, Chang SP, Chu CF, Su YW, Ho HT. Analysis of transfusion reactions in the Mackay Memorial Hospital. *Formosan J Med*, 2005; 9: 1-7.

137. Trejaut JA, Kivisild T, Loo JH, Lee CL, He CL, Hsu CJ, Li ZY, **Lin M***. Traces of archaic mitochondrial lineages persist in Austronesian-speaking Formosan populations. *PLoS Biology*, 2005; 3: e247.

138. 林媽利, 我們流著不同的血液. *Scientific American* (科學人)<多樣性台灣>特刊, 2006; 4: 122-127.

139. Chu CC. Chang HL, Chen ZS, Lee HL, **Lin M***. A novel HLA-B allele, B*5612, identified by sequence-based typing method. *Int J Immunogent*, 2006; 33: 343-345.

140. Chu CC, Lee HL, Chen ZS, **Lin M***. Identification of novel human leukocyte antigen-B allele, B*4048, in Taiwan. *Tissue Antigens*, 2006; 68: 180-181.

141. Chu CC, Lee HL, **Lin M***. A*1126: a novel HLA-A11 variant identified by sequence-based typing method. *Tissue Antigens*, 2006; 68: 263-265.

142. **Lin M***. Taiwan experience suggests that RhD typing for blood transfusion is unnecessary in southeast Asian populations. *Transfusion*, 2006; 46: 95-98.

143. **Lin M**, Hou MJ, Yu LC. A novel *IGnT* allele responsible for the adult i phenotype. *Transfusion*, 2006; 46: 1982-1987.

144. Wang LY, Liang DC, Liu HC, Chang FC, Wang CL, Chan YS, **Lin M***. Alloimmunization among patients with transfusion-dependent thalassemia in Taiwan. *Transfusion Med*, 2006; 16: 200-203.

145. Yang YC, Chang TY, Lee YJ, Su TH, Dang CW, Wu CC, Liu HF, Chu CC, **Lin M***. HLA-DRB1 alleles and cervical squamous cell carcinoma: experimental study and Meta-analysis. *Human Immunology*, 2006; 67: 331-340.

146. Chu CC, Lee HL, **Lin M***. A novel HLA-A2 variant, A*9203, identified by sequence-based typing. *Int J Immunogenetics*, 2007; 34: 13-15.

147. Chu CC, Lin CY, Trejaut JA, Wu MM, **Lin M***. HLA-DQB1*0317 is a novel allele with an unusual DR-DQ haplotypes. *Tissue Antigens*, 2007; 69: 370-372.

148. Dang CW, Chu CC, Liu TYC, **Lin M**, Lee YJ. A novel HLA-DRB1 allele, DRB1*0832, identified by sequence-based typing method. *Tissue Antigens*, 2006; 70: 527-529.

149. Huang FY, Chang TY, Chen MR, Hsu CH, Lee HC, Lin SP, Kao HA, Chiu NC, Chi H, Liu TYC, Liu HF, Dang CW, Chu CC, **Lin M**, Sung TC, Lee YJ. Genetic variations of HLA-DRB1 and susceptibility to Kawasaki disease in Taiwanese children. *Human Immunology*, 2007; 68: 69-74.

150. Liu SC, Chang TY, Lee YJ, Chu CC, **Lin M**, Chen ZX, Liu HF, Dang CW, Chang SC, Lee CS, Chen TL, Huang CH. Influence of HLA-DRB1 genes and the shared epitope on genetic susceptibility to rheumatoid arthritis in Taiwanese. *J Rheumatology,* 2007; 34: 674-680.

151. Su TH, Chang TY, Lee YJ, Chen CK, Liu HF, Chu CC, **Lin M**, Wang PT, Huang WC, Chen TC, Yang YC. CTLA-4 gene and susceptibility to human papillomavirus-16-associated cervical squamous cell carcinoma in Taiwanese women. *Carcinogenesis*, 2007; 28: 1237-1240.

152. Huang FY, Chang TY, Chen MR, Chiu NC, Chi H, Lee HC, Lin SP, Chen CK, Chan HW, Chen WF, Liu HF, Chu CC, **Lin M**, Lee YJ. Genetic polymorphisms in the CD40 ligand gene and Kawasaki disease. *J Clin Immunol,* 2008; 28: 405-410.

153. Huang FY, Chang TY, Chen MR, Lee HC, Chi H, Chiu NC, Hsu CH, Lin SP, Kao HA, Chen WF, Chan HW, Liu HF, Chu CC, **Lin M**, Lee YJ. Lack of association of the vascular endothelial growth factor gene polymorphisms with Kawasaki disease in Taiwanese children. *J Clin Immunol*, 2008; 28: 322-8.

154. Huang FY, Chang TY, Chen MR, Lee HC, Chiu NC, Chi H, Hsu CH, Lin SP, Liu HF, Chen WF, Chu CC, **Lin M**, Lee YJ. The -590 C/T and 8375 A/G interleukin-4 polymorphisms are not associated with Kawasaki disease in Taiwanese children. *Hum Immunol*, 2008; 69: 52-57.

155. Lee HL, Chu CC, Trejaut JA, Yang KL, **Lin M***. Identification of two novel HLA-DRB1 alleles, HLA-DRB1*1214 and HLA-DRB1*1215, in two Taiwanese individuals. *Int J Immunogenetics*, 2008; 35: 423-426.

156. **Lin M**, Yu LC. Frequencies of the *JKnull (IVS5-1g>a)* allele in Taiwanese, Fujian, Filipino, and Indonesian populations. *Transfusion*, 2008; 48: 1768.

157. Wu LLF, Chen YR, **Lin M**, Chern HD, Shen LJ. Variability in the Frequency of Single Nucleotide Polymorphisms of N-acetyl Transferase 2 (NAT2) Gene among the Different Ethnic Groups in Taiwan. *Journal of Food and Drug Analysis*, 2008; 16: 15-20.

158. Soares P, Trejaut JA, Loo JH, Hill C, Mormina M, Lee CL, Chen YM, Hudjashov G, Forster P, Macaulay V, Bulbeck D, Oppenheimer S, **Lin M**, Richards MB. Climate change and post-glacial human dispersals in Southeast Asia. *Molecular Biology and Evolution*, 2008; 25: 1209-1218.

159. Tsai ST, Huang CY, Lo FS, Chang YT, Tanizawa T, Chen CK, Wang ZC, Liu HF, Chu CC, **Lin M**, Lin CH, Li HJ, Lee YJ. Association of CT60 polymorphism of the CTLA4 gene with Graves' disease in Taiwanese children. *J Pediatric Endocrinology & Metabolism*, 2008; 21: 665-671.

160. Chen CG, Lu YT, **Lin M**, Savelyeva N, Stevenson FK, Zhu D. Amplification of immune responses against a DNA-delivered idiotypic lymphoma antigen by fusion to the B subunit of E. coli heat labile toxin. *Vaccine*, 2009; 27: 4289-4296.

161. Chu CC, Chen YF, Lee HL, Lin CY, **Lin M***. Identification of HLA-B*9521 in Taiwan. *Tissue Antigens*, 2009; 74: 445-446.

162. Chu CC, Ho HT, Lee HL, Chan YS, Chang FJ, Wang CL and **Lin M***. Anti-"Mi^a" immunization is associated with HLA-DRB1*0901. *Transfusion*, 2009; 49: 472-478.

163. Chu CC, Lee HL, **Lin M***. A novel HLA-DRB1 allele, DRB*1611, is identified in two Taiwanese individuals. *Tissue Antigens*, 2009; 74: 175-176.

164. Chu CC, H-L Lee, **Lin M***. Identification of novel HLA-B allele, B460102, in three Taiwanese individuals. *Tissue antigens*, 2009; 73: 374-375.

165. Chu CC, Lee HL, **Lin M***. A novel HLA-DRB1 allele, DRB*090202, is identified in a Taiwanese family. *Tissue Antigens*, 2009; 74: 262-263.

166. Chu CC, Lee KC, Lee HL and **Lin M***. Identification of HLA-B*5410 in Taiwan. *Tissue Antigens*, 2009; 73: 611-612.

167. Hsu K, Chi N, Gucek M, Cole RN, Van Eyk JE, **Lin M**, Foster DB. Miltenberger blood group antigen type III (Mi.III) enhances the expression of band 3. *Blood,* 2009; 114: 1919-1928.

168. Pan CF, Wu CJ, Chen HH, Dang CW, Chang F M, Liu HF, Chu CC, **Lin M**, Lee YJ. Molecular analysis of HLA-DRB1 allelic associations with systemic lupus erythematous and lupus nephritis in Taiwan. *Lupus*, 2009; 18: 698-704.

169. Wang LY, Wang CL, Chu CC, Lee HL, Ho HT, Liang DC, Liu HC, **Lin M***. Primary autoimmune neutropenia in children in Taiwan. *Transfusion*, 2009; 49: 1003-1006.

170. Chu CC, Lee KC, Lee HL, Lai SK, **Lin M***. Identification of the novel allele HLA-B*13:01:03 by sequence-based typing method in a Taiwanese individual. *Tissue Antigens*, 2010; 76: 496-497.

171. Chu CC, Lu YT, Lai SK, Lee HL, **Lin M***. Identification of the novel allele HLA-B*51:84 by sequence-based typing method in a Taiwanese individual. *Tissue Antigens*, 2010; 76: 337-338.

172. Hsieh NK, Chu CC, Lee NS, Lee HL, **Lin M***. Association of HLA-DRB1*0405 with resistance to multibacillary leprosy in Taiwanese. *Human Immunology*, 2010; 71: 712-716.

173. Lee, HC, Chang TY, Yeung CY, Chan WT, Jiang CB, Chen WF, Chan HW, Liu HF, **Lin M**, Lee YJ. Association of interferon-gamma gene polymorphisms in Taiwanese children with biliary atresia. *J Clin Immunol*, 2010; 30: 68-73.

174. Tabbada KA, Trejaut J, Loo JH, Chen YM, **Lin M**, Mirazón-Lahr M, Kivisild T, De Ungria MC. Philippine mitochondrial DNA diversity: a populated viaduct between Taiwan and Indonesia? *Mol Biol Evol,* 2010; 27: 21-31.

175. Chen PL, Fann CS, Chu CC, Chang CC, Chang SW, Hsieh HY, **Lin M**, Yang WS, Chang TC. Comprehensive genotyping in two homogeneous Graves' disease samples reveals major and novel HLA association alleles. *PLoS One*, 2011; 6: e16635.

176. Hsu, K, Lin YC, Lee TY, **Lin M**. Miltenberger blood group antigen subtype III (Mi.III) supports Wr^b expression. *Vox Sang,* 2011; 100: 389-394.

177. Loo JH, Trejaut JA, Yen JC, Chen ZS, Lee CL, **Lin M***. Genetic affinities between the Yami tribe people of Orchid Island and the Philippine Islanders of the Batanes archipelago. *BMC Genetics,* 2011; 12: 21.

178. Soares P, Rito T, Trejaut J, Mormina M, Hill C, Tinkler-Hundal E, Braid M, Clarke DJ, Loo JH, Thomson N, Denham T, Donohue M, Macaulay V, **Lin M**, Oppenheimer S, Richards MB. Ancient Voyaging and Polynesian Origins. *Am J Hum Genet*, 2011; 88: 239-247.

179. Trejaut J, Lee CL, Yen JC, Loo JH, **Lin M***. Ancient migration routes of Austronesian-speaking populations in oceanic Southeast Asia and Melanesia might mimic the spread of nasopharyngeal carcinoma. *Chin J Cancer*, 2011; 30: 96-105.

180. Wang LY, Chan YS, Chang FC, Wang CL, **Lin M***. Thomsen-Friedenreich activation in infants with necrotizing enterocolitis in Taiwan. *Transfusion*, 2011; 51: 1972-1976.

181. Yeh CH, Cho W, So EC, Chu CC, **Lin M**, Wang JJ, Hsing CH. Propofol inhibits lipopolysaccharide-induced lung epithelial cell injury by reducing hypoxia-inducible factor-1alpha expression. *Br J Anaesth*, 2011; 106: 590-599.

182. Yu LC, **Lin M***. Molecular genetics of the blood group I system and the regulation of I antigen expression during erythropoiesis and granulopoiesis. *Curr Opin Hematol*, 2011; 18: 421-426.

183. Hsu K, Lee TY, Chao HP, Chan YS, Lin YC, **Lin M**. Expression of the Rh/RhAG complex is reduced in Mi.III erythrocytes. *Vox Sang*, 2011; 102: 221-227.

184. Hsu K, Lin YC, Chang YC, Chan YS, Chao HP, Lee TY, **Lin M**. A direct blood polymerase chain reaction approach for the determination of GP.Mur (Mi.III) and other HiI+ Miltenberger glycophorin variants. *Transfusion*, 2013; 53: 962-71.

185. Hsu K, Lin YC, Chao HP, Lee TY, Chan YS, **Lin M**. Assessing the frequencies of GP.Mur (Mi.III) in several Southeast Asian populations by PCR typing. *Transfusion and Apheresis Science*, 2013; 49: 370-371.

186. Lai SK, Chu CC, **Lin M***. Characterization of the novel HLA-DPA1*02:02:04 allele. *Tissue Antigens*, 2013; 82: 77-78.

187. Loo JH, Trejaut J, Yen JC, Chen ZS, Ng WM, Huang CY, Hsu KN, Hung KH, Hsiao YC, Wei YH, **Lin M***. Mitochondrial DNA association Study of Type 2 Diabetes with or without Ischemic Stroke in Taiwan. *BMC Research Notes*, 2014; 7: 223.

188. Trejaut JA, Poloni ES, Yen JC, Lai YH, Loo JH, Lee CL, He CL, **Lin M***. Taiwan Y-chromosomal DNA variation and its relationship with Island Southeast Asia. *BMC Genet*, 2014; 15: 77.

189. Wu TW, Chu CC, Liao Chang HW, Lin SK, Ho TY, **Lin M**, Lin HH, Wang LY. HLA-DPB1 and anti-HBs titer kinetics in hepatitis B booster recipients who completed primary hepatitis B vaccination during infancy. *Genes Immun*, 2014; 15: 47-53.

190. Dai CS, Chu CC, Chen SF, Sun CY, **Lin M**, Lee CC. Association between human leucocyte antigen subtypes and risk of end stage renal disease in Taiwanese: a retrospective study, *BMC Nephrol*, 2015; 16: 177.

191. Soares PA, Tejaut JA, Rito T, Cavadas B, Hill C, Eng K, Mormina M, Brandao A, Fraser RM, Wang TY, Loo JH, Snell C, Ko TM, Amorim A, Pala M, Macaulay V, Bulbeck D, Wilson JF, Gusmao L, Pereira L, Oppenheimer S, **Lin M**, Richards MB. Resolving the ancestry of Austronesian-speaking populations. *Hum Genet*, 2016; 135: 309-326.

192. Hsu K, Kuo MS, Yao CC, Cheng HC, Lin HJ, Chan YS, **Lin M**. The MNS glycophorin variant GP.Mur affects differential erythroid expression of Rh/RhAG transcripts, *Vox Sang*, 2017; 112: 671-677.

193. Hsu K, Lee TY, Periasamy A, Kao FJ, Li LT, Lin CY, Lin HJ, **Lin M**. Adaptable interaction between aquaporin-1 and band 3 reveals a potential role of water channel in blood CO(2) transport. *FASEB J*, 2017; 31: 4256-4264.

194. Huang JY, Trejaut JA, Lee CL, Wang TY, Loo JH, Chen ZS, Chen LR, Liu KH, Liu YC, Hu CH, **Lin M***. Mitochondrial DNA Sequencing of Middle Neolithic Human Remains of Ling-Ding Site Implication for the Social Structure and the Origin of Northeast Coast Taiwanese. *Journal of Phylogenetics & Evolutionary Biology*, 2018; 6: 6.

195. **Lin M**, Xu X, Lee HL, Liang DC, Santoso S. Fetal/neonatal alloimmune thrombocytopenia due to anti-CD36 antibodies: antibody evaluations by CD36-transfected cell lines. *Transfusion*, 2018; 58: 189-195.

196. Yeh CC, Chang CJ, Twu YC, Chu CC, Liu BS, Huang JT, Hung ST, Chan YS, Tsai YJ, Lin SW, **Lin M**, Yu LC. The molecular genetic background leading to the formation of the human erythroid-specific Xg(a)/CD99 blood groups. *Blood Adv*, 2018; 2: 1854-1864.

197. Chen LR, Trejaut JA, Lai YH, Chen ZS, Huang JY, **Lin M**, Loo JH. Mitochondrial DNA Polymorphisms of the Saisiyat Indigenous Group of Taiwan, Search for a Negrito Signature. *Edelweiss Journal of Biomedical Research and Review*, 2019; 1: 12-18.

198. Trejaut JA, Muyard F, Lai YH, Chen LR, Chen ZS, Loo JH, Huang JY, **Lin M***. Genetic diversity of the Thao people of Taiwan using Y-chromosome, mitochondrial DNA and HLA gene systems. *BMC Evolutionary Biology*, 2019; 19: 64.

199. Chen ZS, Trejaut JA, Loo JH, Lai YH, Huang JY, **Lin M***. Mitochondrial DNA diversity of the Nangan islanders living in the Mazu archipelago of the Taiwan strait. *Edel J Biomed Res Rev*, 2021; 3: 25-27.

200. **Lin M**. Elimination of pretransfusion RhD typing at Mackay Memorial Hospital, Taiwan-30-year experience (1988-2017). *Vox Sang*, 2021; 116: 234-238.

201. Lo YH, Cheng HC, Wang HY, Peng CW, Chen CY, Lin KP, Kang ML, Hsiung CN, Chen CH, Chu HW, Shen CY, Lin CF, Lee MH, Liu QL, Satta Yoko, Lin CJ, **Lin M**, Chaw SM, Loo JH, Ko WY. Detecting genetic ancestry and adaptation in the Taiwanese Han people. *Molecular Biology and Evolution*, 2021; 38: 4149-4165.

202. **Lin M**, Trejaut JA. Diversity and distribution of mitochondrial DNA in non-Austronesian-speaking Taiwanese individuals. *Hum Genome Var*, 2023; 10: 2.

203. 林媽利. 台灣人的來源—DNA的探索. *台灣醫界*, 2023; 66: 261-266.

三、學術研討會摘要集（1983-2009）　　　（粗體：附論文）

1. Lin-Chu M. Antibody screening & blood transfusion. Transaction of the Hematology Society of ROC, 1983.

2. Lin-Chu M, Lee YC, Chen YJ, Huang FY. Hemolytic disease of the newborn due to ABO-incompatibility. Transaction of the Hematology Society of ROC, 1983.

3. Lin-Chu M. Rhesus blood group in Taiwan. The 18th Congress of the International Society of Blood Transfusion. Munich, 1984.

4. Lin-Chu M, Lin SJ, Chen LY. Antibody screening in blood transfusion. Transaction of the Hematology Society of ROC, 1984.

5. Lin-Chu M, Lin SJ, Chen LY. Discrepancy between cell and serum ABO grouping with special reference on A_m variant. Transaction of Hematology Society of ROC, 1984.

6. **Lin-Chu M, Chang FJ, Broadberry RE, Huang FY. An Example of A_{el}, a rare sub-type of blood group A. Transaction of the Hematology Society of ROC, 1984, PP. 44-46.**

7. Lin SJ, Chen LY, Yung GW, Lin-Chu M. Red cell phenotypes and frequencies of Kidd, Duffy, P, Lewis, Lutheran, Kell and MN systems on Chinese. Transaction of the Hematology Society of ROC, 1985.

8. 鮑博瑞，林媽利，張鳳娟. 在台灣地區輸血前最適當的抗體篩檢方法 — Manual Polybrene. Transaction of the Hematology Society of ROC, 1985, P. 40.（中文）

9. Lin-Chu M, Experience of Blood Banking in Taiwan. International Exchange Forum, AABB Annual Meeting, USA, 1985.

10. Lin-Chu M, Broadberry RE, Chang FJ, Yang TF, Huang FY. Blood group antibodies and ABO hemolytic disease of newborn. The 78th Annual Meeting of the Formosan Medical Association, 1985.

11. **Lin-Chu M, Broadberry RE, Yen LS. Deletion of pretransfusion Rh(D) typing in Chinese. *J. Formosan Med. Assoc*, 84: 54-55, 1985.（中文）**

12. Lin-Chu M, Broadberry RE. Reappraisal of pretransfusion Rh(D) typing in Chinese. The 19th Congress of the International Society of Blood Transfusion, Sidney, 1986.

13. Lin-Chu M. Blood Transfusion in Taiwan, Western Pacific Regional Meeting of MWIA, Taipei, 1986.

14. **Lin-Chu M, Hwang FY, Broadberry RE, Lin SP, Hsu ZC. Para-Bombay phenotype and ABO blood group incompatibility between parents and Children in three families. The Pediatric Association of the ROC, the 27th Annual Convention, PP. 25-26, 1986. (中文)**

15. **Lin-Chu M, Broadberry RE, Chyou SC, Hung HY, Shen EY, Hsu CH, Ho MY. Hemolytic disease of the newborn due to maternal irregular antibodies in Taiwan. J Formosan Med Assoc 85: S107, 1986. International Exchange Forum, AABB Annual Meeting, USA, 1987.**

16. **Lin-Chu M. The B$_3$ phenotype in Chinese.** *J Formosan Med Assoc*, **85: 107, 1986. (中文)**

17. **Lin-Chu M, Pi CS, Chuang CK and Lin SP. Maleimide as an inhibitor in measurement of erythrocyte G-6-PD activity with a centrifugal analyzer: on whole blood and the dried blood on filter paper. The Second Joint Annual Conference of Biomedical Sciences (Taipei). P. 162, 1987; ASCP Fall meeting, Chicago, USA, 1987.**

18. **Lin-Chu M and Broadberry RE. The Lewis phenotypes among Chinese in Taiwan. Proceeding of the 2nd International Workshop and Symposium on monoclonal antibody against Human Red Cells and related antigens, Lund Sweden, 1986.**

19. **Broadberry RE, Lin-Chu M. A report on monoclonal anti-M and anti-N. Proceeding of the 2nd International Workshop and Symposium on monoclonal antibody against Human Red Cells and related antigens, Lund Sweden, P. 96, 1986.**

20. **Lin Chu M, Yen LL. The preparation of leukocyte depleted red cells. Transactions of Taiwan Society of Blood Transfusion, P. 26, 1987. (中文)**

21. Chen LY, Yen LS, Wen PW, Lin SJ, Broadberry RE, Lin-Chu M. Irregular antibodies identified by Taipei Blood Donation Center during the period June 1980 to June 1987. Transactions of Taiwan Society of Blood Transfusion, P. 28, 1987.

22. **Lin-Chu M, Broadberry RE. ABO blood group antibodies in the sera of individuals with the paraBombay phenotypes. Transactions of Taiwan Society of Blood Transfusion, PP. 32-32, 1987. (中文)**

23. Lin-Chu M, Broadberry RE, Yang TF, Cheng JC, Hwang CH. Comparisons of two cross-match techniques in platelet transfusion in an alloimmunized AML; lymphocytotoxicity assay and platelet suspension immunofluorescence test. Translocation of Hematology Society of ROC, PP. 106-107, 1987.

24. Lee SS, Tsang KW, Lin-Chu M, Shih CC. Thrombotic thrombocytopenic purpura. Translocation of Hematology Society of ROC, P. 150, 1987.

25. Lin-Chu M, Broadberry RE, Chang FJ, Kuon FC, Tseng H. The phenotype Jk(a-b-) with anti-Jk3. Translocation of Hematology Society of ROC, P. 158, 1987.

26. Lin-Chu M, Loo JH and Lin SP. The newborn screening strategy for G-6-PD deficiency at Mackay Memorial Hospital. The 3rd Joint Annual Conference of Biomedical Science, P. 157, 1988.

27. Loo JH and Lin-Chu M. Determination of the normal range for G-6-PD activity in newborn babies at Mackay Memorial Hospital. The 3rd Joint Annual Conference of Biomedical Science, P. 158, 1988.

28. **Lin-Chu M, Broadberry RE, Yen LS. ABO subgroups among Chinese in Taiwan. Annual Meeting of Hematology Society and Chinese Society of Blood Transfusion, PP. 33-33, 1988. (中文)**

29. **Lin-Chu M, Broadberry RE, Yen LS. ABO subgroups among Chinese in Taiwan. The 20 Congress of International Society of Blood Transfusion, London, Book of Abstracts, P. 78, 1988.**

30. **Broadberry RE, Lin-Chu M, Yen LS. The B_x phenotype in Chinese. The 20 Congress of International Society of Blood Transfusion, London, Book of Abstracts, P. 78, 1988.**

31. Chien SF, Lin-Chu M. The conversion of group B RBC to group O by taro α-glucosidase. The 20 Congress of International Society of Blood Transfusion, London, Book of Abstracts, P. 80, 1988.

32. Lin-Chu M, Tsai SJL, Shieh MF. The prevalence of hepatitis B surface antigen among Chinese voluntary blood donor in Taiwan. The 20 Congress of International Society of Blood Transfusion, London, Book of Abstracts, P. 210, 1988.

33. **Lin-Chu M, Lin SJ and Chang SL. HLA antigens among Chinese in Taiwan and association of Cw1 and Cw3 on the same Haplotype. The 20 Congress of International Society of Blood Transfusion, London, Book of Abstracts, P. 291, 1988.**

34. Broadberry RE, Lin-Chu M, Chang FC. The first example of the Lu(a-b-) phenotype in Chinese. The 20th Congress of International Society of Blood Transfusion, London, Book of Abstracts, P. 301, 1988.

35. Lin-Chu M, Broadberry RE, Chang FC. The distribution of blood group antigens and alloantibodies among Chinese in Taiwan. The 20th Congress of International Society of Blood Transfusion, London, Book of Abstracts, P. 320, 1988.

36. Lin-Chu M, Yen CT. The prevalence of hepatitis B surface antigen among Chinese voluntary blood donor in Taiwan. The Second International Symposium on Viral Hepatitis and Hepatocellular Carcinoma, Taipei, P. 73, 1988.

37. Lin-Chu M, Loo JH. The gene frequencies of PGM1 (phosphorglucomutase) subtypes among Chinese in Taiwan. The Fourth Joint Annual Conference of Biomedical Science, P. 94, 1989.

38. Chien SF, Lin-Chu M. ^{51}Cr survival test for $α$-glucosidase treated red blood cell in monkeys. The Fourth Joint Annual Conference of Biomedical Science, P. 122, 1989.

39. Lin-Chu M, Broadberry RE. Application of lectins to blood group typing. Carbohydrates and Medicine, Institute of Biomedical Sciences, Academia Sinica. P. 16, 1989.

40. Lin-Chu M, Yang TF, Chang SL, Lee CS. Plasma exchange in hyper viscosity syndrome. Transactions of Taiwan Society of Blood Transfusion of ROC, P. 13, 1989.

41. Lin-Chu M, Broadberry RE, Chang FJ. Acute hemolytic transfusion reaction. Transactions of Taiwan Society of Blood Transfusion of ROC, P. 14, 1989. (中文)

42. Lin-Chu M, Yang TF, Chang SL, Chang LF and Cheng JC. Nonhemolytic transfusion reaction. Transactions of Taiwan Society of Blood Transfusion of ROC, P. 17, 1989.

43. Broadberry RE, Lin-Chu M, Chang FC. Manual Polybrene--the recommended method for pretransfusion testing in Taiwan. Transactions of Taiwan Society of Blood Transfusion of ROC, P. 27, 1989.

44. Broadberry RE, Lin-Chu M, and Yen LL. Th-polyagglutination a case report. Transactions of Taiwan Society of Blood Transfusion of ROC, P. 29, 1989. (中文)

45. Lin-Chu M, Chang FJ. Prediposit autologous transfusion. Transactions of Taiwan Society of Blood Transfusion of ROC, P. 42, 1989. (中文)

46. Broadberry RE, Yen LS, Hung MJ, and Lin-Chu M. A_2 and B_x phenotypes in Taiwan. Transactions of Taiwan Society of Blood Transfusion of ROC, P. 30, 1989. (中文)

47. Lin-Chu M. Transfusion reaction. The 36th Regional Meeting of the Formosan Medical Association, P. 54, 1989.

48. Lin-Chu M. Therapeutic Plasma exchange. Transactions of Taiwan Society of Blood of ROC, P. 13, 1989. (中文)

49. Lin-Chu M, Loo JH. PGM1 phenotypes and gene frequencies among Chinese in Taiwan. Symposium of ROC Society of Clinical pathology, 1989.

50. Chen CC, Broadberry RE, Chang FJ, Lin-Chu M. Mackay Memorial Hospital Reference laboratory on blood banking. Transactions of the Society of Blood Transfusion of ROC, 1990.

51. Lin-Chu M, Tsang KW. Mackay Memorial Hospital Transfusion Committee. Transactions of the Society of Blood Transfusion of ROC, 1990.

52. Lin-Chu M, Broadberry RE. The Lewis blood system among Chinese in Taiwan. The 2nd International Workshop and Symposium on Monoclonal Antibodies against Human RBC, Lund, Sweden, 1990.

53. Broadberry RE, Lin-Chu M. A report on monoclonal anti-M and anti-N. The 2nd International Workshop and Symposium on Monoclonal Antibodies against Human RBC, Lund, Sweden, 1990.

54. Hayward MA, Lin-Chu M. The PGM1 phenotyping among Chinese in Taiwan. The First Joint Annual Conference of Biomedical Sciences, P. 169, 1990.

55. Broadberry RE, Lin-Chu M. Further studies on the MiIII (Miltenberger) phenotype in Chinese. Transaction of the Society of Blood Transfusion of ROC, P. 11, 1990.

56. Lin-Chu M, Broadberry RE. The Lewis phenotype among Chinese in Taiwan. Transaction of the Society of Blood Transfusion of ROC, P. 27, 1990.

57. Lin-Chu M, Tsai SJL, Watanabe J, Nishioka K. The prevalence of anti-HCV among Chinese voluntary blood donor in Taiwan. Transaction of the Society of Blood Transfusion of ROC, P. 30, 1990.

58. Lin-Chu M. The blood program of Taiwan, ROC. The First Asian Conference of Clinical Pathology, Sapporo, Japan, 1990.
59. Lin-Chu M, Tsai SJL, Watanabe J, Nishioka K. The prevalence of anti-HCV among Chinese voluntary blood donor in Taiwan. The 1990 International Symposium on viral Hepatitis and Liver Disease, Houston, 1990.
60. Shin MC, Yeh CC, Lin-Chu M. The blood programme of Taiwan, ROC. The 1990 Joint Congress of ISBT and AABB, Los Angeles, P. 234, 1990.
61. **Chang FC, Broadberry RE, Lin-Chu M. Manual Polybrene--the recommended method for detection of clinically significant anti-bodies in Taiwan. The 1990 Joint Congress of ISBT and AABB, Los Angeles, P. 83, 1990.**
62. Lin-Chu M, Broadberry RE, Tanaka M, Okubo Y. The rare I phenotype and congenital catarract among Chinese in Taiwan. The 1990 Joint Congress of ISBT and AABB, Los Angeles, P. 83, 1990.
63. Lin-Chu M. Blood groups among Chinese in Taiwan. Symposium on Hematological Sciences, Taipei, P. 37, 1990.
64. Lin-Chu M. The Blood programme of Taiwan, ROC. The 8th Japanese-Korean Joint Conference of Clinical Pathology and The 1st Asian Conference of Clinical Pathology, Sapporo, 1990.
65. **Chen SH, Liang DC, Lin-Chu M. Treatment of platelet alloimmunization in a child with aplastic anemia during a critical bleeding crisis with intravenous immunoglobulin. Annual Meeting of Hematology Society of ROC, 1991.**
66. Lin-Chu M, Shieh SH. Development of the Lewis antigens. Transactions of ROC Society of Blood Transfusion, 1991.
67. Chen CC, Broadberry RE, Chang FC, Lin-Chu M. The second annual report of the blood bank reference laboratory, Mackay Memorial Hospital. Transactions of ROC Society of Blood Transfusion, 1991.
68. Chen CC, Chang FC, Lin-Chu M. The third annual report of the blood bank reference laboratory, Mackay Memorial Hospital. Transactions of ROC Society of Blood Transfusion, 1991.
69. Lin-Chu M, Shieh SH, Yang TF. Platelet serology in Mackay Memorial Hospital. Transactions of ROC Society of Blood Transfusion, 1991.
70. Lin-Chu M, Chang FC, Chu CF. D^{v1} phenotype (D mosaic) in a Chinese family. Transactions of ROC Society of Blood Transfusion, 1991.

71. Chen CC, Chang FC, Chiou PY, Broadberry RE, Lin-Chu M. Evaluation of clinically significant alloantibodies. Transactions of ROC Society of Blood Transfusion, 1991.

72. Lin-Chu M, Broadberry RE, Chang FC, Ting F. Hemolytic disease of the newborn due to maternal anti-Di^b in a Chinese infant. 2nd Regional Congress of International Society of Blood Transfusion, Western Pacific Region, Hong Kong, 1991.

73. Broadberry RE, Lin-Chu M. The Lewis phenotypes among Chinese in Taiwan. 2nd Regional Congress of International Society of Blood Transfusion, Western Pacific Region, Hong Kong, 1991.

74. Lin M. The Blood programme of Taiwan, ROC. The 2nd Asian Conference of Clinical Pathology, Cheju, Korea, 1992.

75. **Lin M. Paternity testing. Transactions of ROC Society of Blood Transfusion, 1992. (中文)**

76. Chen CC, Chang FC, Lin M. The fourth annual report of the Blood Bank Reference Laboratory, Mackay Memorial Hospital. Transactions of ROC Society of Blood Transfusion, 1992.

77. Wang SL, Lin M, Lee TH, Sun CF, Yung CF. The annual report of the Blood Bank Proficiency Test. Transactions of ROC Society of Blood Transfusion, 1992.

78. Lin M, Chen CC, Chang FJ, Yang TF. Acquired B antigen. Transactions of ROC Society of Blood Transfusion, 1992.

79. Lin YJ, Chang CY, Shieh SH, Chang FJ, Lin M. Detection of human blood group isohemagglutinins by microplate technique. Transactions of ROC Society of Blood Transfusion, 1992.

80. **Lin M, Shieh SH, Yang TF. Frequency of Platelet-specific antigens among Chinese in Taiwan. Proceeding of 22nd Congress of the International Society of Blood Transfusion, Sao Paulo, 1992.**

81. **Chien SF, Lin M, Chen TT. Molecular cloning for taro-α-galactosidase. Proceeding of 22nd Congress of the International Society of Blood Transfusion, Sao Paulo, 1992.**

82. **Lin M, Shieh SF. The development of Lewis antigens in Chinese infants and children. Proceeding of 22nd Congress of the International Society of Blood Transfusion, Sao Paulo, 1992.**

83. Lin M. The blood program of Taiwan, ROC. Proceeding of 2nd Congress of Chinese Society of Blood Transfusion, Harbin, China, 1992.

84. Lin M. Autotransfusion. Transactions of the ROC Society of Blood Transfusion, 1993.
85. Chen CC, Chang FJ, Lin M. The fifth annual report of the Blood Bank Reference Laboratory, Mackay Memorial Hospital. Transactions of the ROC Society of Blood Transfusion, 1993.
86. Wang SL, Lin M, Lee TH, Sun CF, Yung CF. The annual report of the Blood Bank Proficiency Test. Transactions of the ROC Society of Blood Transfusion, 1993.
87. Lin M, Chen CC, Wang CL, Lee HL. The frequencies of neutrophil specific antigens among Chinese in Taiwan. Transactions of the ROC Society of Blood Transfusion, 1993.
88. Broadberry RE, Lin-Chu M. Evaluation of clinically significant alloantibodies in Chinese. Transactions of the ROC Society of Blood Transfusion, 1993.
89. Lin M, Chang SL, Wu LT, Chang YS, Yang TF. The hemolytic disease of the newborn due to anti-Jk3. Transactions of the ROC Society of Blood Transfusion, 1993.
90. Lin YJ, Chen YF, Wu KW, Chang CF, Lin M. Investigation of isoagglutinin formation in Chinese children by microplate method. Transactions of the ROC Society of Blood Transfusion, 1993.
91. Lin M, Shieh S. Postnatal development of red cell Lea and Leb antigens in Chinese infants. Proceeding of the 4th European Regional Congress, International society of Blood Transfusion, Barcelona, Spain, 1994.
92. Lin M. The national blood program of Taiwan, ROC. *Jap J Transf med*, 1994; 40: 278.
93. Lin M. Blood groups in Taiwan. The 3rd Asian Conference of Clinical Pathlogy, Taipei, 1994.
94. Lin M, Cheng YP. Safety of blood and blood products in the ROC. The 3rd Asian Conference of Clinical Pathology, Taipei, 1994.
95. Broadberry RE, Chang SL, Chang FC, Shieh MC, Chang WB, Lin-Chu M. The clinical significance of anti-"Mi[a]" in Taiwan. Transactions of the ROC Society of Blood Transfusion, 1994.
96. Lin M, Shieh, Yang TF, Shibata Y, Liang DC. Neonatal alloimmune thrombocytopenia in Taiwan due to an antibody against a labile component(s) of HPA-3a (Bak[a]). Transactions of the ROC Society of Blood Transfusion, 1994.

97. Lin M, Chen CC, Hong CC, Lin WS, Cheng YP. Transfusion-associated respiratory distress. Transactions of the ROC Society of Blood Transfusion, 1994.

98. Sun CF, Lin M, Wang SL, Lin TC, Yung CF. The annual report of the Blood Bank Proficiency Test. Transactions of the ROC Society of Blood Transfusion, 1994.

99. Chen CC, Broadberry RE, Lin-Chu M. The sixth annual report of the Blood bank Reference laboratory, Mackay Memorial Hospital. Transactions of the ROC Society of Blood Transfusion, 1994.

100. Lin M, Yang TF, Chang SL. HLA haplotype frequencies in Taiwan. *Vox Sang*, 1994; 67(S2): 57.

101. Lin M, Chen CC, Hong CC, Lin WS, Cheng YD. Transfusion-associated respiratory distress in Taiwan. *Vox Sang*, 1994; 67(S2): 85.

102. Broadberry RE, Chan YS, Lin-Chu M. The distribution of the GP.Mur (MiIII) Phenotype among different population groups in Taiwan. Transactions of the ROC Society of Blood Transfusion, 1995; Proceeding of 24th Congress of the International Society of Blood Transfusion, Tokyo, 1996.

103. Lin M, Chang SL. Current status of HLA study in Mackay Memorial Hospital. Transactions of the ROC Society of Blood Transfusion, 1995.

104. Lin M, Shieh SH, Liang DC, Yang TF, Shibata Y. Neonatal alloimmune thrombocytopenia in Taiwan due to an antibody against a labile component(s) of HPA-3a(Bak[a]). Proceeding of 5th Regional (IV European) Congress of the International Society of Blood Transfusion, Venezia, Italy, 1995.

105. Lin M, Shieh SH, Lee FL, Liang DC. Neonatal alloimmune thrombocytopenia (NAIT) due to anti-Naka. Transactions of the ROC Society of Blood Transfusion, 1995.

106. Yu LC, Yang YH, Broadberry RE, Chan YS, Lin M. A potential molecular basis for the Lewis(a+b+) phenotype. Proceeding of 24th Congress of the International Society of Blood Transfusion, Tokyo, 1996.

107. Lin M, Broadberry RE. Variation in the incidence of the MiIII phenotype in Taiwan. Proceeding of 24th Congress of the International Society of Blood Transfusion, Tokyo, 1996.

108. Lin M, Chen ST, Lee HL, Chang SL. Distribution of HLA class I and class II antigens among the Bunun tribe, one of the indigenous groups of Taiwan. *Human Immunology*, 1996; 47 (1/2).

109. Lin M, Broadberry RE, Chang YS. The distribution of various blood groups among the different population groups of Taiwan. Transactions of the ROC Society of Blood Transfusion, 1996.

110. Broadberry RE, Chang YS, Lin M. Comparison of the Lewis phenotypes among the different population groups of Taiwan. Transactions of the ROC Society of Blood Transfusion, PP. 2-3, 1996.

111. Yu LC, Broadberry RE, Lin M. Molecular basis for the Lewis(a+b+) and Lewis(a+b-) non-secretor phenotype. Transactions of the ROC Society of Blood Transfusion, P. 4, 1996.

112. Lin M, Broadberry RE, Chang YS. The distribution of various blood groups among the different population groups of Taiwan. Transactions of the ROC Society of Blood Transfusion, P. 1, 1996.

113. Broadberry RE, Lin M. A report on glycophorin (GP) associated monoclonal antibodies (Mabs). Transion Clinigue at Biologique (France), 1996, 3: 48s.

114. Chen CC, Tsou CC, Lu SH, Lin M. RFLP analysis for parentage testing. Transactions of the ROC Society of Blood Transfusion, 1997.

115. Chu CC, Lee HL, Chang SL, Lin M. HLA antigen distribution in the population of Ami tribe, Rukai tribe and Atayal tribe. Transactions of the ROC Society of Blood Transfusion, 1997.

116. Yu LC, Lee HL, Lin M. Heterogeneity of the secretor and H-α (1,2) fucosyltransferase genes. Transactions of the ROC Society of Blood Transfusion, 1997.

117. Broadberry RE, Chan YS, Chang FC, Lin M. The distribution of the St[a] phenotype among the different population groups in Taiwan. Transactions of the ROC Society of Blood Transfusion, 1997.

118. Yu LC, Liu SM, Chan YS, Lin M. Molecular genetic analysis of the B(A) allele. Proceeding of 25th Congress of the International Society of Blood Transfusion, Oslo, 1998; *Vox Sang* 74 (supp 1), 1998.

119. Lin M, Chu CC, Lee HL, Chang SL. Distribution of HLA class I antigens among the Paiwan, Tsou and Puyuma tribes, the indigenous groups of Taiwan. Proceeding of 25th Congress of the International Society of Blood Transfusion, Oslo, 1998; *Vox Sang* 74 (supp 1), 1998.

120. Chan YS, Hong CC, Wang CL, Lin M. Hemolytic transfusion reaction due to overheating of blood by blood warmer. Transactions of Taiwan Society of Blood Transfusion, P. 32, 1998.

121. Chu CC, Lee HL, Chang SL, Lin M. HLA antigen distribution in the population of Tsou, Paiwan, Puyuma and Pazeh tribes. Transactions of Taiwan Society of Blood Transfusion, P. 41, 1998.

122. Lin M. Neonatal transfusion. Transactions of Taiwan Society of Blood Transfusion, P. 78, 1998.

123. Lin M. Paternity testing in Mackay Memorial Hospital. Annual Meeting of Chinese Medical Association, Taipei, 1999.

124. Lin M, Chu CC, Broadberry RE, Lee HL, Chan YS, Chang SL. Blood group and HLA class I studies on the indigenous groups of Taiwan. Proceeding of VI Regional Congress of the International Society of Blood Transfusion, Jerusalem, 1999.

125. Lin M. Immunohematology in Taiwan. Proceeding of 10th Regional Congress of the International Society of Blood Transfusion, Taipei, P. 3, 1998.

126. Lin M, Chu CC, Lee HL, Chang SL, Ohashi J, Tokunaga K, Akaza T, Juji T. Heterogeneity of Taiwan's indigenous population: Possible relation to prehistoric Mongoloid dispersals. Proceeding of 10th Regional Congress of the International Society of Blood Transfusion, Taipei, P. 113, 1999.

127. Wan HL, Lin M. Standardization of the manual Polybrene reagents for pretransfusion test. Proceeding of 10th Regional Congress of the International Society of Blood Transfusion, Taipei, P. 140, 1999.

128. Yu LC, Lin M. Molecular genetic study of the ABH and Lewis histo-blood group systems in Taiwan. Proceeding of 10th Regional Congress of the International Society of Blood Transfusion, Taipei, P. 250, 1999.

129. Chu CC, Lee HL, Chang SL, Lin M. HLA-DRB1 alleles in six Taiwan indigenous tribes. Proceeding of 10th Regional Congress of the International Society of Blood Transfusion, Taipei, P. 260, 1999.

130. Chu CC, Lee HL, Chu TW, Lin M. Genotyping of human platelet antigen system 1-5 and neutrophil antigen in Taiwan. Proceeding of 10th Regional Congress of the International Society of Blood Transfusion, Taipei, P. 266, 1999.

131. Huang WF, Yang CC, Tsai SJL, Lin M. Fresh frozen plasma and frozen plasma utilization in Taiwan. Proceeding of 10th Regional Congress of the International Society of Blood Transfusion, Taipei, P. 287, 1999.

132. Yang CC, Huang WF, Lin M, Tsai SJL. Red blood cells utilization in Taiwan. Proceeding of 10th Regional Congress of the International Society of Blood Transfusion, Taipei, P. 288, 1999.

133. Yu LC, Lin M. Different enhancer elements and their transcriptional regulation activities of the blood group A and B glycosyltransferase genes. Proceeding of 10th Regional Congress of the International Society of Blood Transfusion, Taipei, P. 309, 1999.

134. Yu. LC, Lee HL, Chan YS, Lin M. The A- and B- transferase activities of the glycosyltransferase encoded by the B(A) Allele. Proceeding of 10th Regional Congress of the International Society of Blood Transfusion, Taipei, P. 310, 1999.

135. Chan YS, Wang CL, Chang FJ, Broadberry RE, Ho HT, Lin M. The incidence and distribution of alloantibodies among patients in Taiwan. Proceeding of 10th Regional Congress of the International Society of Blood Transfusion, Taipei, P. 316, 1999.

136. Lin M, Chang SL, Loo JH, Chu CF, Chu CC. Paternity testing in Mackay Memorial Hospital. Proceeding of 10th Regional Congress of the International Society of Blood Transfusion, Taipei, P. 334, 1999.

137. Loo JH, Hong IB, Chu CC, Lin M. The estimation of Rh and MNSs MilII haplotype frequency by maximum likelihood method in Taiwan. Proceeding of 10th Regional Congress of the International Society of Blood Transfusion, Taipei, P. 337, 1999.

138. Chu CC, Chang SL, Lee HL, Lin M. HLA haplotypes of Taiwan population based on family study. Proceeding of 10th Regional Congress of the International Society of Blood Transfusion, Taipei, P. 339, 1999.

139. Liu HC, Chu CC, Lee HL, Wang CL, Lin M. Autoimmune neutropenia caused by anti-NA1 autoantibody in Taiwan: one case report. Proceeding of 10th Regional Congress of the International Society of Blood Transfusion, Taipei, P. 350, 1999.

140. Lin M, Chang SL, Chen CC, Loo IH, Chu CF, Chu CC. Paternity testing in Mackay Memorial hospital. Workshop for Paternity Testing in Taiwan, P. 11, 1999.

141. Chu CC, Lee HL, Wang CL, Lin M. Antibodies in chronic autoimmune neutropenia were found against neutrophil antigen (NA) system in Taiwan. Transactions of Taiwan Society of Blood Transfusion, P. 34, 2000.

142. Wan HL, Sun CF, Lin M. Standardization of the 3-step manual Polybrene test. Transactions of Taiwan Society of Blood Transfusion, P. 35, 2000.

143. Yu LC, Twu YC, Chang CY, Lee HL, Chang HL, Lin M. Molecular basis for the adult i phenotype. Transactions of Taiwan Society of Blood Transfusion, P. 36, 2000.

144. Lin M, Wang CL, Yu LC, Chang LC, Chang SL, Hong CC, Ho HT, Chu CT. Rare blood group Ko phenotype with transfusion reaction due to anti-Ku. Transactions of Taiwan Society of Blood Transfusion, P. 34, 2000.

145. Chu CC, Lee HL, Chu TW, Lin M. Genotyping of human platelet antigen system 1-5 and neutrophil antigen in Taiwan. *Vox Sang* 78 (Suppl 1), 2000. Proceeding of 26th Congress of the International Society of Blood Transfusion, Vienna, 2000.

146. Yu LC, Chu CC, Twu YC, Chang CY, Lee HL, Lin M. Heterogeneity and distribution of the secretor fucosyltransferase gene among Taiwanese populations. *Vox Sang* 78 (Suppl 1), 2000. Proceeding of 26th Congress of the International Society of Blood Transfusion, Vienna, 2000.

147. Lin M, Chu CC, Lee HL, Chang SL. HLA-DRB1 alleles in Taiwan indigenous tribes. *Vox Sang* 78 (Suppl 1), 2000. Proceeding of 26th Congress of the International Society of Blood Transfusion, Vienna, 2000.

148. Chu CC, Lee HL, Lin M. HLA-DRB1 gene distribution among Taiwan indigenous tribes. Transactions of Taiwan Society of Blood Transfusion, P. 219, 2000.

149. Lin M, Chu CC, Broadberry RE, Lee, HL, Chan YS, Chang SL, Yu LC. The origin of Taiwan indigenous tribes inferred by HLA study and the disease association. Proceeding of 93rd annual meeting of the Formosan Medical Association. P. 105, 2000.

150. Lin M, HLA alleles and medical implications among Taiwan's indigenous tribes. NHRI Conference on new perspectives in molecular diagnosis of genetic disorders, Taipei, 2001.

151. Chen TL, Lin M, Lee CS. Plasmapheresis in the treatment of rheumatic disease: a nine year experience. Proceeding of the 3rd World Congress of International of Society of Apheresis, Taipei, P. 86, 2001.

152. Lin M, Chang SL, Chu CF, Chang FC. Therapeutic plasma exchange in infant. Proceeding of the 3rd World Congress of International of Society of Apheresis, Taipei, P. 93, 2001.

153. Flower RLP, Chen Q, Sakuldamrongpanich T, Lin M. Morel-Kopp M-C, Sztynda T, Woodland N and Ward CM. Detection of antibodies to peptides defining Miltenberger antigens in an ELISA in which streptavidin is used to capture the peptide antigens. *Transfusion Medicine*, 2001; 11: 227.

154. Lin M. Immunohematology in Taiwan (Key note speaker). Proceeding of the HSANZ/ASBT Annual Scientific Meeting, Adelaide, Australia, 2002.

155. Lin M. Blood groups study in Taiwan. Proceeding of the HSANZ/ASBT Annual Scientific Meeting, Adelaide, Australia, 2002.

156. Lin M. Terminology of red cell surface Antigens. Proceeding of the HSANZ/ASBT Annual Scientific Meeting, Adelaide, Australia, 2002.

157. Chang FJ, Chan YS, Wang CL, Pan SH, Chiou PY, HO KN, Lin M. Frequency of alloantibodies in Taiwan with special reference to anti-D. Transaction of Taiwan Society of Blood Transfusion, 2002.

158. Wu IC, Hong CC, Chang SP, Lee MC, Su YW, Lin M. Transfusion reaction analysis (1999-2002) in the Mackay Memorial Hospital. Transaction of Taiwan Society of Blood Transfusion, 2002.

159. Trejaut JA, Loo JH, Lee ZY, Li HL, Chang HL, Chu CC, Lin M. Mitochondrial DNA analysis of migration of nine Taiwan indigenous tribes. Transaction of Taiwan Society of Blood Transfusion, 2002.

160. Flower RLP, Lin M, Kamhieh S, Chen-Q and Ward CM. Characterisation of antibodies to variant MNS red cell antigens by peptide ELISA. *Vox Sang* 2002 (Suppl 2); 83: 24.

161. Flower RLP, Lin M, Kamhieh S, Chen-Q, Morel-Kopp M-C, Sztynda T and Ward C. Antibodies to variant MNS (Miltenberger) antigens detected in Australia and Asia: are some cases of "anemia of prematurity" undiagnosed haemolytic disease of the newborn? *Transfusion Medicine*, 2002; 12: 159.

162. Yu LC, Twu YC, Chou ML, Lin M. Molecular genetic analysis for the B_3 allele. *Vox Sang* 2002 (Suppl 2); 83: 23.

163. Chu CC. Lee HL, Trejaut J, Lin M. A new HLA-Cw allele found in one of Taiwan indigenous tribes with frequency of 5%. *Tissue Antigens* 2002 (Suppl); 59: 51.

164. Lin M, Chu CC, Lee HL, Chang SL. Taiwan HLA-A, B serology typing tray. *Tissue Antigens* 2002 (Suppl); 59: 144.

165. Chen ZX, Chu CC, Lee HL, Chang SL, Lin M. Two new HLA-B alleles found in Taiwan. Transactions of Taiwan Society of Blood Transfusion, 2003.

166. Lin M, Shu WT, Wang CL, Liang TC. Serological study of autoimmune neutropenia. Transactions of Taiwan Society of Blood Transfusion, 2003.

167. **Lin M, Chan YS, Chang FJ, Wang CL. Frequency of alloantibodies in Taiwan. Proceeding of 12 Asia Pacific Conference of International Society of Blood Transfusion, New Delhi, India, 2003.**

168. Chu CC, Chen ZX, Trejaut JA, Lin M. Sequence analysis of the ATP6G and NFKB1L 1 gene in four HLA haplotypes commonly seen in the Ami tribe. Proceeding of 7th Asia-Oceania Histocompatibility Workshop and Conference, Karuizawa, Japan, 2003.

169. Lin M, Trejant JA. Severity of infection of serve acute respiratory syndrome (SARS) Coronavirus could be related to human leukocyte antigen (HLA). Proceeding of 7th Asia-Oceania Histocompatibility Workshop and Conference, Karuizawa, Japan, 2003.

170. 陸中衡，張小琳，林媽利。馬偕紀念醫院親子鑑定的經驗談。台灣輸血學會會刊，2003。

171. Lin M. Multigenetic analysis of Taiwan populations. Transactions of Taiwan Society of Blood Transfusion, 2004.

172. Chu CC, Lee HL, Chen ZX, Lin M. Two new HLA-Cw alleles found in Taiwan. Transactions of Taiwan Society of Blood Transfusion, 2004.

173. 王昌玲，詹詠絜，張鳳娟，林媽利。疑捐血人 G-6-PD 缺乏導致病人溶血性輸血反應，二病歷報告。台灣輸血學會會刊，2004。

174. Lin M. A multigenetic analysis of Taiwan populations. Proceedings of Human Migration in Continental East Asia and Taiwan: Genetic, Linguistic and Archeological Evidence, Geneva, 2004.

175. Lin M. Miltenberger phenotypes among Taiwanese. Proceedings of XV International Society of Blood Transfusion, Regional Congress Europe, Athens, 2005.

176. 陳文發，朱正中，張小琳，李慧玲，林媽利。HLA-B27 分型法比較 (PCR-SSP 與血清學法)。台灣輸血學會會刊，2005。

177. 張小琳，朱正中，李慧玲，林媽利。 HLA-A$_{null}$ allele(A*0253N) 血清學即 DNA based 的分析。台灣輸血學會會刊，2005。

178. 王昌玲，詹詠絜，張鳳娟，何信重，林媽利。馬偕紀念醫院稀有血型細胞及血清庫。台灣輸血學會會刊，2005。

179. 詹詠絜，林媽利。可使用於開發中國家的配合試驗，凝聚胺玻片法。台灣輸血學會會刊，2005。

180. 詹詠絜，王昌玲，張鳳娟，羅君維，何信重，林媽利。疑似血小板輸注引起的紅血球異體抗體。台灣輸血學刊，2005。

181. 朱正中，李慧玲，林媽利。使用核酸定序分型法確認八個新的 HLA 對偶基因。台灣輸血學會會刊，2006。

182. Lin M, Chan YS, Wang CL, Hsueh EJ. Transfusion of normal blood to patients with rare adult i phenotype. XXIX International Congress of the International Society of Blood Transfusion, Cape Town, South Africa, 2006.

183. 林媽利。台灣族群遺傳基因的過去與現在。台灣歷史與文化國際會議,台北國立圖書館,2006。

184. 王麟燕,王昌玲,朱正中,李慧玲,梁德城,劉希哲,何信重,林媽利。Autoimmune neutropenia among children in Taiwan-Report of 58 cases。台灣輸血學會會刊,2007。

185. 林媽利,Jean Trejaut,陸中衡,朱正中,李建良,何俊霖,李慧玲,簡炯仁。永恆的西拉雅族,遺傳基因的研究。再現西拉雅研討會,台南縣政府文化局,2007。

186. Lin M. Pretransfusion compatibility testing in Taiwan. Proceedings of Securing Safe Blood (V), The fifth Red Cross and Red Crecent Symposium on Blood Programs in the Asian Region, Bangkok, Thailand, 2007.

187. Lin M, Trejaut JA, Loo JH, He CL, Lee CL, Chu CC, Lee HL, Lin CS. Genetic profile of "non" Aboriginal Taiwanese. HUGO-Pacific Meeting, Cebo, Philippines, 2008. (www.HUGO-AP2008.ph).

188. Lee CL, Trejaut JA, Loo JH, He CL, Lin M. Odyssey of a new DNA laboratory for the study of ancient human remains in Taiwan. HUGO-Pacific Meeting, Cebo, Philippines, 2008. (www.HUGO-AP2008.ph).

189. He CL, Trejaut JA, Loo JH, Lee KH, Lin M. Y chromosome structure of Taiwan Aborigines and Non Aboriginal populations. HUGO-Pacific Meeting, Cebo, Philippines, 2008. (www.HUGO-AP2008.ph).

190. Trejaut JA, Loo JH, Lee CL, Lin M. Antiquated mtDNA lineages found in ISEA trace back to first modern human migrations. HUGO-Pacific Meeting, Cebo, Philippines, 2008. (www.HUGO-AP2008.ph).

191. Loo JH, Trejaut JA, Lee CL, Lin CS, Lin M. Ivatan and Orchid islands. Genetic relationship to Taiwan and the Philippines. HUGO-Pacific Meeting, Cebo, Philippines, 2008. (www.HUGO-AP2008.ph).

192. 詹詠絮,王昌玲,張鳳娟,何信重,林媽利。血庫檢驗案例分析。台灣輸血學會會刊,2009。

193. Loo JH, Trejaut JA, Chen XZ, Yen RC, Lee CL, He CL, Lin CH, Lin M. Yami and Batanese: mtDNA and Y chromosome study. 2009 International Symposium of Austronesian studies. National Museum of Prehistory, Taiwan.

194. Trejaut JA, Lee CL, Yen RC, Loo JH, Lin M. Mitochondria, Y chromosome and an ancient DNA molecular genetic analysis of Taiwan and Island Southeast Asia. 2009 International Symposium of Austronesian studies. National Museum of Prehistory, Taiwan.

195. Yen HC, Trejaut JA, He CL, Loo JH, Lin M. Higher definition of Y chromosome typing in Taiwan and Island Southeast Asia. 2009 International Symposium of Austronesian studies. National Museum of Prehistory, Taiwan.

196. Lee CL, Trejaut JA, Lin M. Three ancient DNA studies from different sites in Taiwan. 2009 International Symposium of Austronesian studies. National Museum of Prehistory, Taiwan.

197. Trejaut J, Lee CL, Yen JC, Loo JH, Lin M. Mitochondrial, Y chromosome and an ancient DNA molecular analysis in Taiwan and Island Southeast Asia. 19th Indo-Pacific Prehistory Association Congress, Hanoi, Vietnam, 2009.

198. **Lin M, Lee CL, Loo JH, Yen JC, Chu CC, Lee HL, Trejaut JA. More genetic sharing among the populations of Taiwan than expected: a plain tribe (Pinpu) perspective. PNC 2009 Annual Conference, Taipei, Taiwan.**

199. 張小琳，詹詠絮，李佳玲，楊茜淳，許玉妃，林奐綺，林媽利。由 **HPA-3** 抗原系統的抗體引起的新生兒異體免疫血小板缺乏症。台灣輸血學會會刊，**2019**。

國家圖書館出版品預行編目(CIP)資料

豐富多彩的台灣：林媽利醫師談台灣特有血型及血緣研究 = Abundant and colorful Taiwan : blood groups, heritage and ups and downs of life / 林媽利著. -- 初版. -- 臺北市：前衛出版社, 2025.05
288面；15×21公分
中英對照
ISBN 978-626-7463-98-7(平裝)

1.CST: 輸血醫學 2.CST: 血型 3.CST: 種族遺傳 4.CST: 臺灣

415.652　　　　　　　　　　　　　　　　114004386

豐富多彩的台灣

林媽利醫師談台灣特有血型及血緣研究

作　　者	林媽利
責任編輯	周俊男
美術編輯	Nico
封面設計	兒日設計

出 版 者　前衛出版社
　　　　　地　　址｜10468 台北市中山區農安街 153 號 4 樓之 3
　　　　　電　　話｜02-25865708｜傳　　真｜02-25863758
　　　　　郵撥帳號｜05625551
　　　　　購書・業務信箱｜a4791@ms15.hinet.net
　　　　　投稿・編輯信箱｜avanguardbook@gmail.com
　　　　　官方網站｜http://www.avanguard.com.tw

出版總監　林文欽
法律顧問　陽光百合律師事務所
經 銷 商　紅螞蟻圖書有限公司
　　　　　地　　址｜11494 台北市內湖區舊宗路二段 121 巷 19 號
　　　　　電　　話｜02-27953656｜傳　　真｜02-27954100

出版日期　2025 年 5 月初版一刷
定　　價　新台幣 420 元

Ｉ Ｓ Ｂ Ｎ：　978-626-7463-98-7 (平裝)
E-ISBN：　978-626-7463-96-3 (PDF)
　　　　　978-626-7463-97-0 (EPUB)

©Avanguard Publishing House 2025
Printed in Taiwan.

＊請上『前衛出版社』臉書專頁按讚，獲得更多書籍、活動資訊 https://www.facebook.com/AVANGUARDTaiwan